Clinical Advances in Psychiatry

Clinical Advances in Psychiatry

Edited by Fernando Hogan

AMERICAN
MEDICAL PUBLISHERS
www.americanmedicalpublishers.com

American Medical Publishers,
41 Flatbush Avenue,
1st Floor, New York,
NY 11217, USA

Visit us on the World Wide Web at:
www.americanmedicalpublishers.com

ISBN: 978-1-63927-436-9

Cataloging-in-Publication Data

Clinical advances in psychiatry / edited by Fernando Hogan.
p. cm.
Includes bibliographical references and index.
ISBN 978-1-63927-436-9
1. Psychiatry. 2. Psychology, Pathological--Diagnosis. 3. Mental illness--Treatment.
4. Psychotherapy patients. I. Hogan, Fernando.
RC454.4 .D53 2022
616.89--dc23

Table of Contents

Preface

This book aims to highlight the current researches and provides a platform to further the scope of innovations in this area. This book is a product of the combined efforts of many researchers and scientists, after going through thorough studies and analysis from different parts of the world. The objective of this book is to provide the readers with the latest information of the field.

Psychiatry is a speciality of medical science that is concerned with the diagnosis, prevention and treatment of mental disorders. Various maladaptations related to mood, behavior, cognition and perceptions are included in this domain. The most common mode of psychiatric treatment is psychiatric medication and psychotherapy. The other contemporary practices include a wide variety of modalities such as assertive community treatment, community reinforcement and supported employment. The domain of psychiatry uses research in the field of neuroscience, psychology, medicine, biology, biochemistry and pharmacology. The disorders treated under this domain are broadly classified into personality disorders, mental illnesses and severe learning disabilities. Some of the specialities within this area are addiction psychiatry, neuropsychiatry, sleep medicine, child and adolescent psychiatry, social psychiatry, etc. The objective of this book is to give a general view of the different areas of psychiatry and its applications. It strives to provide a fair idea about this discipline and to help develop a better understanding of the latest advances within this field. This book is a vital tool for all researching and studying this field.

I would like to express my sincere thanks to the authors for their dedicated efforts in the completion of this book. I acknowledge the efforts of the publisher for providing constant support. Lastly, I would like to thank my family for their support in all academic endeavors.

Editor

1

FT4 and TSH, relation to diagnoses in an unselected psychiatric acute-ward population, and change during acute psychiatric admission

Yuki Sakai[1], Valentina Iversen[1,2] and Solveig Klæbo Reitan[1,2*]

Abstract

Background: Alteration in thyroid activity is a well-known cause of symptoms mimicking psychiatric disorders. There are reports on altered levels of thyroid hormones in patients with certain psychiatric disorders compared to healthy controls; still, the magnitude and importance of the phenomenon is not known. We wanted to explore the level of thyroid hormones in different diagnostic groups in an acute-psychiatric population. We also wanted to follow any change during their stay.

Methods: Patients aged 18 years and older admitted to a closed, psychiatric inpatient ward were eligible if giving informed consent. For 539 patients representing all main psychiatric diagnostic groups and with equal gender distribution, data for FT4 were available for 539 patients, and data for TSH were available from 538 patients at admittance. For 239 patients, data for FT4 were available at both admittance and discharge, and the corresponding number for TSH was 236 patients.

Results: A significantly higher share of patients had higher levels of FT4 and TSH at admittance than expected for healthy individuals. No significant effect of gender or most diagnostic groups was seen.
For female patients with substance-use disorder (SUD), the level of TSH was significantly lower than that for all other diagnostic groups. No other difference in the levels of FT4 and TSH was seen between the main diagnostic groups, and the effect in SUD was not seen in males.
For the population with available markers at both admittance and discharge, in total, there was a significant reduction of FT4 from admittance to discharge, not followed by any change in TSH.

Conclusions: In acutely admitted psychiatric patients there seems to be an increased FT4 and TSH. FT4 is normalized during the inpatient stay independently of TSH. This indicates somatic effects of psychiatric stress that may be of clinical importance and the phenomenon should be further explored. Mainly different diagnostic groups did not differ in level of FT4 and TSH. Thus future studies on thyroid activity in psychiatric patients should focus on function and level of stress and suffering rather than diagnostic groups.

Keywords: Thyroid, TSH, FT4, Psychiatric, Stress, Acute, The HPT axis

* Correspondence: Solveig.Reitan@ntnu.no
[1]Faculty of Medicine and Health sciences, Institute for Mental Health, Norwegian University of Science and Technology, Trondheim, Norway
[2]Department of Mental health, St. Olav's University Hospital, Trondheim, Norway

Background

Clinical thyroidal disorders mimicking depression and anxiety are well known. Further, thyroid hormones (T3/T4) and thyroid-stimulating hormone (TSH) have been suggested to play a critical role in the regulation of neuronal growth and development, as well as in the alteration of neurocognitive functions including mood and cognition in the mature brain [1]. Although it is established that hypothalamic-pituitary-thyroid (HPT) axis abnormalities may be associated with psychiatric pathophysiology [2–4], the HPT pattern in psychiatric patients with non-thyroidal illness is still inconsistent. Altered concentrations of free thyroxine (FT4) have been described in patients with psychiatric disorders such as schizophrenia and affective disorders [3, 5–8], but findings are inconsistent; for example, other reports on personality disorder and alcoholism are negative [6]. In addition, an association between thyroid hormones within reference range and cognitive dysfunction in older people has been indicated [1]. The levels of TSH as well as TSH responses to thyrotropin - releasing hormone (TRH) have been described to be different in healthy controls compared to patients with psychiatric disorders, including major depression, bipolar mania, alcoholism, and borderline personality disorder [9, 10]. Thyroid disorders have been described as a risk factor for treatment resistant depression [11]. However, other studies do not find an association between the levels of thyroidal components and neuropsychiatric disorders [1, 12]. Dickerman and Barnhill [13] hypothesized that these considerable variations in thyroid alterations in psychiatric patients may be caused by a response to an underlying systemic illness or by the acute psychiatric illness itself. In line with this, altered levels of FT4 from acute state to remission have been described in schizophrenic patients in one study and attributed to medications [5], although it is far from being clear. To our knowledge, there are no studies on levels of thyroid hormones in a general psychiatric population at acute admittance.

To summarize, the connection between thyroid status and different psychiatric disorders is not consistently clear, and although an important effect of thyroid hormones on brain function is suggested, it is not clear whether acute psychiatric suffering has an effect.

Thus, the aim of this study was to investigate the relation between the levels of thyroid hormones and different psychiatric diagnoses in a general psychiatric acute inpatient population. In addition, we wanted to study the variation in thyroid status over an acute admission.

Methods

Aim

The first aim was to explore the prevalence of deviating thyroid levels in an unselected psychiatric acute-ward population and potential relations to diagnoses.

The second aim was to study whether there was a change in thyroid levels from admittance to discharge.

Ethics

The study was part of a large study approved by the Norwegian Regional Committee for Ethics (REC, identification number 199/04) and by Middle Norway and Norwegian Social Science Data Services (NSD, identification number 11771).

Design and setting of the study

The study was a cross-sectional study on the prevalence of thyroid levels and a follow up for change in thyroid levels in some of the participants.

Participants were recruited among patients admitted to the only closed, inpatient acute psychiatric ward for a population of 150.000 above the age of 18 years in South-Trøndelag county in the Middle of Norway in the period from 19.10.2004 to 30.11.2006. Clinical data and laboratory data according to standard clinical procedures in the hospital were available in the patients' files. Patients were given information and asked to consent to participation in a study collecting data on several fields including thyroid status. For patients giving informed consent, the data were collected in a research database, and participants were made anonymous.

Patients and patient characteristics

A total of 585 persons among the 1771 patients admitted in the study period gave written informed consent to participate. Some patients were excluded from these analyses because of disorders of the thyroid gland (International Classification of Diseases version 10 (ICD-10): E00–07) or because of the presence of anti-thyroid peroxidase antibodies (Anti-TPO). Also, patients for whom no measurements of FT4 or TSH were registered were excluded. As shown in Fig. 1, we included 539 patients with measurement for FT4 and 538 patients for TSH at admittance, and 254 and 252 patients at discharge, respectively. Data were available at both admittance and discharge for 239 patients for FT4 and for 236 patients for TSH.

Upon discharge, the patients' psychiatric diagnoses were set according to ICD-10 research criteria. Final diagnoses were set in a consensus meeting with the physician or psychologist in charge of the patient's treatment and at least two psychiatrists and/or senior clinical psychologist of whom at least one had personally examined the patient. In this study, the main diagnosis was used if multiple diagnoses were set. Diagnoses were categorized into 8 groups based on ICD-10 codes: Substance use disorder (SUD) (F10–19), schizophrenia spectrum disorder (F20–29), mania (F30–F31.2), bipolar depression (F31.3–31.5), unipolar depression (F32–F33), neurotic disorders (F40–49),

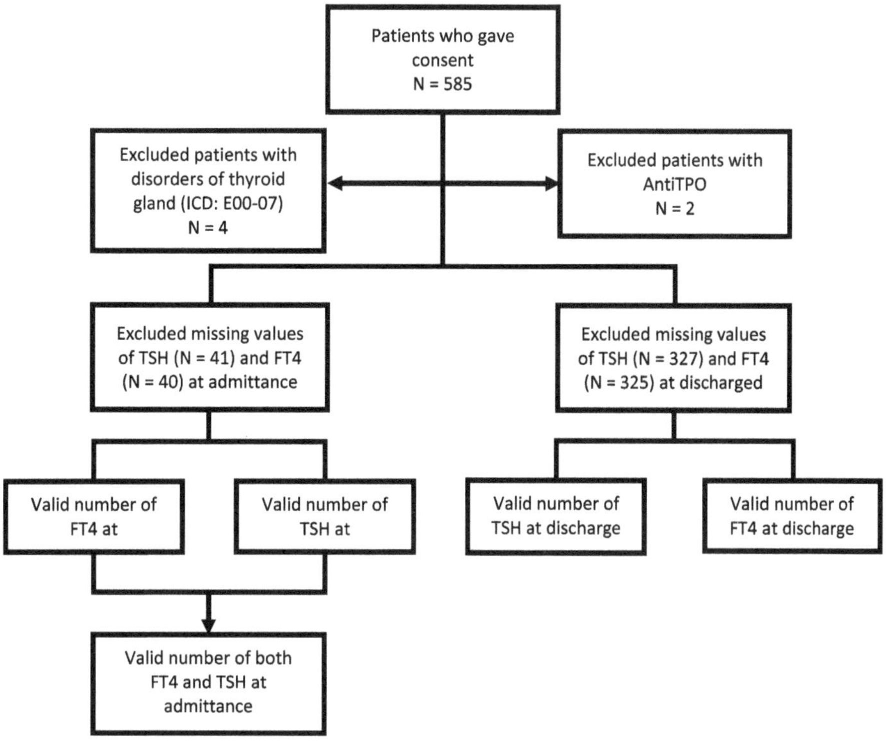

Fig. 1 Inclusion and exclusion of patients

and personality disorders (F60–69), and all other diagnoses were labeled as 'other'.

Patient characteristics are shown in Table 1. Mean and median patient ages were 41 and 39 years, respectively. Mean and median days of duration of stay were 12 and 6, respectively. The patient distribution in diagnostic groups is shown in Table 2. After Bonferroni correction for multiple testing, still significantly more males than females were having SUD diagnoses ($x^2(df) = 19.528$ (7), $p = 0.007$). For the other diagnostic groups, there was no difference in the gender distribution of diagnoses.

Table 1 Characteristics of patients at admittance

	FT4 (*N* = 539)	TSH (*N* = 538)
Gender		
Male	255	255
Female	284	283
Age		
years, mean ± SD	41.15 ± 16.93	41.09 ± 16.909
median	39.0	39.0
Duration of Stay		
days, mean ± SD	12.66 ± 35.320	12.69 ± 35.442
median	6.0	6.0

FT4 free thyroxin, *TSH* thyroid-stimulating hormone

Blood samples and laboratory assays

As part of the standard clinical procedure, FT4 and TSH were measured in blood collected between 7:00 am and 10:00 am the first working day after admission. For some of the participants, the same analyses were done at discharge. Blood was analyzed the same day by immunochemiluminescent procedures at the clinical laboratory at St Olav's University Hospital, Trondheim, Norway on Siemens ADVIA Centaur XPT. The reference ranges for TSH were between 0.56–4.89 mIU/L for persons 16–20 years old and 0.24–3.78 mIU/L for those above 20 years of age. The reference range for FT4 was 11.6–19.1 pmol/L.

Statistics

Characteristics of patients at admittance, shown separately for TSH and FT4, were described as number of samples, age, gender, and duration of stay and were analyzed by descriptive analysis shown in frequencies, mean, standard deviation, and median. In this study, biological variables such as TSH and FT4 were used as continuous scales. The variable for diagnostic groups was used as categorical variable which contained 8 groups. A chi-Square test was conducted to examine the relationship between gender and diagnostic groups. Because the normality of continuous variables assessed by the Kolmogorov–Smirnov test were all skewed, non-parametric statistical analyses were chosen for further analysis. The

Table 2 Summary of the diagnostic groups distribution

Diagnostic Group	ICD	FT4 (N, Male/Female)	TSH (N, Male/Female)
SUD	F10–19	82 (51/31)[b]	83 (51/32)[b]
Schizophrenia	F20–29	92 (45/47)	91 (44/47)
Bipolar Mania	F30–31.2	32 (17/15)	32 (17/15)
Bipolar Depression	F31.3–31.5	18 (8/10)	18 (8/10)
Unipolar Depression	F32 - F33	115 (45/70)	114 (44/70)
Neurotic Disorders	F40–49	51 (17/34)	52 (18/34)
Personality Disorders	F60–69	33 (11/22)	34 (11/23)
Others	–	115 (61/54)	115 (62/53)
Statistics[a]		$x^2(df)$ = 19.528 (7), p = **0.007**	$x^2(df)$ = 18.613 (7), p = **0.009**

SUD substance use disorder, *ICD* International Classification of Diseases, *FT4* free thyroxin, *TSH* thyroid-stimulating hormone
[a]Chi-Square Test was conducted to examine a relationship between gender and diagnostic groups
[b]After Bonferroni correction, only SUD reaches significant
Entries in bold are significant at 0.05 level

levels of TSH and FT4 at admittance and at discharge were analyzed by descriptive statistics shown in frequencies, mean, median, and range, in addition to the Wilcoxon signed-ranks test which compares the levels of neuroendocrine biomarkers before and after hospitalization by using TSH or FT4 samples which are available at both admittance and discharge. As preliminary analysis, differences in the levels of TSH and FT4 across the diagnostic groups were assessed by a Kruskal-Wallis H-test both in total and for gender-separated samples. Lastly, the association between a specific psychiatric diagnostic group and the effect of TSH and FT4 in the model was assessed by binary logistic regression for psychiatric diagnostic groups including SUD, schizophrenia, bipolar mania, bipolar depression, unipolar depression, neurotic disorders, and personality disorders, both in total and for gender-separated samples.

If there was a statistically significant difference in any analysis, the Dunn-Bonferroni correction was used for *post-hoc* test to avoid multiple test problems. For statistical analysis, IBM-SPSS version 22 was used to assess all data. The results were considered significant when the p value was lower than 0.05.

Results

Deviation outside reference ranges of TSH and FT4 in total sample and in different genders and different diagnostic groups

1.7% of the participants had FT4 levels below reference range and 21.9% above. For TSH numbers were 2.6 and 5.8%, respectively. The deviation from the expected value of 2.5% both above and below each reference range is significant for both FT4 ($p < 0.000$) and TSH ($p < 0.000$) (calculations not shown). Comparing differences in distribution between diagnostic groups and thyroid hormone ranges did not reveal significant association for FT4 (p = 0.281), while there was a slightly significant difference regarding TSH (p = 0.047). There were no significant differences between genders regarding frequency of patients with levels of FT4 or TSH outside reference levels (Table 3).

Differences in the levels of TSH or FT4 across psychiatric diagnosis in total and for gender-separated samples

Analyzing the total sample did not indicate any association between diagnoses and level of FT4 ($x^2(df)$ = 2.307(7), p = 0.941). For TSH however, an association was indicated ($x^2(df)$ = 14.062(7), p = 0.05, Additional file 1: Table S1). Separating the population into genders revealed significant differences in the levels of TSH between the diagnostic groups among females. SUD had the lowest mean score (mean score = 1.30 mIU/L), followed by schizophrenia (1.63 mIU/L), unipolar depression (1.70 mIU/L), neurotic disorders (1.85 mIU/L), bipolar mania (1.90 mIU/L), bipolar depression (2.10 mIU/L), other (2.27 mIU/L), and personality disorders (2.32 mIU/L) (Additional file 2: Table S2). A post hoc comparison by the Dunn-Bonferroni approach with adjusted p-value, confirmed significant difference among females between SUD and 'other', of which 'other' had significantly higher TSH levels (Z = – 3.202, SE = 18.321, p = 0.038) and this was confirmed in the regression model (Additional file 3: Table S3). No significant difference in the levels of TSH between different diagnostic groups was found for male patients.

Variation in thyroid hormones from admittance to discharge

Data for FT4 were available at both admittance and discharge for 239 patients. Mean (median) levels of FT4 were 17.09 (16.75) pmol/L at admittance, and 16.07 (16.00) pmol/L at discharge. There was a statistically significant reduction from admittance to discharge (n = 239, Z = – 5.680, p = 0.00, Table 4).

Data for TSH were available at both admittance and discharge for 236 patients. Mean (median) levels of TSH

Table 3 The relationship between FT4 and TSH levels in different ranges and gender as well as diagnostic groups

	FT4 Reference Range (≤ 11.6–19.1 ≤ (pmol/L))			TSH Reference Range (≤ 0.24–3.78 ≤ (mIU/L))		
	Below (n, %)	Within Reference Range (n, %)	Above (n, %)	Below (n, %)	Within Reference Range (n, %)	Above (n, %)
Total	9 (1.7%)	412 (76.4%)	118 (21.9%)	14 (2.6%)	493 (91.6%)	31 (5.8%)
Gender						
Male	6 (2.3%)	184 (72.2%)	65 (25.5%)	4 (1.6%)	240 (94.1%)	11 (4.3%)
Female	3 (1%)	228 (80.3%)	53 (18.7%)	10 (3.5%)	253 (89.4%)	20 (7.1%)
	$x^2(df) = 5.375$ (2), $p = 0.068$			$x^2(df) = 4.081$ (2), $p = 0.13$		
Diagnoses						
SUD	4 (5%)	64 (79%)	13 (16%)	4 (4.9%)	75 (91.5%)	3 (3.6%)
Schizophrenia	–	68 (73.9%)	24 (26.1%)	5 (5.5%)	84 (92.5%)	2 (2%)
Mania	–	22 (68.8%)	10 (31.2%)	–	30 (93.8%)	2 (6.2%)
Bipolar Depression	1 (2.9%)	26 (76.5%)	7 (20.6%)	1 (2.9%)	29 (85.3%)	4 (11.8%)
Unipolar Depression	–	90 (78.3%)	25 (21.7%)	1 (0.9%)	110 (96.5%)	3 (2.6%)
Neurotic Disorders	2 (3.9%)	41 (80.4%)	8 (15.7%)	1 (2%)	49 (94.2%)	2 (3.8%)
Personality Disorders	1 (3%)	25 (73.5%)	8 (23.5%)	1 (3%)	27 (81.8%)	5 (15.2%)
Others	1 (1%)	76 (76%)	23 (23%)	1 (1%)	89 (89%)	10 (10%)
	$x^2(df) = 16.543$ (14), $p = 0.281$			$x^2(df) = 23.946$ (14), $p =$ **0.047**		

SUD substance use disorder, *TSH* thyroid-stimulating hormone, *FT4* free thyroxine
Chi-Square Test was conducted to examine a relationship between FT4 and TSH in above and below the reference ranges and gender as well as diagnostic groups
Reference range was set by 95% of healthy population
Entries in bold are significant at 0.05 level

at admittance were 1.85 (1.86) mIU/L, and 1.81 (1.62) mIU/L at discharged. As seen in Table 4, there was no significant difference in the levels of TSH at admittance and discharge ($n = 236$, $Z = -0.268$, $p = 0.789$) (Table 4).

Discussion

In a general psychiatric acute closed inpatient population with equal gender distribution, levels of FT4 and TSH at admittance deviated from levels expected in the general population with significantly more patients than expected having levels above reference range. There were no differences between neither genders nor different diagnostic groups regarding number of patients outside reference ranges for FT4 and TSH apart from a slight difference for TSH between diagnostic groups. Comparing absolute levels of TSH and FT4 revealed a significantly lower level of TSH in the group SUD compared to other diagnostic groups in females. No significant differences were seen between other diagnostic groups in females, and no significant difference between diagnostic groups was seen in males. Comparing levels of hormones at admittance and discharge (mean 12 / median 6 days later) showed a significant reduction in the level of FT4 during stay, whereas no significant change in the level of TSH was seen.

Table 4 Descriptive statistics of FT4 and TSH (Admittance and Discharge)

	FT4 (pmol/L)		TSH (mIU/L)	
	Admittance	Discharge	Admittance	Discharge
N	538	252	539	254
Levels of Biomarkers				
mean	17.094	16.069	1.846	1.805
median	16.750	16.0	1.56	1.615
range	9.3–31.3	9.0–25.7	0.01–9.87	0.04–8.45
Statistics[a]	$Z = -5.680$, $p =$ **0.00**		$Z = -0.268$, $p = 0.789$	

FT4 free thyroxin, *TSH* thyroid-stimulating hormone
[a]Wilcoxon Signed-Ranks Test was conducted to compare difference between admittance and discharged
Entries in bold are significant at 0.05 level

Hypo- and hyperthyroidism as a cause of symptoms mimicking depression and other psychiatric problems is a well-known clinical phenomenon. We find an increase in both FT4 and TSH over all psychiatric diagnostic groups (maybe except female SUD) without gender differences. Previous studies comparing specific diagnostic groups with healthy controls have found an increased FT4 in depression [5, 8, 14], bipolar disorders [3], and panic disorders [7]. Findings are however deviating [12]. Simultaneously, a decrease in FT4 has been described in patients with chronic alcohol use [15–18]. FT4 and TSH are linked. Associations between depression and level of TSH compared to healthy controls have been found in previous studies [8, 10]. In studies on cannabis users reduced levels of TSH have been reported [19, 20]. There was no significant association between FT4 and any of the diagnostic groups in our cohort. Only TSH showed a significant difference for one diagnostic group (SUD) and only in females. To our knowledge there are not many other studies on altered thyroid function in patients with substance use disorders except for alcohol and cannabis. As TSH was actually higher than expected in our cohort, the interpretation of our finding may simply be that women with SUD were the ones with most normal levels of TSH, all other diagnostic groups having increased levels. There is no obvious explanation for the absence of this effect in the male group. There are however gender differences regarding hormones [8] and this might contribute to altered sensitivity to stress as well as to psychoactive substances.

Psychotropic medication is of relevance in many psychiatric patients. Glucocorticoids, l-dopa and dopamine may reduce TSH-activity, while Li and dopamine-antagonists may increase it [21, 22]. Unfortunately, we did not register data on participants' use of medications. The majority of patients would however not be on medications increasing thyroid function at admittance.

Our study comparing a broad variety of psychiatric diagnostic groups thus supplements the field indicating that the altered levels of thyroid hormones found in specific diagnostic groups compared to healthy controls is a broad psychiatric phenomenon reflecting psychic stress in general, not specific to certain diagnoses. This also is in line with the findings by Spratt in a general psychiatric acute inpatient population [23], although the potential variation over different diagnoses was not studied there. One explanation for the lack of relation between FT4 and diagnostic groups in our study could be the lack of power (small groups) or the acute-stress effect masking any differences between diagnostic groups, emphasizing the strength and potential clinical importance of the acute stress. This also emphasizes that altered thyroid function is not only potentially a cause of psychiatric symptoms but also, as postulated by Parry in 1825 [24], can be a result of emotional stress.

At admittance a higher number of patients than expected had FT4 above reference range. There then was a significant reduction in the level of FT4 from admittance to discharge. No significant change in TSH was seen. In a study with longer follow up (mean 21 days) in 22 acutely ill patients [23], a decrease in FT4 was seen, and in another longer follow up (mean 29 days) on acutely ill psychotic patients, both a decrease in FT4 and an increase in TSH were seen. However, despite a longer follow up than in our study, the increase in TSH was seen in fewer patients than those with a decrease in FT4 (41% vs 66%) [25]. Together, the findings indicate that the change in FT4 is not primarily driven by the central TSH as one could expect according to theories on the effect of psychiatric stress on the pituitary gland. Bunevicius suggests that the reduction in FT4 [25] is due to the use of antipsychotics. This would be in line with the mood stabilizer Li^+ known to cause hypothyroidism by reducing production in the thyroid gland [26]. Bunevicius et al. however have no control group without medication preventing the disclosure of an effect independent of medications. Unfortunately we have not recorded use of medications in patients. However, as the whole diagnostic specter was represented no single group of medication would be used and not all patients would have medications. Besides, the significant number of patients with FT4 above reference range at admittance increases likelihood that a reduction for normalization is expected. The mechanism for this peripheral effect of stress on the thyroid gland could involve receptors for stress hormones such as cortisol and adrenaline in the thyroid gland; this, however, remains to be explored further.

Taken together, our findings do not link alterations in TSH / FT4 to any specific diagnoses but rather to psychiatric suffering in general. In line with this, there is a significant reduction in the level of FT4 over a mean 12-day (median 6-day) stay in a psychiatric acute ward.

Limitations and strengths

There are several limitations to our study. The duration of stay was relatively short, lowering the possibility to detect a variation over time. However, at the same time, the registered variation in FT4 from admittance to discharge is thus more important because it reveals a dramatic change over a short time.

The number of participants is not large compared to epidemiological studies, although it is rather high for this kind of population and compared to other studies in acute-ward populations.

We do not have a group of healthy controls that could improve clarification of findings.

Data on patients' use of medications is not included. As discussed above this is a weakness. However, our aim was to study the thyroid status in the psychiatric patients independent of the etiology of any deviation. This is interesting as deviating thyroid status may cause problems for the patients and need attention and treatment independently of its etiology.

All main psychiatric diagnostic groups were included in the study, and the wards represented the only closed, acute psychiatric inpatient service in the area, reducing the likelihood of social selection and loss of important groups. The possibility to use data for persons at the time they are acutely ill at admittance is a strength.

Conclusion

Our study indicates that there is an overall increase in the level of FT4 and TSH in the acute psychiatric ill population independent of diagnoses and that there is a reduction (normalization) during the acute stay. There is no significant change in TSH, and the change in FT4 is quick (median duration of stay was 6 days), indicating that the change in FT4 is not driven by TSH. The effect of psychological stress via hypothalamus and TSH has been suggested previously; our study indicates that another mechanism must be causing this. Cortisol and adrenaline binding directly to the thyroid gland are candidates, although the mechanisms are, to our knowledge, not known.

The findings indicate that psychological stress may affect somatic functions in ways not known so far, a phenomenon that may have implications for treatment and somatic follow up of severely ill psychiatric patients.

Abbreviations

Anti-TPO: Anti-thyroid peroxidase antibodies; FT4: Free thyroxine; HPT: Hypothalamic–Pituitary–Thyroid; ICD: International classification of diseases; SUD: Substance use disorder; T3: Triiodothyronine; T4: Thyroxine; TCA: Tricyclic antidepressants; TRH: Thyrotropin-releasing hormone; TSH: Thyroid Stimulating hormone

Acknowledgements

We want to thank Øyvind Husøy and Marit Vik for skillful assistance in handling laboratory samples. We also want to thank the staff at the psychiatric acute wards at St Olav's hospital Department Østmarka as well as the patients for cooperation in collecting the data.

Authors' contributions

SKR designed the study including writing all protocols and taking care of all applications. SKR lead the inclusion of participants and the registration of data. SKR took an equal part in analyzing and interpreting the data and lead the writing of the manuscript. YS did the statistical analyses and took an equal part in interpreting the data. YS wrote the first draft for the manuscript. VI supervised and took an equal part in statistical analyses and took an equal part in writing the manuscript. All authors read and approved the final manuscript.

Consent for publication

Not applicable

Competing interests

Not applicable

References

1. Ritchie M, Yeap BB. Thyroid hormone: influences on mood and cognition in adults. Maturitas. 2015;81(2):266–75.
2. Bauer M, Goetz T, Glenn T, Whybrow PC. The thyroid-brain interaction in thyroid disorders and mood disorders. J Neuroendocrinol. 2008;20(10):1101–14.
3. Chakrabarti S. Thyroid functions and bipolar affective disorder. J Thyroid Res. 2011;2011:306367.
4. Brand SJ, Moller M, Harvey BH. A review of biomarkers in mood and psychotic disorders: a dissection of clinical vs. preclinical correlates. Curr Neuropharmacol. 2015;13(3):324–68.
5. Baumgartner A, Pietzcker A, Gaebel W. The hypothalamic-pituitary-thyroid axis in patients with schizophrenia. Schizophr Res. 2000;44(3):233–43.
6. Hein MD, Jackson IM. Review: thyroid function in psychiatric illness. Gen Hosp Psychiatry. 1990;12(4):232–44.
7. Fardella C, Gloger S, Figueroa R, Santis R, Gajardo C, Salgado C, Barroilhet S, Foradori A. High prevalence of thyroid abnormalities in a Chilean psychiatric outpatient population. J Endocrinol Investig. 2000;23(2):102–6.
8. Forman-Hoffman V, Philibert RA. Lower TSH and higher T4 levels are associated with current depressive syndrome in young adults. Acta Psychiatr Scand. 2006;114(2):132–9.
9. Loosen PT. The TRH-induced TSH response in psychiatric patients: a possible neuroendocrine marker. Psychoneuroendocrinology. 1985;10(3):237–60.
10. Jia Y, Zhong S, Wang Y, Liu T, Liao X, Huang L. The correlation between biochemical abnormalities in frontal white matter, hippocampus and serum thyroid hormone levels in first-episode patients with major depressive disorder. J Affect Disord. 2015;180:162–9.
11. Kautzky A, et al. A new prediction model for evaluating treatment resistant depression. J Clin Psychiatry. 2017;78(2):215–22. https://doi.org/10.4088/JCP.15m10381.
12. Olff M, Guzelcan Y, de Vries GJ, Assies J, Gersons BP. HPA- and HPT-axis alterations in chronic posttraumatic stress disorder. Psychoneuroendocrinology. 2006;31(10):1220–30.
13. Dickerman AL, Barnhill JW. Abnormal thyroid function tests in psychiatric patients: a red herring? Am J Psychiatry. 2012;169(2):127–33.
14. Sim K, Chong SA, Chan YH, Lum WM. Thyroid dysfunction in chronic schizophrenia within a state psychiatric hospital. Ann Acad Med Singap. 2002;31(5):641–4.
15. Balhara YP, Deb KS. Impact of alcohol use on thyroid function. Indian J Endocrinol Metab. 2013;17(4):580–7.
16. Valeix P, et al. Effects of light to moderate alcohol consumption on thyroid volume and thyroide function. Clin Endocrinol. 2008;68(6):988–95.
17. Rachdaoui N, Sarkar DK. Pathophysiology of the effects of alcohol abuse on the endocrine system. Alcohol Res. 2017;38(2):255–76.
18. Honnamurthy JB, Shivashankara AR, Avinash SS, John Mathai P, Malathi M. Effect of interaction between duration of alcohol consumption and alcohol dependence on thyroid function test: cross sectional observational study. Indian J Clin Biochem. 2018;33(1):61–8.
19. Bonnet U. Chronic cannabis abuse, delta-9-tetrahydrocannabinol and thyroid function. Pharmacopsychiatry. 2013;46(1):35–6.
20. Malhotra S, Heptulla RA, Homel P, Motaghedi R. Effect of marijuana use on thyroid function and autoimmunity. Thyroid. 2017;27(2):167–73.
21. Sauvage MF, Marquet P, Rousseau A, Raby C, Buxeraud J, Lachatre G. Relationship between psychotropic drugs and thyroid function: a review. Toxicol Appl Pharmacol. 1998;149(2):127–35.
22. Bou Khalil R, Richa S. Thyroid adverse effects of psychotropic drugs: a review. Clin Neuropharmacol. 2011;34(6):248–55.
23. Spratt DI, Pont A, Miller MB, McDougall IR, Bayer MF, McLaughlin WT. Hyperthyroxinemia in patients with acute psychiatric disorders. Am J Med. 1982;73(1):41–8.
24. Wheeler MH. A tale of two celts. World J Surg. 2010;34(6):1151–6.
25. Bunevicius R, Steibliene V, Prange AJ Jr. Thyroid axis function after in-patient treatment of acute psychosis with antipsychotics: a naturalistic study. BMC Psychiatry. 2014;14:279.
26. Engin A, Altan N, Isik E. Erythrocyte glutathione levels in lithium-induced hypothyroidism. Drugs R D. 2005;6(1):35–40.

2

Selected psychiatric problems among college students in two Arab countries: comparison with the USA

Ziad Kronfol[1,5*], Batoul Khalifa[2], Brigitte Khoury[3], Omar Omar[1], Sariah Daouk[3], J. P. deWitt[4], Nourehan ElAzab[1] and Daniel Eisenberg[4]

Abstract

Background: Psychiatric problems among college students on USA campuses are common. Little is known about similar problems in developing countries, particularly the Arab region. The goal of this study was to assess the frequency of selected psychiatric problems among college students in two Arab countries: Qatar and Lebanon, and to compare them to the USA.

Methods: The Healthy Minds Study, an online confidential survey of common psychiatric symptoms designed for college campuses was used. We used the Patient Health Questionnaire-9 (PHQ-9) to screen for major depression, the Generalized Anxiety Disorder-7 (GAD-7) to screen for generalized anxiety and the SCOFF questionnaire to screen for eating disorders. Comparisons were made using ANOVA, Chi-Square tests and logistic regressions.

Results: A total of 1841 students participated in the study. The rates of depression (PHQ-9 ≥ 12), generalized anxiety (GAD-7 ≥ 10) and eating disorders (SCOFF≥3) at the combined Arab universities were 34.6, 36.1 and 20.4% respectively. The corresponding rates in the USA were: 12.8, 15.9 and 6.8% ($p < 0.001$ for all measures). The impact of psychiatric problems on functioning in general and academic performance in particular was more severe in the Arab countries compared to the USA ($p < 0.001$). Independent predictors of psychiatric problems in general included location, female gender, financial difficulties and poor grades. Being religious had a protective association with mental health.

Conclusion: The rates of depression, anxiety and eating disorders were significantly higher among college students in Qatar and Lebanon compared to the USA. Additional research is needed to determine whether these results reflect methodological limitations or true differences in psychopathology across these populations. If replicated, the results indicate that the psychiatric problems on college campuses in the USA are a microcosm of a global problem that needs global solutions.

Keywords: College students, Arab countries, Depression, Anxiety, Eating disorders, Cultural psychiatry

Background

The college experience is a highly desirable experience worldwide and is often associated with independence, creativity, achievements and youth. It is often seen as a rite of passage from an often tumultuous adolescence to a more stable young adulthood. However the college experience can also be very challenging to many students who are living away from home for the first time and are often facing academic pressure, financial difficulties, problems in relationships and career choices. In the USA, three quarters of all lifetime cases of mental illness begin by age 24 [1]. It is therefore not surprising that surveys of mental health problems among college students in the USA indicate a high rate of depression, anxiety and other psychiatric disorders [2]. There is also a high rate of suicidal ideation and occasional reports of completed suicide, which has led many colleges and

* Correspondence: zik2002@qatar-med.cornell.edu
[1]Weill Cornell Medicine-Qatar, Doha, Qatar
[5]Weill Cornell Medicine, 445 E 69th St. Suite 432, New York, NY 10021, USA
Full list of author information is available at the end of the article

universities across the USA to take preventive measures and increase access to counseling [2]. The success of such measures in reducing psychological morbidity and preventing suicide has not yet been firmly established.

While mental health problems among college students in developed countries such as the USA and Europe are well recognized and efforts are underway to deal with them, very little information is available from developing countries and particularly Arab countries such as Qatar, which boasts one of the highest per capita income in the world and where about half of the population is under the age of 25 [3].

The topic of college students' mental health is not adequately covered in the Arabic literature. Substance use among college students was the topic of several reports, mostly from Lebanon [4, 5]. Anxiety symptoms among university students in the United Arab Emirates UAE were assessed using the Arabic Version of the Beck Anxiety Inventory [6]. Female students in general scored higher than their male counterparts. In a cross-national study of anxiety symptoms among college students in Beirut, Lebanon and Calgary, Canada, Lebanese students obtained higher scores than their Canadian counterparts [7]. Using the Zagazig Depression Scale (ZDS), Ibrahim and colleagues surveyed undergraduate college students at Assiut University in Egypt for depressive symptoms. They found that 37% of the students had symptoms scored above the threshold for moderate depression [8]. They also found an association between depression and low socioeconomic indices such as father's occupation, family income and number of persons per room. The survey was done face-to-face while confidentiality of the response was assured. The same group of researchers conducted a similar survey in 6 different universities in the UK, using online methodology. They found practically the same results, pointing to the strength of the association between low socioeconomic status and depressive symptomatology in different regions and cultures [9]. To our knowledge, no comprehensive assessment of various aspects of college students' mental health using validated instruments and modern online secure survey techniques across countries has ever been done in the Arab world. This research project is designed in part to fill this gap. We conducted a confidential online survey of selected psychiatric disorders, lifestyles, attitudes towards mental illness, and mental service utilization among college students at three universities in two Arab countries, and compared the results to a college campus in the USA.

Methods

Sample and data collection

The study included four universities: Education City (EC) and Qatar University (QU) in Doha, Qatar, the American University of Beirut (AUB) in Lebanon, and the University of Michigan (UM) in Ann Arbor, Michigan, USA. EC [10] is a modern hub for branches in Doha for several major universities in the USA and Europe. EC at present includes branches from Weill Cornell Medical College (medicine), Carnegie Mellon University (business and computers), Georgetown University (foreign affairs), Northwestern University (communication, journalism), Virginia Commonwealth University (art history and design), Qatar Faculty of Islamic Studies (religion), Hautes Etudes Commerciales (business) and University College London (archeology). Together EC has about 1500 students, many of them foreigners coming to study in Qatar. They come mostly from Arab or other Middle Eastern countries, Eastern European countries, or the Indian subcontinent. They also speak a variety of languages. Teaching at EC is in English. Men and women attend the same classes. QU [11], on the other hand, is a more traditional campus. Teaching is mostly in Arabic but most students speak English as well. Classes are often segregated, with men and women studying in separate classrooms. The student population is just over 17,000, the majority of whom are Qatari. AUB [12] is a private, secular and independent university. Originally founded in 1866 by Quaker missionaries as the Syrian Protestant College, it presently has about 8000 students about half of whom are Lebanese while the rest come from various, mostly Arab or Middle Eastern countries. AUB is chartered in the USA in the state of New York. The rationale for the choice of these universities is that QU represents a traditional university in a conservative Islamic country (Qatar), EC represents a more western-style, more liberal model of education in the same traditional country, while AUB offers the same model of western education in a more open and liberal Arab society (Lebanon). UM [13] on the other hand is a large, public American University located in the American Midwest. In 2017 UM celebrated its 200th anniversary.

Students were selected by simple randomization at QU, AUB and UM. The recruited sample was 6000 at QU, 3000 at AUB, and 4000 at UM. Because of the smaller population at EC, we tried to recruit all students enrolled at this site. Carnegie Mellon University-Qatar declined participation. All other universities participated, resulting in a sample size of 1200 students. The surveys were run in parallel during the spring of 2015. The selected students were sent emails inviting them to participate. All participants indicated their informed consent at the beginning of the survey. The study was approved by the institutional review board of each of the four sites.

Sample weights

To address potential nonresponse bias, we constructed sample weights for each site's sample, based on a small number of demographic characteristics for which the population distribution was known. For the samples at the Arab universities, these weights adjusted for the lower participation rates of men compared to women, by weighting participants by the inverse of the overall participation rate by gender. For the sample at UM, we had additional demographic information, and constructed sample weights based on gender, academic level, and grade point average. In our experience surveying university student populations, gender is the strongest predictor of survey response and therefore our estimates of the US sample do not change much if we use only gender rather than the larger set of demographics used.

Key measures

We used the Patient Health Questionnaire-9 (PHQ-9) to measure symptoms of depression over the last 2 weeks period. This self-report scale, which is based on the DSM-IV, has been used to measure both the severity of depressive symptoms as well as the diagnosis of major depression [14]. The scale has been shown to have good sensitivity and specificity [15]. It has been used in different settings and has been translated into different languages including Arabic and validated in different cultures including Saudi Arabia [16] and Lebanon [17]. Scores on the PHQ-9 are usually interpreted as follows: score 0–4: no depression; score 5–9: mild depression; score 10–14: moderate depression and score ≥ 15: severe depression. We have used the PHQ-9 as a screen for the diagnosis for major depression. Although different cutoff points have been suggested, we used the cutoff of 12 as the best cutoff both for sensitivity and specificity in an Arab country [18].

We used the Generalized Anxiety Disorder-7 (GAD-7) to measure symptoms of anxiety over the last 2 weeks. Like the PHQ-9, the GAD-7 is a self-report questionnaire based on DSM-IV criteria of generalized anxiety disorder [19]. This scale was also shown to have good sensitivity but specificity has been variable [20]. This scale has also been used in different settings and in different countries including Lebanon [17]. Scores on the GAD-7 were interpreted as follows: score 0–4: no anxiety; score 5–9: mild anxiety; score 10–14: moderate anxiety and score ≥ 15: severe anxiety. As with the PHQ-9, we also used the GAD-7 for the diagnosis of generalized anxiety disorder. We also chose a cutoff of 10 for this diagnosis, in line with similar studies conducted in Arab countries [17].

We used the SCOFF questionnaire [21] as a screening tool for eating disorders at the time of the study. The SCOFF is comprised of 5 leading questions covering different aspects of an eating disorder. A "yes" answer to 3 questions or more is highly suggestive of the presence of anorexia nervosa or bulimia. The SCOFF has been used in a variety of settings and in different countries, and has been validated for use in Lebanon [22].

We also included other demographic and personal measures such as living arrangements, financial situation and religiosity. Many of these measures are self-explanatory (e.g. living in dorms, off-campus single or sharing or off-campus with parent, spouse or other relative), Some measures require a certain amount of subjectivity (e.g. current financial situation: "it's a financial struggle"; "tight but doing fine" or "finances aren't a problem" and religiosity: "very religious"; "fairly religious"; "not too religious" or "not religious at all"). For measurement of functional impairments caused by mental health problems we used two items. First, we included an item that usually follows the PHQ-9: "If you checked off any problems, how difficult have these problems made it for you to do your work, take care of things at home, or get along with other people?" Second, we included a question about impairment in academic performance: "In the past 4 weeks, how many days have you felt that emotional or mental difficulties have hurt your academic performance?" These measures complement the PHQ-9 and the GAD-7 screens for clinical depression and anxiety and have frequently been used in college surveys screening for mental health problems among students [2].

Statistical analysis

Chi-squared tests were used to determine the differences between schools (Arab and USA) for binary outcomes. Differences between schools for ordinal outcomes were calculated by using chi-squared test for trend. Multivariable logistic regression with random intercept models was used to test for independent associations between outcomes (depression/ anxiety/ eating disorders) and variables of interest taking account of the clustering effect of schools by using Stata 13 command *xtlogit.* Main effects and interactions between correlates and schools were examined for each outcome. All analyses were done using Stata 13 (Stata Corp, College Station, Texas, USA) and using the svy commands to account for the sampling weights as discussed above.

Results

Basic sample characteristics

Fourteen thousand two-hundred students were recruited during the spring of 2015. Participation rates were as follows: EC 351/1200 (29%); QU: 434/6000 (7.2%); AUB: 167/3000 (5.6%) and UM: 889/4000 (22.2%) for a total participation rate of 1841/14,200 (13.0%). Participants' characteristics are shown in Table 1. As expected, there were major differences in the basic profile of the students at the different sites. This was our intention, as we wanted to compare campuses with different cultural, ethnic, and socioeconomic characteristics.

Table 1 Participants characteristics, in weighted percentages (Standard error)

Characteristic	Education City ($n = 351$)	Qatar University ($n = 434$)	American University of Beirut ($n = 167$)	University of Michigan ($n = 889$)	*P*-value
Age in years					
18–20	36.5 (3.5)	33.8 (2.3)	64.0 (3.9)	35.7 (1.8)	< 0.001
21–25	42.1 (3.5)	46.7 (2.5)	30.8 (3.7)	42.3 (1.8)	
> =26	21.4 (2.5)	19.5 (2.0)	5.3 (1.9)	22.0 (1.4)	
Gender					
Female	58.3 (3.5)	71.9 (2.3)	50.3 (4.1)	47.4 (1.8)	< 0.001
Nationality					
Nationals of the host country	47.3 (3.6)	71.5 (2.3)	83.5 (3.0)	86.6 (1.2)	< 0.001
Program					
Undergraduate	76.7 (2.6)	83.6 (2.0)	93.7 (1.8)	65.2 (1.7)	< 0.001
Living arrangements					
On campus Dorms	25.7 (3.2)	1.2 (0.6)	16.8 (3.1)	21.8 (1.6)	< 0.001
Off-campus, single or sharing	7.7 (1.5)	3.8 (1.0)	18.0 (3.2)	71.2 (1.7)	
Off-campus, parents, spouse or other relatives	66.7 (3.4)	95.1 (1.2)	65.3 (3.9)	7.0 (0.9)	
In a relationship					
Yes	31.7 (3.4)	29.7 (2.5)	23.7 (3.5)	46.0 (1.8)	0.0259
Current financial situation					
It's a financial struggle	10.6 (2.3)	3.6 (1.0)	9.4 (2.4)	10.2 (1.1)	< 0.001
Tight but doing fine	46.5 (3.8)	42.3 (2.6)	54.2 (4.1)	50.7 (1.8)	
Finances aren't a problem	42.9 (3.7)	54.1 (2.6)	36.4 (3.9)	39.2 (1.8)	
GPA					
A+ to A-	55.8 (3.9)	22.2 (2.2)	33.5 (3.9)	59.2 (1.9)	< 0.001
B+ to B-	39.6 (3.9)	50.6 (2.7)	56.8 (4.1)	37.2 (1.9)	
C+ and below	4.5 (1.6)	27.2 (2.4)	9.7 (2.5)	3.7 (0.8)	
Religiosity					
Fairly/Very religious	87.0 (2.3)	94.7 (1.2)	43.7 (4.0)	32.5 (1.7)	< 0.001
Not too religious/Not religious at all	13.0 (2.3)	5.3 (1.2)	56.3 (4.0)	67.5 (1.7)	

The students in the Arab universities tended to be slightly younger, likely because of the higher proportion of undergraduates, particularly at AUB. Interestingly, there was also a higher representation by women. The universities in Qatar had fewer nationals compared to both AUB and UM. More students in the Arab universities lived with their parents or relatives and fewer at the dorms. Also, more students at UM reported being in a relationship. Financially, the students in Qatar reported being better off than students both in Lebanon and the USA. Academically, the students both in EC and at UM reported having somewhat better grades. Also, the students in Qatar identified as being more religious than their counterparts in Lebanon or the USA. Many of these differences were expected as the sites were chosen to reflect different cultures and sensitivities.

Overall prevalence of depression, anxiety and eating disorders

The prevalence rates for major depression (PHQ-9 ≥ 12), generalized anxiety (GAD≥10) and eating disorders (SCOFF≥3) in EC, QU, AUB and UM are shown in Table 2. The rates of major depression, generalized anxiety and eating disorder were very similar in EC, QU and AUB compared to UM. The corresponding rate (SE) for major depression in EC was 40.5% (4.1), in QU was 32.0% (2.7), and at AUB was 38.6% (4.1). The rate at UM was much smaller at 12.8%.(1.3)), a difference which is statistically significant ($p < 0.001$). The corresponding rate (SE) for generalized anxiety disorder in EC was 38.3%, (3.6), in QU was 34.2%,(2.8) and at AUB was 39.4% (4.2), significantly higher than at UM where the rate was 15.9% (1.4), a difference which was statistically significant ($p < 0.001$). Similar trends were also

Table 2 Prevalence of psychiatric problems and consequences in Qatar, Lebanon and the USA, in weighted percentage (Standard error)

	Education City (*n* = 351)	Qatar University (*n* = 434)	American University of Beirut (*n* = 167)	Arab Universities combined (*n* = 952)	University of Michigan (*n* = 889)	*p*-value
Major Depression (PHQ-9)						
No (0–11)	59.5 (4.1)	68.0 (2.7)	61.4 (4.1)	65.4 (2.1)	87.2 (1.3)	< 0.001
Yes (≥12)	40.5 (4.1)	32.0 (2.7)	38.6 (4.1)	34.6 (2.1)	12.8 (1.3)	
Generalized Anxiety (GAD-7)						
No (0–9)	61.7 (4.2)	65.8 (2.8)	60.6 (4.2)	63.9 (2.2)	84.1 (1.4)	< 0.001
Yes (≥10)	38.3 (4.2)	34.2 (2.8)	39.4 (4.2)	36.1 (2.2)	15.9 (1.4)	
Eating disorder (SCOFF)						
No (0–2)	81.2 (4.2)	78.6 (2.4)	81.4 (3.2)	79.6 (1.8)	93.2 (0.9)	< 0.001
Yes (≥3)	18.8 (4.2)	21.4 (2.4)	18.6 (3.2)	20.4 (1.8)	6.8 (0.9)	
Function impairments caused by depression						
Not at all difficult	20.6 (3.1)	26.1 (2.5)	24.1 (3.7)	25.2 (1.9)	40.9 (1.9)	< 0.001
Somewhat difficult	51.7 (4.2)	59.0 (2.8)	54.6 (4.2)	57.3 (2.2)	48.6 (2.0)	
Very difficult	18.4 (3.3)	11.3 (1.8)	15.0 (3.1)	12.9 (1.5)	9.2 (1.2)	
Extremely difficult	9.3 (2.7)	3.5 (1.0)	6.2 (1.9)	4.7 (0.9)	1.3 (0.4)	
MH affected academic performance						
0 days	25.4 (3.3)	21.5 (2.5)	21.4 (3.5)	21.7 (1.9)	45.6 (1.9)	< 0.001
1–2 days	23.0 (3.6)	32.4 (2.8)	25.9 (3.8)	29.7 (2.1)	28.2 (1.7)	
3–5 days	19.0 (3.2)	24.4 (2.6)	23.2 (3.6)	23.7 (2.0)	16.1 (1.4)	
≥ 6 days	32.6 (4.1)	21.6 (2.5)	29.5 (3.8)	24.8 (2.0)	10.2 (1.1)	

noted for eating disorders, with corresponding rates (SE) of 18.8% (4.2), 21.4% (2.4) and 18.6% (3.2) at EC, QU and AUB respectively, rates significantly higher than at UM, with a rate of only 6.8% (0.9). These differences were also statistically significant ($p < 0.001$). Questions regarding functional impairment caused by depression and academic performance being affected by mental health problems are also shown in Table 2. The functional impairment was higher in EC, QU and AUB than at UM ($p < 0.001$). Similarly, the students at EC, QU and AUB report their academic performance has been more seriously affected than students at UM ($p < 0.001$).

Because of the similarities in the rates of depression, anxiety and eating disorders in the three Arab sites (none of the differences were statistically significant), we combined the three Arab universities together and compared them with the one University in the USA. The results are shown graphically in Fig. 1. These results show that the rates of major depression of 34.6% (2.1), generalized anxiety 36.1% (2.2) and eating disorder 20.4% (1.8) on college campuses in Arab countries are significantly higher ($p < 0.001$) than corresponding rates in the USA of 12.8% (1.3), 15.9% (1.4) and 6.8% (0.9) respectively.

Independent correlates of psychiatric problems on university campuses

We then looked at independent predictors of major depression, generalized anxiety and eating disorder in our entire sample (both Arab campuses and the USA) (Table 3). Significant predictors of major depression included location in the two Arab countries (OR: 4.82; CI: 4.01, 5.79), being a woman (OR: 1.88; CI: 1.72, 2.05), having financial difficulties (OR: 7.63; CI: 3.50, 16.65) and having low grades (OR: 2.79; CI: 0.74, 10.55). Being in a relationship was a protective factor (OR: 0.90; CI: 0.83, 0.97). Being fairly or very religious was another independent protective factor (OR: 0.57; CI: 0.38, 0.86).

Significant predictors for generalized anxiety again included location in the two Arab countries (OR: 1.98; CI: 1.16, 3.40), being a woman (OR: 2.40; CI: 2.17, 2.67) and having financial difficulties (OR: 12.10; CI: 7.45, 19.64). Other predictors of generalized anxiety include older age (OR: 1.46; CI: 1.14, 1.86) and living off campus with a parent, relative or a spouse (OR: 1.86; CI: 1.03, 3.36) and being a B student (OR: 1.35; CI: 1.11, 1.64). Protective factors against anxiety include again being religious (OR: 0.46: CI: 0.31, 0.71), but also being a graduate student (OR: 0.52; CI: 0.35, 0.78).

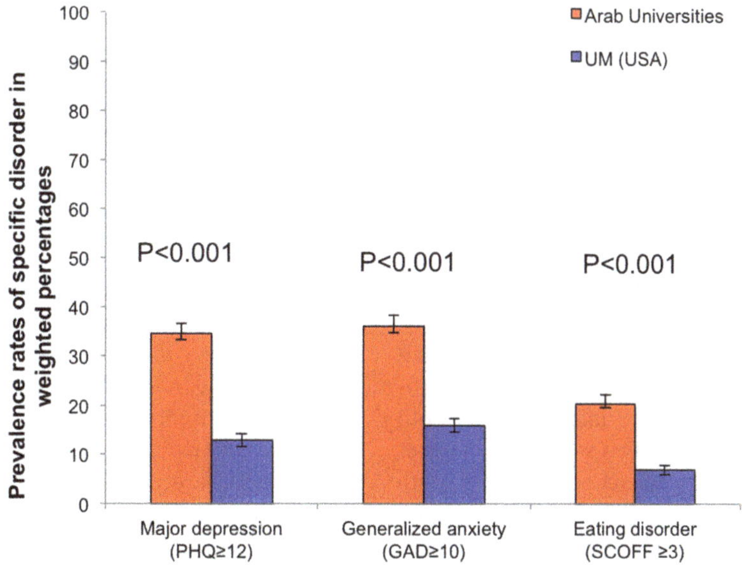

Fig. 1 Prevalence rates (in weighted percentages +/− SE) of major depression, generalized anxiety and eating disorders among college students in Arab countries and the USA

Table 3 Adjusted Odds Ratios (OR) and 95% Confidence Intervals (CIs) for predictors of psychiatric problems

	Depression (PHQ ≥ 12) (*n* = 1312)	Anxiety (GAD ≥ 10) (*n* = 1266)	Eating disorders (*n* = 571)
	OR (95% CI)	OR (95% CI)	OR (95% CI)
UM	1.00	1.00	1.00
Arab	4.82 (4.01, 5.79)[b]	2.72 (1.52, 4.86)[b]	1.98 (1.16, 3.40)[a]
Age 18–20	1.00	1.00	1.00
Age 21–25	1.13 (0.77, 1.66)	0.75 (0.36, 1.54)	1.04 (0.60, 1.79)
Age 26–30	1.23 (0.76, 1.97)	1.46 (1.14, 1.86)[b]	2.19 (0.63, 7.62)
Female	1.88 (1.72, 2.05)[b]	2.40 (2.17, 2.67)[b]	2.52 (1.40, 4.51)[b]
Dorms	1.00	1.00	1.00
Off-campus, single or sharing	1.33 (0.61, 2.89)	1.18 (0.90, 1.55)	0.82 (0.46, 1.46)
Off-campus, parent, relative or spouse	1.07 (0.51, 2.24)	1.86 (1.03, 3.36)[a]	1.69 (1.00, 2.85)
Graduate	0.78 (0.57, 1.08)	0.52 (0.35, 0.78)[b]	0.31 (0.10, 0.97)[a]
Finances aren't a problem	1.00	1.00	1.00
Tight but doing fine	1.57 (1.16, 2.13)[b]	1.86 (1.79, 1.94)[b]	1.35 (0.79, 2.30)
It's a financial struggle	7.63 (3.50, 16.65)[b]	12.10 (7.45, 19.64)[b]	2.83 (1.11, 7.24)[a]
In a relationship	0.90 (0.83, 0.97)[b]	0.93 (0.63, 1.38)	1.31 (0.80, 2.13)
GPA			
A+ to A-	1.00	1.00	1.00
B+ to B-	1.60 (1.08, 2.38)[a]	1.35 (1.11, 1.64)[b]	0.78 (0.38, 1.60)
C+ and below	2.79 (0.74, 10.55)[b]	1.51 (0.74, 3.09)	0.94 (0.49, 1.79)
Not religious or not religious at all	1.00	1.00	1.00
Fairly or very religious	0.57 (0.38, 0.86)[b]	0.46 (0.31, 0.71)[b]	0.89 (0.67, 1.18)
National of country	1.00 (0.78, 1.29)	0.98 (0.79, 1.21)	1.19 (0.67, 2.13)

[a]significant at 5% level
[b]significant at 1% level

Predictors for eating disorders again include location in the two Arab countries (OR: 1.98; CI: 1.16, 3.40), female gender (OR: 2.52; CI: 1.40, 4.51) and having financial difficulties (OR: 2.83; CI: 1.11, 7.24). One protective factor is being a graduate student (OR: 0.31; CI: 0.10, 0.97).

We also looked at interactions (data not shown) between the different variables, the outcome measures (depression, anxiety and eating disorders) and school location (Arab vs USA). We found interesting significant interactions ($p < 0.05$) between gender and school for all three outcomes, with female gender being more closely associated with psychopathology in the three Arab universities compared to the USA. There were also significant interactions between financial difficulties and both depression ($p < 0.001$) and anxiety ($p < 0.001$) but not eating disorders with respect to school location, with more than double the rates of both depression and anxiety among students who are struggling financially and living in Arab countries compared to those living in the USA. We also found significant interactions between academic performance, the various outcomes and school location, with low grades again being more strongly associated with psychopathology in the Arab countries ($p < 0.001$) compared to the USA.

Discussion

The most notable finding from this study is the high prevalence of probable major depression (34.6%), generalized anxiety (36.1%), and eating disorders (20.4%) reported by a sample of college students in Arab countries compared to the USA, with corresponding rates of 12.8, 15.9 and 6.8% respectively. It is also important to note that these disorders seem to cause more functional impairment and are more likely to affect academic performance in Arab countries compared to the USA. These results are of particular interest when put in context: the three universities in the Arab countries are quite different in terms of history, location, educational philosophy and student population. We therefore expected the rate of psychopathology for instance in Lebanon to be somewhat halfway between the corresponding rates in Qatar and the USA. Yet the prevalence of three of the most common psychiatric disorders among the students in the two Arab countries is very similar. The prevalence of these disorders among the students in Qatar and Lebanon is 2–3 times larger than in the USA. Furthermore, the survey was done online using the same survey format at approximately the same time in all four locations, adding to the validity of the findings.

How do results from this survey compare with other surveys from Arab countries? In a recent study on the prevalence of depression and anxiety among Saudi university students using the PHQ-9 and the standard algorithm for depression, the authors report symptoms of major depression in 9.9% of the students, symptoms of other depression in 19.4%, and any depression in 24.4% of the students [23]. Again using the PHQ, they report generalized anxiety in 14.0% of the students. Part of the discrepancy with our results may be related to gender differences, as their sample consisted mostly of men who reported significantly lower rates of both major depression and generalized anxiety than women. Again using the PHQ-9 with a cut-off of 12, Al-Ghafri and colleagues estimated the prevalence of depression among medical trainees in Oman to be 11.4%. [18]. As to the prevalence of depression in Saudi primary care adult patients, the rates for depression using PHQ-9 were 49.9%, of which 31% had mild symptoms, 13.4% moderate, 4.4% moderate to severe and 1.0% severe symptoms [24]. As mentioned earlier, using the ZDS rating scale, Ibrahim and colleagues reported a depression rate of 37% among undergraduate students at Assiut University in Egypt [8].

Regarding the behavioral rating scales we used, namely the PHQ-9, the GAD-7 and the SCOFF, although they have all been validated for use in Arab countries, there is still some controversy regarding the cut-off point to be used for diagnostic purposes, particularly with the PHQ-9 for depression. In general, the lower the cutoff point, the larger the rate of a particular diagnosis. In our study, we used these instruments both for severity measurements and disease prevalence. However, because this is a comparative study, the conclusion that the rates of depression, anxiety and eating disorders are higher in Arab countries remains valid regardless of the cutoff point used. Some researchers have used the standard algorithm for interpreting the PHQ-9 [25], and accordingly diagnosed the subjects with major depression, minor depression or no depression. We examined our data along these lines and reached the same conclusion: that although the rates for specific disorders could change, these disorders are substantially more common in Arab countries compared to the USA (data not shown).

In a systematic review of depression prevalence among university students worldwide [26], the rates of depression varied between 10.3 and 84.5% with a mean weighted prevalence of 30.6%. The most common scales used were the Beck Depression Inventory BDI [27] followed by the Center for Epidemiological Studies-Depression CES-D [28] and the PHQ-9. The authors concluded that the rates of depression experienced by university students are substantially higher than those found in the general population [26]. In a recent validation study of the PHQ-9 and GAD-7 in a Lebanese psychiatric clinic, the authors conclude that both the PHQ-9 and the GAD-7 are reliable screening tools for depression and anxiety in an Arabic population, but that the diagnostic specificity of these instruments is not very robust. Furthermore, the authors believe the PHQ-9 tends to exaggerate depressive symptomatology in the Arabic population or that it may be sensitive to subthreshold symptoms [17].

Direct comparison of psychiatric symptoms between Arab and American universities is rare but results similar to our own have been reported by Abdel-Khalek and Lester who found anxiety among Kuwaiti college students to be higher than in their American counterparts [29]. One possible explanation could be the high rate of comorbidity in the Arab sample. Co-occurrence rates (at least two occurrences) were elevated, both in the Arab countries and the USA but were more elevated among students in Arab countries. This could account, at least in part, for the inflation seen in the Arab countries. Among students with an eating disorder, for instance, 64.0% reported a co-occurring condition (depression or anxiety) in Arab countries. The corresponding rate was 38.2% at UM.

When we looked at independent risk factors that may be associated with depression, anxiety and eating disorders among college students on all campuses, several interesting findings were noted. First, location (being in the two Arab countries) was a significant predictor for all three outcomes, consistent with data presented in Table 2. Similarly, being a woman was a significant risk factor associated with all three conditions, a finding in line with most epidemiological studies regarding these conditions [23, 30]. Another major predictor of mental health problems across countries seems to be financial difficulties, which is associated with depression, anxiety and eating disorders on all campuses. This is somewhat surprising as many students, particularly in Qatar, described their current financial situation as “finances aren’t a problem”, yet for those who struggle financially there is an increased risk for depression, anxiety and eating disorder both in Arab countries and the USA. In that regard, our results seem to agree with Amr and colleagues who reported that female gender, financial and personal problems were significant predictors of depression in Saudi university students [23]. Another interesting predictor of psychopathology is the effect of academic performance [31]: low grades (C+ and below) constitute an independent risk factor for depression while being a B student increases the risk for anxiety. Perhaps the B performance keeps many students on their guards, producing more anxiety, while the C and below performance is more likely to lead to despair and depression.

There were also factors that seem to provide some protection against psychopathology. For instance, being a graduate student seems to be associated with a lower risk for both anxiety and eating disorder. This could be a sign of better adaptation to college life but more data are needed in that regard. Similarly, being in a relationship could reduce the risk for depression, as loneliness is a factor that is frequently associated with depression. Religiosity is another factor that seems to be associated with a lower risk for both depression and anxiety. This is consistent with other reports from both Arab countries [32] and the USA [33] as religiosity can be understood as providing a sense of purpose and support for students everywhere [34].

This study has a number of limitations. First, the survey participation rate was very low (under 10%) at two of the sites (AUB and QU). The rate was substantially higher at EC, however, and the prevalence estimates were similar across all three Arab universities. We expected the participation to be lower in Arab countries as the students are not used to this type of research. Our sample weights can at least correct for a limited set of demographic characteristics that predict participation, such as gender. Second, the universities we surveyed may not be representative of the regions we cover. We chose three very different universities in two very different Arab countries. The demographic characteristics were very different. Yet the prevalence of depression, anxiety and eating disorder were very similar. Obviously more countries need to be included in future studies using similar methodologies to better map-out the prevalence of these common psychiatric disorders. There is also the possibility that UM does not adequately represent all US universities, although previous studies suggest that it is near the middle of the national distribution in terms of mental health prevalence [2]. Lastly, we used measures of mental health that although validated in the different countries, were based on brief self-reported instruments that may not correlate perfectly with clinicians’ diagnoses.

Conclusions

In summary, our work shows that psychiatric problems so common on college campuses in Western countries are not limited to those countries. In fact, these problems may be even more common and more serious in developing countries, where students often face greater financial, political and/or other psychosocial challenges and lack the services and/or resources to deal with them. We are presently looking at mental health service utilization in those countries and the reasons why the people who need them the most are not accessing them the way they should. Some answers may be local in nature and call for specific legislation in a specific country or region while others may be more general in nature and call for more global attention and intervention.

Abbreviations
AUB: American University of Beirut; EC: Education City; GAD-7: Generalized Anxiety Disorder-7; PHQ-9: Patient Health Questionnaire-9; QU: Qatar University; UM: University of Michigan

Funding
This study was made possible by NPRP Grant 5-618-5-087 from the Qatar National Research Fund (a member of Qatar Foundation). The findings achieved herein are solely the responsibility of the authors.

Authors' contributions
ZK and DE conceived of the study and participated in its design and coordination and drafted the manuscript. BK1 and BK2 participated in the design and coordination at different sites; SD, JPW and NEA coordinated data collection and analysis; OO performed the statistical analysis; all authors made intellectual contributions and approved the final manuscript.

Competing interests
The authors declare that they have no competing interests.

Author details
[1]Weill Cornell Medicine-Qatar, Doha, Qatar. [2]Qatar University, Doha, Qatar. [3]American University of Beirut, Beirut, Lebanon. [4]University of Michigan, Ann Arbor, USA. [5]Weill Cornell Medicine, 445 E 69th St. Suite 432, New York, NY 10021, USA.

References
1. Kessler RC, Berglund P, Demler O, Jin R, Merikangas KR, Walters EE. Lifetime prevalence and age-of-onset distributions of DSM-IV disorders in the National Comorbidity Survey Replication. Arch Gen Psychiatry. 2005;62:593.
2. Eisenberg D, Hunt J, Speer N. Mental health in American colleges and universities: variation across student subgroups and across campuses. J Nerv Ment Dis. 2013;201:60.
3. Qatar Population (2017) – World Population Review. http://worldpopulation review.com/countries/qatar-population/. Accessed 8 Mar 2017.
4. Tamim H, Terro A, Kassem H, Ghazi A, Khamis TA, MMA H. Tobacco use by university students, Lebanon, 2001. Addict. 2003;98:933.
5. Karam EG, Maalouf WE, Ghandour LA. Alcohol use among university students in Lebanon: prevalence, trends and covariates. The IDRAAC university substance use monitoring study (1991 and 1999). Drug Alcohol Depend. 2004;76:273.
6. Al-Issa I, Al Zubaidi A, Bakal A, Fung TS. Beck anxiety inventory symptoms in Arab college students. Arab J Psychiatry. 2000;11:41.
7. Al-Issa I, Al Zubaidi A, Bakal A, Fung TS. Beck anxiety inventory symptom comparisons between students in Lebanon and Canada. Arab J Psychiatry. 1999;10:24.
8. Ibrahim A, Kelly S, Glazebrook C. Analysis of an Egyptian study on the socioeconomic distribution of depressive symptoms among undergraduates. Soc Psychiatry Psychiatr Epidemiol. 2012;47:927.
9. Ibrahim A, Kelly S, Glazebrook C. Socioeconomic status and the risk of depression among UK higher education students. Soc Psychiatry Psychiatr Epidemiol. 2013;48:149.
10. Qatar Foundation Education. http://www.qf.org.qa/education. Accessed 8 Mar 2017.
11. Qatar University about. Http://www.qu.edu.qa/about. Accessed 8 Mar 2017.
12. American University of Beirut About Us. http://www.aub.edu.lb. Accessed 8 Mar 2017.
13. University of Michigan. http://umich.edu. Accessed 8 Mar 2017.
14. Kroenke K, Spitzer RL. The PHQ-9: a new depression diagnostic and severity measure. Psychiatr Ann. 2002;32:509.
15. Kroenke K, Spitzer RL, Williams JB. The PHQ-9: validity of a brief depression severity measure. J Gen Intern Med. 2001;16:606.
16. Becker S, Al Zaid K, Al FE. Screening for somatization and depression in Saudi Arabia: a validation study of the PHQ in primary care. Int J Psychiatry Med. 2002;32:271.
17. Sawaya H, Atoui M, Hamadeh A, Zeinoun P, Nahas Z. Adaptation and initial validation of the patient health questionnaire - 9 (PHQ-9) and the generalized anxiety disorder - 7 questionnaire (GAD-7) in an Arabic speaking Lebanese psychiatric outpatient sample. Psychiatry Res. 2016;239:245.
18. Al-Ghafri G, Al-Sinawi H, Al-Muniri A, Dorvlo ASS, Al-Farsi YM, Armstrong K. Prevalence of depressive symptoms as elicited by patient health questionnaire (PHQ-9) among medical trainees in Oman. Asian J Psychiatry. 2014;8:59.
19. Spitzer RL, Kroenke K, Williams JBW, Löwe B. A brief measure for assessing generalized anxiety disorder: the GAD-7. Arch Intern Med. 2006;166:1092.
20. Kertz S, Bigda-Peyton J, Bjorgvinsson T. Validity of the generalized anxiety Disorder-7 scale in an acute psychiatric sample. Clin Psychol Psychother. 2013;20:456.
21. Morgan JF, Reid F, Lacey JH. The SCOFF questionnaire: assessment of a new screening tool for eating disorders. BMJ. 1999;319:1467.
22. Aoun A, Azzam J, Jabbour FE, Hlais S, Daham D, Amm CE, et al. Validation of the Arabic version of the SCOFF questionnaire for the screening of eating disorders. East Mediterr Health J. 2015;21:326.
23. Amr M, Amin T, Saddichha S, Al Malki S, Al Saail M, Al Qahtani N, AlAbdulhadi A, Al Shoaibi A. Depression and anxiety among Saudi university Students : prevalence and correlates. Arab J Psychiatry. 2013;24:1.
24. Al-Qadhi W, Ur Rahman S, Ferwana MS, Abdulmajeed IA. Adult depression screening in Saudi primary care: prevalence, instrument and cost. BMC Psychiatry. 2014;14:190.
25. Spitzer RL, Kroenke K, Williams JBW. Validation and utility of a self-report version of PRIME-MD: the PHQ primary care study. JAMA. 1999;282:1737.
26. Ibrahim AK, Kelly SJ, Adams CE, Glazebrook C. A systematic review of studies of depression prevalence in university students. J Psychiatr Res. 2013;47:391.
27. Beck AT, Steer RA, Garbin MGJ. Psychometric properties of the Beck depression inventory twenty-five years of evaluation. Clin Psych. 1988;8:77.
28. Radloff LS. The CES-D scale: a self-report depression scale for research in the general population. Appl Psychol Meas. 1977;1:385.
29. Abdel-Khalek AM, Lester D. Anxiety in Kuwaiti and American college students. Psychol Rep. 2006;99:512.
30. Black D, Andreason N. Introductory textbook of psychiatry. 6th ed: American Psychiatric Association; 2014.
31. Eisenberg D, Golberstein E, Hunt JB. Mental health and academic success in college. B E J Econ Anal Policy. 2009;9
32. Abdel-Khalek AM. Subjective well-being and religiosity in Egyptian college students. Psychol Rep. 2011;108:54.
33. Abdel-Khalek AM, Lester D. Constructions of religiosity, subjective well-being, anxiety, and depression in two cultures: Kuwait and USA. Int J Soc Psychiatry. 2012;58:138.
34. Miller L, Wickramaratne P, Gameroff MJ, Sage M, Tenke CE, Weissman MM. Religiosity and major depression in adults at high risk: a ten-year prospective study. Am J Psychiatry. 2012;169:89.

Prevalence of psychiatric diagnoses in asylum seekers with follow-up

Kneginja Richter[1,2,3*], Lukas Peter[1], Hartmut Lehfeld[1], Harald Zäske[4], Salina Brar-Reissinger[1] and Günter Niklewski[1,2]

Abstract

Background: In the study, the frequency and nature of asylum seekers' psychiatric diagnoses in a German admission center were examined. Additional aims were to identify changes in those diagnoses over time and to investigate health care utilization of mentally ill asylum seekers in the community.

Methods: The sample for the study "Psychiatric Examination of Asylum Seekers" in Bavaria consisted of a total of 283 asylum seekers and included 2 subsamples: help-seeking individuals and a randomly selected group. 34 of all asylum seekers were part of an extensive psychiatric follow-up examination (t2) about six months after the first examination (t1). Here, we used psychometric tools and a psychiatric interview by a medical doctor and a psychologist with the help of translators.

Results: 79% of help-seekers and 45% of the random group received at least one psychiatric diagnosis at t1. The most frequent diagnoses were trauma- and stress-related disorders, affective disorders, and insomnia. Men and Muslims were underrepresented in the help-seeking group. In the follow-up subsample, the rate of psychiatric diagnoses went down from 74% at t1 to 38% at t2. In contrast, the number of PTSD cases increased from 4 at t1 to 7 at t2. The severity of PTSD symptoms such as hyperarousal and avoidance also increased. Of the 13 persons in the follow-up-sample diagnosed with depression at t1, only 2 still fit the criteria of the disease at t2. Only 5 subjects had received some sort of psychotherapy or counseling.

Conclusion: The prevalence of mental illness in asylum seekers reported here corresponds to the usual range in the literature. It is significantly higher than in European civil society, especially regarding PTSD. At t2, the diagnoses of PTDS had increased within several months without evident additional traumatic events. Asylum seekers' psychiatric diagnoses soon after arrival should be recorded carefully and examination should be repeated after six months. The psychiatric and psychotherapeutic treatment of asylum seekers is still insufficient. Psychoeducative steps should be taken to relieve the stigma on mental illness, especially among males and Muslims.

Keywords: Asylum seekers, Refugees, Mental health, PTSD, Depression, Insomnia

Background

Asylum seekers are among the most vulnerable, marginalized and powerless groups in society with a high risk for psychiatric disturbances. They have most likely only recently fled difficult living conditions [1–8] and now live in constant fear of deportation and under permanent strain in admission centers, which contributes to their psychological distress.

* Correspondence: kneginja.richter@gmx.de
[1]Clinic Nuremberg, University Clinic for Psychiatry and Psychotherapy, Paracelsus Private Medical University, Nuremberg, Germany
[2]Faculty for Social Sciences, Technical University for Applied Sciences Georg Simon Ohm, Nuremberg, Germany
Full list of author information is available at the end of the article

Germany was the country with the highest number of applications for asylum (65,000) within the European Union in the Year 2012, recording an increase of 41% in application numbers as compared to 2011 [9].

This study was conducted in one of Bavaria's biggest admission centers, the Admission Center for Asylum Seekers (ZAE) – Zirndorf. The goals were to examine asylum seekers' psychiatric diagnoses in the first weeks after their arrival in the country, to verify the diagnoses a few months after their discharge from the center and to examine whether mentally ill asylum seekers had received appropriate psychiatric and psychological treatment after discharge.

Most studies on mental disorders in asylum seekers focus on posttraumatic stress disorder (PTSD), reporting a range of prevalence rates between 32 and 46% [4, 10–16]. Others report numbers as high as 74% [17] or as low as 14% [18]. Affective and anxiety disorders were found to be the most frequent comorbidities with PTSD [19–21].

A review of published studies on the prevalence of mental disorders in asylum seekers shows a fundamental problem which makes a comparison of results difficult: the sampling methods used are very heterogeneous and led to samples that range from a randomly selected group of subjects to an examination of a rigidly selected group such as the population using counselling or other services [22].

Trying to build on and extend the reviewed research, we formulated the following questions: What are the prevalence rates of mental illness in groups of randomly selected and help-seeking asylum seekers? Which socio-demographic groups will be represented in these two groups? How will psychiatric diagnoses develop over time? And finally, in what ways will mentally ill asylum seekers receive treatment in the German public health system?

Methods

Within the project "Psychiatric Examination of Asylum Seekers" supported by the Bavarian Ministry of Labour, Social Affairs, Family and Women [23], a psychiatric center was installed in an admission center in southern Germany. Here, two samples of asylum seekers underwent examination for mental disorders in a preliminary study (t1) between 01/2011 and 05/2012. The first sample consisted of help-seekers, i.e. individuals who had contacted the center of their own impetus. Information regarding psychiatric services was freely available to the residents of the admission center in the form of flyers which had been translated into ten different languages. As a result of close working relationships with local services, medical practitioners, and volunteer services, the project coordinators were able to widely disseminate information about the psychiatric services offered. The random sample consisted of randomly selected residents of the center. As part of the randomization process, a cross-check procedure was used to ensure that no participants from the help seeking group were invited to the random group. All of the invited individuals agreed to participate in the initial screening and all participants provided their consent in written form. Following written agreement from the Ethical Committee, participants were interviewed within the first six weeks of their residence in the center. The most common countries of origin in both samples were Iran (30.4%), Afghanistan (20.1%), Russia (19.4%), Iraq (14.5%), and Azerbaijan (5.7%). Islam (66.5%) and Christianity (13.9%) were the most common religious denominations.

Participants were interviewed by trained bilingual specialists who administered questionnaires to assess the frequency of mental disorders in the 12 months before the interview. Where possible, patients' preferences with regard to the examiner's gender were accommodated. Diagnoses were made in accordance with the International Classification of Diseases, 10th revision (ICD 10; [24]) using the Mini-International Neuropsychiatric Interview (MINI; [25]). We assessed psychiatric symptoms by use of the Brief Symptom Inventory (BSI), a culturally sensitive 53-item self-report symptom checklist. Based on BSI results, nine primary symptom dimensions can be computed: somatic symptoms, obsessive-compulsive symptoms, feelings of personal inadequacy, depression, clinical anxiety, anger and hostility, phobic anxiety, paranoid ideation, and social alienation [26]. To measure suicidal thoughts, item 10 of the Montgomery Asberg Depression Rating Scale (MADRS) was used, explicitly asking on a seven point scale for the feeling that life is not worth living, death would be welcome, suicidal thoughts are present or that a suicidal act is being prepared [27]. PTSD symptoms were measured using the Essen Trauma Inventory (ETI), a screening inventory consisting of 35 items for a broad range of traumatic events and 23 symptom based items for posttraumatic stress symptoms on four subscales: intrusion, avoidance, hyperarousal, and peritraumatic dissociation [28]. To assess sleep disturbances, we used the Pittsburg Sleep Quality Index (PSQI), concentrating on the first three of its seven subscores, i.e. subjective sleep quality, sleep latency, and sleep duration [29]. In addition, the interview included questions about the asylum seekers' use of health services, as well as on social, economic and cultural factors since the migration.

The examinations were performed over a 3-h period during which a psychiatric history was taken by a psychiatry specialist and psychometric testing was carried out by a psychologist. The psychologist/psychiatrist provided detailed information to the participants on the background of the study and the examination procedure. In all cases, the psychiatric-psychological examination was carried out fully after the person selected for examination had given their written consent.

One week after the first interview, subjects that had received a psychiatric diagnosis were asked to return for a second interview (see fig. 1). In this second consultation, therapeutic recommendations for future treatment were made after a discussion of the results and the diagnosis with the patient. Persons without a psychiatric diagnosis were not invited to the second interview.

Four to ten months later, after the asylum seekers had been discharged from the admission center to steadier

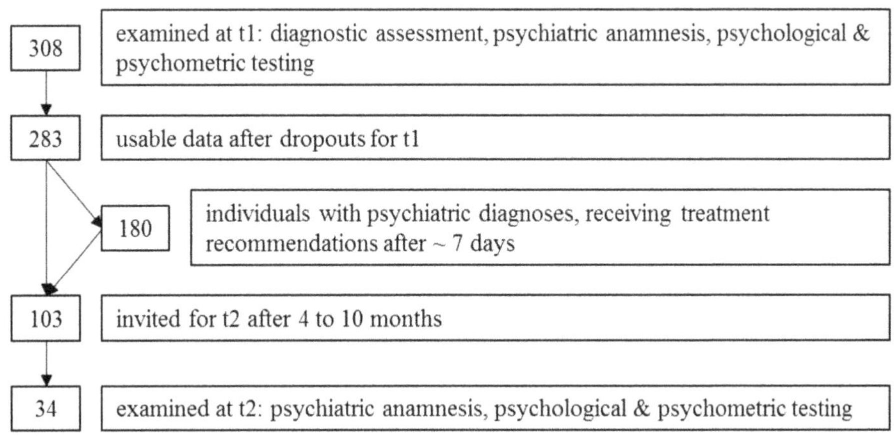

Fig. 1 Steps of examination

accommodations, a follow-up examination (t2) was carried out. Our aim was to interview subsamples of both initially examined groups in their new homes. At t2, most individuals in the sample were either of Iranian (44.1%), Afghan (26.5%), or Russian (11.8%) nationality.

Statistical Analyses were performed using the program SPSS 20. Chi-square tests and variance analysis methods were used for interference statistical comparisons of the two subsamples in addition to the descriptive presentation of results by frequency charts and mean values. Missing data was excluded from the statistical analysis.

Results

Preliminary examination (t1)

In total, 308 individuals were examined. After dropouts, data for 283 asylum seekers (125 women, 158 men, age 31.9 ± 10.6 years) was analysed (see fig. 2). The most common reasons for dropout were fatigue or decompensation during the examination and refusal of the psychological examination after the psychiatric interview. 158 of the examined individuals were part of the help-seeking sample, 125 formed the random group.

Women (51.9% vs. 34.4%, Chi-square test $p < .01$), Christians (22.4% vs. 17.7%, $p < .05$), Russians (27.8% vs 8.8%, $p < .000$) and Afghans (24.1% vs. 15.2%, $p < .000$), as well as those with previous migration experience (13.9% vs. 1.6%, $p < .001$) were significantly overrepresented in the help-seeking group as compared to the random group. We also found a tendency of those arriving with children prevailing among help-seekers (55.1% vs. 44.8%, $p = .088$), most likely because of the higher amount of women in this group. Men (48.1% vs 65.5%; $p < .01$) and Muslims (50.4% vs. 66.5%; $p < .05$) were underrepresented among help-seekers. There were no significant differences regarding age, marital status, education, or professional status.

Significantly more psychiatric diagnoses were made in the help-seeking group than in the random group (78.5%

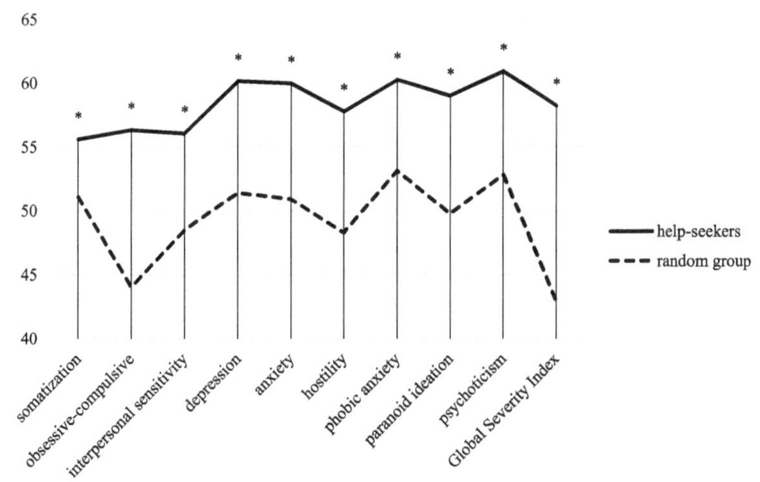

Fig. 2 BSI profile plots for both groups at t1 (t-scores). $N = 283$. All differences $p < .000$

vs. 44.8%, $p < .000$, see Table 1). The most common primary diagnoses were stress-related and anxiety disorders (F4 and F3; 53.3% of diagnoses), affective disorders (34.4%) and insomnia (7.2%). There was no significant difference between the groups in the relative frequency of diagnoses (see Table 2). The most frequent diagnosis was PTSD with 17.6% of all subjects in the random group and 22.8% in the help seeking group fulfilling the criteria (see Table 1).

Help-seekers also showed significantly more psychiatric symptoms compared to the random group across all scales of the BSI (see fig. 2), as well as the MADRS, and the PSQI (ANOVA all $p < .000$). These differences persisted after excluding all individuals without a psychiatric diagnosis from the analysis. In external assessment, at least temporary thoughts of suicide were documented in 26% of the help-seeking group and in 6% of the random group ($p < .000$). Likewise, the number of potentially traumatizing events in an individual's previous history reported in ETI was 1.1 in the random sample and almost double this number in the help-seeking group (1.9, $p < .000$).

In the help-seeking group, 50.6% received a drug prescription from the psychiatrist as compared to 25.6% in the random group. Most of these prescriptions were for mild sedatives and antidepressants. 18 individuals were referred to psychiatric inpatient treatment, 13 to psychiatric outpatient, and 18 to non-psychiatric outpatient treatment.

Table 1 Frequencies of diagnose-clusters, including most frequent specific diagnoses, in both subsamples at t1

ICD 10 chapter	help seekers	random
diagnosis	124 (78.5%)	56 (44.8%)
F0	1 (0.6%)	0 (0.0%)
F1	1 (0.6%)	1 (0.8%)
F2	2 (1.3%)	1 (0.8%)
F3	46 (29.1%)	16 (12.8%)
F32.1	14 (8.9%)	5 (4.0%)
F33.1	9 (5.7%)	4 (3.2%)
F33.2	12 (7.6%)	2 (1.6%)
F4	65 (41.1%)	31 (24.8%)
F43.1	36 (22.8%)	22 (17.6%)
F43.2	14 (8.9%)	7 (5.6%)
F5	8 (5.1%)	5 (4.0%)
F6	1 (0.6%)	2 (1.6%)
no diagnosis	34 (21.5%)	69 (55.2%)
total	158 (100%)	125 (100%)

Note. F0 = Organic, including symptomatic, mental disorders. F1 = Mental and behavioural disorders due to psychoactive substance use. F2 = Schizophrenia, schizotypal and delusional disorders. F3 = Mood (affective) disorders. F32.1 = Moderate depressive episode. F33.1 = Recurrent depressive disorder, current episode moderate. F33.2 = Recurrent depressive disorder, current episode severe without psychotic symptoms. F4 = Neurotic, stress-related and somatoform disorders. F43.1 = Posttraumatic stress disorder. F43.2 = Adjustment disorders. F5 = Behavioural syndromes associated with physiological disturbances and physical factors. F6 = Disorders of adult personality and behavior

Table 2 Relative frequencies of F3 and F4 diagnoses in both subsamples at t1

psychiatric disorder	help-seekers $n = 124$	random $n = 56$
F3	45 (36.3%)	16 (28.6%)
F31.0	1 (0.8%)	0 (0.0%)
F32.0	1 (0.8%)	3 (5.4%)
F32.1	14 (11.3%)	5 (8.9%)
F32.2	6 (4.8%)	1 (1.8%)
F32.3	1 (0.8%)	0 (0.0%)
F33.1	9 (7.3%)	4 (7.1%)
F33.2	12 (9.7%)	2 (3.6%)
F33.3	0 (0%)	1 (1.8%)
F34.1	2 (1.6%)	0 (0%)
F4	65 (52.4%)	31 (55.4%)
F41.0	8 (6.5%)	1 (1.8%)
F41.1	3 (2.4%)	0 (0%)
F41.2	1 (0.8%)	1 (1.8%)
F43.0	1 (0.8%)	0 (0%)
F43.1	36 (39.3%)	22 (29%)
F43.2	14 (11.3%)	7 (12.5%)
F44.0	1 (0.8%)	0 (0%)
F45.8	1 (0.8%)	0 (0%)

Note. F31.0 = Bipolar affective disorder, current episode hypomanic. F32.0 = Mild depressive episode. F32.1 = Moderate depressive episode. F32.2 = Severe depressive episode without psychotic symptoms. F32.3 = Severe depressive episode with psychotic symptoms. F33.1 = Recurrent depressive disorder, current episode moderate. F33.2 = Recurrent depressive disorder, current episode severe without psychotic symptoms. F33.3 = Recurrent depressive disorder, current episode severe with psychotic symptoms. F34.1 = Dysthymia. F41.0 = Panic disorder (episodic paroxysmal anxiety). F41.1 = Generalized anxiety disorder. F41.2 = Mixed anxiety and depressive disorder. F43.0 = Acute stress reaction. F43.1 = Posttraumatic stress disorder. F43.2 = Adjustment disorders. F44.0 = Dissociative amnesia. F45.8 = Other somatoform disorders. F51.0 = Nonorganic insomnia

Follow-up (t2)

103 individuals were invited for a follow-up examination. For practical reasons, those that had moved away over 100 km from the study center in Nuremberg, Germany, were excluded from the follow-up. By the end of the study, 34 subjects (11 from the help-seeking group, 23 from the random group, age 32.50 ± 11.14 years) could be identified and examined. When controlling for group and gender, the follow-up sample did not differ significantly from the rest of the initial sample regarding symptoms on the BSI, MADRS or PSQI.

The average time lag between t1 and t2 was 214.6 ± 86.4 days. There were no significant differences between former help seekers and members of the random group regarding sociodemographic characteristics.

The total amount of psychiatric diagnoses decreased from 25 at t1 to 13 at t2. At t1, 41.2% had been diagnosed with an affective disorder from the F3 chapter of the ICD 10. At t2, 8.8% fit the criteria of such a disorder. All 7 cases of severe depressive episodes (F32.2, F33.2) had receded. Diagnoses of trauma and stress-related disorders stayed at 20.6% at both points in time. However, there was a shift, and arguably an increase, in severity: while there were four cases of adjustment disorder less, four new cases of PTSD were diagnosed (see Table 2). All three initial cases of non-organic insomnia either persisted or shifted to a more severe diagnose at follow-up.

More than half of the sample ($n = 19$) reported having been in contact with the public health system since t1, either receiving medical treatment (12), prescription drugs (2), psychotherapy (2), or other forms of therapy and counseling (3) (Table 3).

Discussion

Our results show a high prevalence of psychiatric disorders in asylum seekers with a significantly higher prevalence in the help-seeking group of patients as opposed to the random group. The most frequent primary diagnosis in both groups was PTSD (F43.1). Compared to the research provided by Wittchen and colleagues [30], the prevalence is clearly higher in our random sample than in the European population (17.6% vs. 2.9%). This might be explained by the potentially traumatic circumstances that may have led this population to seek asylum in the first place, in combination with post migration stress [31–33]. The second most frequent diagnosis found was a depressive episode (light to severe) followed by insomnia. When we combine the prevalence of stress-related and affective disorders, the results are similar to those shown in the research on refugees by Lindert and colleagues [5] (37.6% vs. 40%). In total, the prevalence rates in our random sample falls into the mid-range of values reported in literature on this topic [4, 12, 14–16].

Table 3 Overview of psychiatric diagnoses at t1 and t2 in the follow-up sample. $N = 34$

diagnosis	t1	t2
F3	14	3
F32.1	4	1
F32.2	3	0
F33.1	3	1
F33.2	4	0
F34.1	0	1
F4	7	7
F43.1	3	7
F43.2	4	0
F51.0	3	3
F60.8	1	0
none	9	21

Note. F32.1 = Moderate depressive episode. F32.2 = Severe depressive episode without psychotic symptoms. F33.1 = Recurrent depressive disorder, current episode moderate. F33.2 = Recurrent depressive disorder, current episode severe without psychotic symptoms. F34.1 = Dysthymia. F43.1 = Posttraumatic stress disorder. F43.2 = Adjustment disorders. F51.0 = Nonorganic insomnia. F60.8 other specific personality disorder

From the collected data we conclude that asylum seekers tend to be more vulnerable to psychiatric illness. This reflects the assumption by Lindert and colleagues [5] that within the heterogeneous group of migrants there is a higher prevalence of depression and anxiety in asylum seekers than in other groups, such as labor migrants.

From t1 to t2, the prevalence of PTSD increased without evident additional traumatic events. According to the diagnostic criteria for PTSD in ICD 10 [24], there is a time latency of several weeks or months for the manifestation of the main symptoms. These results suggest that asylum seekers' psychiatric diagnoses soon after arrival should be recorded carefully and that examination should be repeated after six months. Otherwise, PTSD symptoms might remain undiscovered and grow even more severe. Considering the diagnoses of depression, the disease receded in 11 of 13 cases. We assume that the improvement of social circumstances and living conditions after leaving the crowded admission center might be contributing to this, as only five subjects in the follow-up sample had received some sort of psychotherapy or counselling. The authors conclude that the psychological and psychiatric treatment of mentally ill asylum seekers after discharge from the admission center is insufficient.

The typical subjects in the help-seeking group were Russian women of Christian denomination with previous migration experience. In the random group, there was a higher proportion of male asylum seekers of Muslim denomination coming mainly from Iraq and Iran, of which 45% fulfilled the criteria for a psychiatric diagnosis. They, however, were not seeking help. The cause for this appears to be due to gender as well as cultural, ethnic and religious differences in how psychiatric symptoms are understood and ultimately expressed. Moreover, they could be a starting point for the targeted treatment of risk groups. In order for public health systems to cope with this problem, the authors suggest psychoeducation and information for asylum seekers with the aim to relieve stigmatization from mental illness.

Implications

From our perspective, a multi-professional and multilingual team with a background in cultural psychiatry is necessary to optimally diagnose and treat a population as heterogenous and burdened as asylum seekers. In the help-seeking group, 21.5% did not fulfill the criteria for a psychiatric illness. We assume that they may have suffered from psychological problems such as anxiety or sleep problems, but their symptoms were not distinct enough to fulfil the criteria for a psychiatric diagnosis. The second reason could be simulation of symptoms wishing to be granted asylum, which we can only assume. We believe, however, that by having two examiners (a psychiatrist and a psychologist) we were able to minimize false positives.

The diagnosis of recurrent depression (F33) was at 9.7% of the random and 17% of the help-seeking group. This means that a high number of asylum seekers are likely to have suffered from depression in the past, which could impact on individual help-seeking behavior.

The fourth most frequent psychiatric diagnosis in our study was insomnia. In order to be able to make a difference between insomnia and insomnia symptoms, we asked for the severity of sleep difficulties. Usually, the subject reported that their insomnia bothered them much more than the depressive or anxious mood and that better sleep would also improve their mood [34]. Our experience was that for some asylum seekers words such as *psychiatry*, *psychology*, or *stress* were not familiar. However, asking how they slept opened the door for better understanding of their psychological status. For this reason, sleep could provide an effective avenue for treatment [35].

We did not diagnose an 'Enduring personality change after catastrophic experience' in any of the participants – one explanation for this fact was that not enough time had passed from the time of trauma.

Our final recommendation for further research on the evaluation of mental disorders in the population of asylum seekers is to always include a randomized control group – this is especially important to help gain representative data for this very diverse population.

Limitations and weaknesses

The random sample could have been structured differently so as to mirror the sociodemographic make-up of the residents at the ZAE Zirndorf more closely and to be more representative of this unit. At the same time, however, the high fluctuation of residents might have counteracted this approach. This means that the random sample only represents a snapshot of the situation at a given moment in time. A more long-term comparison including the statistics for the years 2011 and 2012 might provide further insights in this respect. What remains unclear is whether the site of interview had an impact on help seeking behavior because all of our interviews occurred onsite at the ZAE. Future studies should investigate help seeking behavior in other locations, such as hospitals. Finally, due to administrative and economic reasons, the follow-up group was a lot smaller than intended and may not have produced entirely representative results.

Conclusions

On the basis of current research, we recommend the establishment of outpatient psychiatric-psychological services for those who need treatment as well as short psychiatric screenings for all asylum seekers immediately upon their arrival in the host country. Screening and supportive consultation should be available as part of the first wave of medical screening/treatment with an option for pharmacotherapy if appropriate and necessary. Psychotherapeutic treatments could be offered as a second step in a hierarchy of treatment model. With regard to post migration stress, a helpful step would be to reduce the temporal duration of the application procedure for asylum status - this should also include limiting the time spent in an admission center.

Abbreviations

BSI: Brief Symptom Inventory; ETI: Essen Trauma Inventory; ICD 10: International Classification of Diseases, 10th revision; MADRS: Montgomery Asberg Depression Rating Scale; MINI: Mini-International Neuropsychiatric Interview; PSQI: Pittsburg Sleep Quality Index; PTSD: Posttraumatic Stress Disorder; ZAE: Admission Center for Asylum Seekers (*"Zentrale Aufnahmeeinrichtung"*)

Funding

This study was funded by the Bavarian State Ministry of Employment and Social Order, the Family and Women with the explicit aim to examine prevalence rates of mental illness and the demand for psychiatric care in the ZAE Zirndorf.

Authors' contributions

KR, HL, SBR, and GN were involved in designing and implementing the study. KR and LP wrote the manuscript. HL and HZ provided statistical evaluation and interpretation. All authors have revised the manuscript critically and have agreed to be accountable for all aspects of the work in ensuring that questions related to the accuracy or integrity of any part of the work are appropriately investigated and resolved.

Consent for publication

Not applicable.

Competing interests

The authors declare that they have no competing interests.

Author details

[1]Clinic Nuremberg, University Clinic for Psychiatry and Psychotherapy, Paracelsus Private Medical University, Nuremberg, Germany. [2]Faculty for Social Sciences, Technical University for Applied Sciences Georg Simon Ohm, Nuremberg, Germany. [3]Faculty for Medical Sciences, University Goce Delcev, Stip, Macedonia. [4]Department of Psychiatry and Psychotherapy, Medical Faculty, Heinrich-Heine-University, Düsseldorf, Germany.

References

1. Abebe DS, Lien L, Hjelde KH. What we know and don't know about mental health problems among immigrants in Norway. J Immigr Minor Health. 2014;16:60–7.

2. Bhugra D. Migration and mental health. Acta Psychiatr Scand. 2004;109:243–58.
3. Grüsser SM, Wölfling K, Mörsen CP, Albrecht U, Heinz A. Immigration-associated variables and substance dependence. J Stud Alcohol Drugs. 2005;66:98–104.
4. Iversen VC, Morken G. Differences in acute psychiatric admissions between asylum seekers and refugees. Nord J Psychiatry. 2004;58:465–70.
5. Lindert J, Priebe S, Penka S, Napo F, Schouler-Ocak M, Heinz A. Depression and anxiety in labor migrants and refugees: a systematic review and meta-analysis. Soc Sci Med. 2009;69:246–57.
6. Machleidt W, Calliess IT. Transkulturelle Psychiatrie und Migration: Psychische Erkrankungen aus ethnischer Sicht. Psychiatrie (Stuttg). 2005;2:77–84.
7. Ryan DA, Kelly FE, Kelly BD. Mental health among persons awaiting an asylum outcome in western countries. Int J Ment Health. 2009;38:88–111.
8. Tribe R. Mental health of refugees and asylum-seekers. Adv Psychiatr Treat. 2002;8:240–7.
9. Bundesamt für Migration und Flüchtlinge. Migrationsbericht 2012. 2014. http://www.bamf.de/SharedDocs/Anlagen/DE/Publikationen/Migrationsberichte/migrationsbericht-2012.pdf. Accessed 23 Aug 2017.
10. Gäbel U, Ruf M, Schauer M, Odenwald M, Neuner F. Prävalenz der posttraumatischen Belastungsstörung (PTSD) und Möglichkeiten der Ermittlung in der Asylverfahrenspraxis. Z Klin Psychol Psychother. 2006;35:12–20.
11. Gerritsen AA, Bramsen I, Devillé W, van Willigen LH, Hovens JE, Van Der Ploeg HM. Physical and mental health of afghan, Iranian and Somali asylum seekers and refugees living in the Netherlands. Soc Psychiatry Psychiatr Epidemiol. 2005;66:98–104.
12. Karunakara UK, Neuner F, Schauer M, Singh K, Hill K, Elbert T, Burnham G. Traumatic events and symptoms of post-traumatic stress disorder amongst Sudanese nationals, refugees and Ugandans in the West Nile. Afr Health Sci. 2004;4:82–93.
13. Laban CJ, Gernaat HB, Komproe IH, Schreuders BA, de JJT. Impact of a long asylum procedure on the prevalence of psychiatric disorders in Iraqi asylum seekers in the Netherlands. J Nerv Ment Dis. 2004;192:843–51.
14. Peltzer K. Trauma and mental health problems of Sudanese refugees in Uganda. Cent Afr J Med. 1999;45:110–4.
15. Roodenrijs T, Scherpenzeel R, de Jong J. Traumatic experiences and psychopathology among Somalian refugees in the Netherlands. Tijdschrift voor Psychiatrie. 1998;40:132–42.
16. Silove D, Sinnerbrink I, Field A, Manicavasagar V, Steel Z. Anxiety, depression and PTSD in asylum-seekers: assocations with pre-migration trauma and post-migration stressors. Br J Psychiatry. 1997;170:351–7.
17. Sieberer M, Ziegenbein M, Eckhardt G, Machleidt W, Calliess IT. Psychiatrische Begutachtung im Asylverfahren. Psychiatr Prax. 2011;38:38–44.
18. Bradley L, Tawfiq N. The physical and psychological effects of torture in Kurds seeking asylum in the United Kingdom. Torture. 2006;16:41–7.
19. Bogic M, Njoku A, Priebe S. Long-term mental health of war-refugees: a systematic literature review. BMC Int Health Hum Rights. 2015;15:29. https://doi.org/10.1186/s12914-015-0064-9.
20. Breslau N, Davis GC, Schultz LR. Posttraumatic stress disorder and the incidence of nicotine, alcohol, and other drug disorders in persons who have experienced trauma. Arch Gen Psychiatry. 2003;60:289–94.
21. Ehlers A, Steil R, Winter H, Foa EB. German translation of the posttraumatic stress diagnostic scale (PDS): unpublished manuscript; 1996.
22. Schwarz-Nielsen KH, Elklit A. An evaluation of the mental status of rejected asylum seekers in two Danish asylum centers. Torture. 2009;19:51–9.
23. Richter K, Lehfeld H, Niklewski G. Warten auf Asyl: Psychiatrische Diagnosen in der zentralen Aufnahmeeinrichtung in Bayern. Gesundheitswesen. 2015; 77:834–8.
24. World Health Organization. The ICD-10 classification of mental and behavioural disorders: clinical descriptions and diagnostic guidelines. Geneva: World Health Organization; 1992.
25. Hergueta T, Baker R, Dunbar GC. The MINI-international neuropsychiatric interview (MINI): the development and validation of a structured diagnostic psychiatric interview for DSM-IV and ICD-10. J Clin Psychiatry. 1998;59(Suppl 20):2233.
26. Derogatis LR, Spencer PM. Brief symptom inventory: BSI. Upper Saddle River, NJ: Pearson; 1993.
27. Montgomery SA, Asberg M. A new depression scale designed to be sensitive to change. Br J Psychiatry. 1979;134:382–9.
28. Tagay S, Erim Y, Möllering A, Stoelk B, Mewes R, Senf W. Das Essener Trauma-Inventar (ETI): Ein Screeninginstrument zur Identifikation traumatischer Ereignisse und posttraumatischer Störungen. Psychother Psychosom Med Psychol. 2006;56:A98.
29. Buysse DJ, Reynolds CF, Monk TH, Berman SR, Kupfer DJ. The Pittsburgh sleep quality index: a new instrument for psychiatric practice and research. Psychiatry Res. 1989;28:193–213.
30. Wittchen HU, Jacobi F, Rehm J, Gustavsson A, Svensson M, Jönsson B, et al. The size and burden of mental disorders and other disorders of the brain in Europe 2010. Eur Neuropsychopharmacol. 2011;21:655–79. https://doi.org/10.1016/j.euroneuro.2011.07.018.
31. Heeren M, Mueller J, Ehlert U, Schnyder U, Copiery N, Maier T. Mental health of asylum seekers: a cross-sectional study of psychiatric disorders. BMC Psychiatry. 2012;12:114. https://doi.org/10.1186/1471-244X-12-114.
32. Silove D, Steel Z, McGorry P, Mohan P. Trauma exposure, postmigration stressors, and symptoms of anxiety, depression and post-traumatic stress in Tamil asylum-seekers: comparison with refugees and immigrants. Acta Psychiatr Scand. 1998;97:175–81.
33. Sönmez E, Jesuthasan J, Abels I, Nassar R, Kurmeyer C, Schouler-Ocak M. Study on female refugees – a representative research study on refugee women in Germany. European Psychiatry. 2017;41:S251. https://doi.org/10.1016/j.eurpsy.2017.02.038.
34. Ohayon MM, Reynolds CF. Epidemiological and clinical relevance of insomnia diagnosis algorithms according to the DSM-IV and the international classification of sleep disorders (ICSD). Sleep Med. 2009;10:952–60. https://doi.org/10.1016/j.sleep.2009.07.008.
35. Bronstein I, Montgomery P. Sleeping patterns of afghan unaccompanied asylum-seeking adolescents: a large observational study. PLoS One. 2013;8:e56156. https://doi.org/10.1371/journal.pone.0056156.

4

Suicidal patients presenting to secondary and tertiary emergency departments and referral to a psychiatrist

Izumi Chihara[1], Ryusuke Ae[1], Yuka Kudo[1,2], Ritei Uehara[1], Nobuko Makino[1], Yuri Matsubara[1], Teppei Sasahara[1], Yasuko Aoyama[1], Kazuhiko Kotani[1] and Yosikazu Nakamura[1*]

Abstract

Background: In Japan, although many suicidal studies were previously conducted in tertiary emergency department (ED) settings, no published studies have reported on suicidal patients presenting to the secondary EDs. The aim of the study was to describe the characteristics of suicidal patients and the referral rates to a psychiatrist overall and by type of facility.

Methods: Questionnaires were sent to all secondary and tertiary EDs in Tochigi prefecture, Japan. Data were collected for cases who presented in September 2009. Chi-square, Fisher's exact, and t-tests compared the results by gender and type of ED.

Results: All 74 EDs responded to the survey. There were 81 patients who attempted or died by suicide (36 men and 45 women). The most common method of suicide attempt was drug overdose (57%) followed by stabbing (17%). About a half used prescription drugs to attempt or die by suicide. The majority had a history of psychiatric disorders, and 35% had previous suicide attempt. About a half were admitted to medical or surgical unit; 33% were discharged home; and 9% died. After excluding those who died, 53% were referred to a psychiatrist, but 47% were not referred to a psychiatrist. The referral rate was lower for cases seen at secondary EDs (38%) compared to tertiary EDs (67%).

Conclusion: Although professional organizations suggest that suicidal patients are seen by a psychiatrist, many were not, especially at secondary EDs. Further research is needed to assure that suicidal patients presenting to EDs receive appropriate psychiatric assessment and follow-up after discharge.

Keywords: Psychiatry, Suicide, Suicide attempt, Emergency medical service, Emergency hospital, Referral, Suicide prevention, Japan

Background

In Japan, suicide is a major public health problem. The number of suicide deaths increased from 23,494 in 1997 to 31,755 in 1998, and remained high around 30,000 per year for about a decade [1]. More recently, mortality rate of suicide decreased from 23.4 per 100,000 population in 2010 to 18.5 per 100,000 population in 2015 [1], which may be attributed to measures taken by the Japanese government, local government, and private organizations to reduce suicide rates in Japan [2]. However, suicide remained to be the eighth leading cause of death of all ages, and it was among the top three leading causes of death among men and women aged 15 to 54 in 2015 [1].

A suicide attempt is one of the most important risk factors for future suicide [3–8]. Studies have shown that 40 to 60% of suicides have previous deliberate self-harm [3, 7–10]. Because medically serious or potentially lethal suicidal patients are likely to present to emergency departments (EDs) [11], and research has shown that about 16 to 24% of them will repeat the attempts with more

* Correspondence: nakamuyk@jichi.ac.jp
[1]Division of Public Health, Center for Community Medicine, Jichi Medical University, 3311-1 Yakushiji, Shimotsuke, Tochigi 329-0498, Japan
Full list of author information is available at the end of the article

lethal methods [12, 13], it is important to study the characteristics of suicidal patients presenting to EDs. EDs can serve as important sites of suicide prevention [14], and the information on who visits the ED for a suicide attempt would be needed to develop intervention strategies tailored toward them [15].

Previous studies on suicidal patients conducted in Japan have been clinical studies at a single medical institution, such as a university hospital or a community hospital [16–23]. All of these studies were conducted in tertiary ED settings; thus, research is limited regarding suicidal patients who visit the secondary EDs. Secondary EDs in Japan are generally small hospitals with 50—200 beds, likely to be understaffed, and likely be an institution without a psychiatric department. Secondary EDs are designed to provide care for moderately-acute patients, who may require inpatient care. Because emergency care system in Japan is not as centralized as in western countries, there are more small emergency hospitals (i.e., secondary EDs) in Japan than in western countries [24]. Several secondary EDs do not have specialists around the clock, and as a result, some have suggested that secondary EDs in Japan may lack the capacity to care for all types of emergencies [24, 25]. However, research is lacking regarding the current status of ED visits by suicidal patients and their characteristics in Japan.

Furthermore, research is limited with regard to how often the suicidal patients are referred to mental health professionals for psychiatric assessment in Japan despite the fact that professional organizations in Japan recommend or suggest that ED physicians refer suicidal patients presenting to EDs to psychiatric departments before patients are discharged home from the ED [26–28]. Suicide prevention opportunities may be missed if appropriate psychiatric assessments for suicidal patients are lacking in the EDs [29]. One study from the US has shown that 90% of pediatric patients who visited one of four EDs in Ohio for psychiatric-related illnesses had a mental health consult in the ED [30]. However, another study from the US reported that psychiatrists evaluate the majority of suicidal patients in only 10% of EDs in California [31]. The current situation has not been rigorously examined in Japan.

To our knowledge, there are no published studies that investigated the number and the characteristics of suicidal patients at secondary EDs in Japan, and how they may differ from patients presenting to tertiary EDs. There is also a gap in knowledge regarding referral rates to a psychiatrist in the EDs, and whether referral rates to psychiatric departments differ by type of facility (i.e., secondary vs. tertiary EDs).

Therefore, we conducted a population-based descriptive epidemiological study to investigate the characteristics of suicidal patients presenting to secondary and tertiary EDs in Tochigi prefecture, and to examine the referral rates to the psychiatric department overall and by type of facility. Specific purposes of the study were (1) to describe the characteristics of ED facilities that treat suicidal patients in Tochigi prefecture; (2) to describe the demographic, social, and clinical characteristics of suicidal patients (including attempted and completed suicide cases) presenting to secondary and tertiary EDs in Tochigi prefecture overall and by type of facility; and (3) to describe the rate of referral to a psychiatrist by ED physicians overall and by type of facility. Our main objective was to understand the population of suicidal patients presenting to EDs, and whether there may be missed opportunities at the EDs related to psychiatric referrals.

Methods

Data collection

Tochigi prefecture is located in Kanto Area, north of Tokyo, and has a population of about two million and an area of about 6408 km^2. Tochigi is about mid-size in terms of population and area among 47 prefectures of Japan, and has experienced a higher suicide mortality rate (27.8 per 100,000 population; ranked 11th of 47 prefectures in 2009) compared to the national average (24.4 per 100,000 population) [1, 32]. There are 69 secondary EDs and 5 tertiary EDs in Tochigi prefecture.

A pen-and-pencil questionnaire survey was sent to all 74 secondary and tertiary EDs in Tochigi prefecture in August 2009, asking the directors, the administrative and/or clinical staff to collect information prospectively on suicidal patients (i.e., attempted suicide and suicide cases) that presented to the ED in the month of September 2009. Questionnaires asked about the characteristics of each institution as well as demographic, social, and clinical characteristics of all attempted suicide and suicide patients presenting to the ED for the study period, patient outcomes (e.g., death, discharged home), and services that they received. We asked that the clinical staff in charge of patient care fill out the part on each patient. A reminder to complete the survey was mailed in September and October. Questionnaires were sent again in October to institutions that had not returned the survey. All responses were collected via mail by the end of November.

Definition of cases

This study used a broad definition of attempted suicide and suicide, with or without the intention to die [33]. The study aimed to capture all cases of attempted and completed suicide, regardless of suicidal intent, for the following three reasons. First, although we acknowledge that patients who engage in self-harm are a heterogeneous group [33], it is still important to describe this population as a whole since there is increased risk of later suicide among self-harm patients [34–37]. Second, it is difficult to differentiate between the different subgroups (e.g., those with and without intent), and the literature is divided on how to define subgroups of self-harm [33, 38, 39]. It would be even more challenging for the ED physicians to categorize cases into different subgroups of self-harm because they are not trained to do so. Finally, it is known that there is substantial overlap between suicides and serious suicide attempts [40]. Since cases presenting to secondary and tertiary EDs would be alive (at least at the time of presentation to ED) but will include medically serious cases [31], it is expected that there will be substantial overlap between attempted suicide (who present to the ED) and suicide cases (who may or may not present to the ED).

Questionnaires

The questionnaires consisted of two parts, which are shown in Additional files 1 and 2. The first part asked about the participating medical institution, such as the number of beds, number of psychiatrists, and the number of total patients seen in the ED during the month of the study. The first part also asked about the number of attempted and completed suicide cases presenting to the ED during the month of September 2009. If there was any case identified by the administrative and/or clinical staff, they were asked to go on to the second part of the survey. The second part collected information on each suicidal patient (i.e., attempted or completed suicide case) that presented to the EDs during the same period, without reference to suicidal intention. The first part of the questionnaire was to be filled out by either administrative and/or clinical staff (either a physician or a nurse) while the second part was to be filled out by ED physicians in charge of patient care. The survey collected demographic and medical information of the suicidal patients as well as their outcomes and services provided.

Data analysis

Descriptive analyses were conducted to describe the characteristics of EDs that treat suicidal patients. Descriptive analyses further described the demographic distributions of suicidal patients. Bivariate analyses, using Student's t-test for numerical data and Chi-Square Tests or Fisher's Exact Tests for categorical data as appropriate, were conducted to assess whether the characteristics of cases, patient outcomes, and referral rates differed by gender or by the type of institution (secondary vs. tertiary). Complete case analysis was used when data were missing on a variable. An alpha level of 0.05 was used to determine statistical significance. Due to small sample size, p values of less than 0.20 are also reported. All data management and analyses were conducted using Statistical Analysis System® (SAS, version 9.3; SAS Institute, Cary, NC). This study was approved by the Ethical Committee on Epidemiologic Research at Jichi Medical University (July 21, 2009, Eki09–09).

Results

All 74 EDs in Tochigi prefecture responded to the survey (100% response rate). Overall, nine EDs (12%) had psychiatry departments in their facilities, of which, four EDs had on-site psychiatrists at night. There were a total of 51 full-time equivalent psychiatrists within all ED facilities. The total number of patients seen at all secondary and tertiary EDs in Tochigi was 19,939 in the month of September 2009.

Of all the 74 EDs, 19 facilities (26%) received at least one suicidal patient in the month of September 2009 (Table 1). A total of 81 suicidal patients were transferred to the 19 EDs. Of the 81 cases, 45 cases presented to one of five tertiary EDs while 36 cases presented to one of 14 secondary EDs. The rest of the 55 EDs (all were secondary EDs) reported that the number of suicidal patients was zero during the observed month. The average number of cases seen at the 19 facilities during September was 4.3. Overall, there were 4.1 attempted suicide/suicide cases per 1000 ED visits. There were 4.0 attempted suicide/suicide cases presenting to EDs per month per 100,000 population during the month of the study.

The demographic and clinical characteristics of suicidal patients ($N = 81$) are shown in Table 2. The average age of the cases was 46 years old, and the age ranged from 15 to 96. There was significant difference in age distribution between men ($n = 36$) and women ($n = 45$) ($p = 0.003$; Table 2). Men were older (average 55 years) compared to women (average 38 years). Majority (59%) of men were 50 years or older while 42% of women were in their teens or twenties. Overall, the majority were unemployed and resided with other family members. Over a quarter of cases had a previous suicide attempt as reported by the healthcare providers. More than half (60%) of them had the recent episode within a year (data not shown in table). Women were more likely than men to have a history of suicide attempt. There was no significant difference regarding sociodemographic and clinical characteristics between cases presenting to secondary or tertiary ED (Table 2).

Most suicidal patients ($n = 48$) had a history of psychiatric disorders in the past. Overall, 38% of the cases either had a history of depressive disorders or had seen a psychiatrist due to depressive symptoms in the past (Table 3). There were no differences in the distributions of past psychiatric illnesses by gender or by type of institution (secondary vs. tertiary ED; data not shown).

Table 1 Characteristics of 19 emergency departments (secondary vs. tertiary)

	Secondary EDs ($n = 14$)	Tertiary EDs ($n = 5$)	P-value [a]
Mean number of beds in the facility (SD)	212 (176)	819 (302)	< .001
Mean number of emergency department visits (SD)	444 (371)	1589 (554)	< .001
Mean number of suicidal patients (SD)	2.6 (2.2)	9.0 (0.7)	< .001
Presence of psychiatrists in the facility			
At least one psychiatrist in the facility, n (%)	3 (21)	4 (80)	0.04
No psychiatrist in the facility, n (%)	11 (79)	1 (20)	
Mean number of psychiatrists in the facility (SD)	0.7 (1.7)	7.8 (9.5)	0.17

Emergency departments with at least one suicidal patient received in the month of September 2009 (of the total 74 facilities)
Abbreviation: *ED* emergency department, *SD* standard deviation
[a]Using Student's t-test for numerical data and Fisher's Exact Tests for categorical data, respectively

There were three national holidays and four weekends (four Saturdays and four Sundays) in the month of September 2009 in Japan. For both men and women, the average numbers of cases were the highest for Mondays and the days after a holiday (Table 4). Men were more likely to attempt/die by suicide on weekdays than on weekends/holidays while women were more likely to attempt/die by suicide on holidays or weekends, although this difference by gender was not statistically significant ($p = 0.11$; Table 4).

The most common method of suicide attempt was drug overdose (57%) followed by stabbing (17%), hanging (7%), and jumping from height (7%; Table 5). A half (49%) used prescription drugs to attempt suicide. Many of them (42% of total) used minor tranquilizers, of which, all were benzodiazepines. Antidepressants were

Table 2 Sociodemographic and clinical characteristics of suicidal patients by gender, and by facility type ($N = 81$)

	Overall ($N = 81$)	Male ($n = 36$)	Female ($n = 45$)	P-value [a]	Secondary EDs ($n = 36$)	Tertiary EDs ($n = 45$)	P-value [a]
Gender, n (%)							NS
Male	36 (44)				18 (50)	18 (40)	
Female	45 (56)				18 (50)	27 (60)	
Age, years, n (%)				0.003			NS
15–29	22 (27)	3 (8)	19 (42)		12 (33)	10 (22)	
30–49	26 (32)	12 (33)	14 (31)		10 (28)	16 (36)	
50–69	17 (21)	10 (28)	7 (16)		8 (22)	9 (20)	
70+	16 (20)	11 (31)	5 (11)		6 (17)	10 (22)	
Occupational status, [b] n (%)				NS			NS
Unemployed	38 (67)	19 (68)	19 (66)		15 (68)	23 (66)	
In Occupation	19 (33)	9 (32)	10 (34)		7 (32)	12 (34)	
Residential status, [b] n (%)				NS			NS
Living with family	69 (90)	32 (94)	37 (86)		28 (88)	41 (91)	
Living alone	8 (10)	2 (6)	6 (14)		4 (13)	4 (9)	
History of previous suicide attempt, [b] n (%)				0.02			0.12
Yes	20 (35)	5 (19)	15 (48)		6 (24)	14 (43)	
No	37 (65)	21 (81)	16 (52)		19 (76)	18 (56)	
History of psychiatric disorder, [b] n (%)				0.06			NS
One or more psychiatric disorders	48 (71)	17 (59)	31 (79)		20 (77)	28 (67)	
None	20 (29)	12 (41)	8 (21)		6 (23)	14 (33)	

Percentages may not add up to 100% because of rounding
Abbreviation: *ED* emergency department, *NS* not significant
[a]Chi-Square Tests or Fisher's Exact Tests [b]Analyzed excluding unknown status: Occupational status (unknown $n = 24$), Residential status (unknown $n = 5$), History of previous suicide attempt (unknown $n = 24$), and History of psychiatric disorder (unknown $n = 13$), respectively

Table 3 Prevalence of previously diagnosed psychiatric disorders among suicidal patients ($N = 81$)

Diagnosis	n (% of all patients)
Depressive disorder and/or depressive symptoms	31 (38)
Bipolar disorder	2 (2)
Schizophrenia	2 (2)
Anxiety disorder	2 (2)
Eating disorder	2 (2)
Personality disorder	1 (1)
Development disorder	1 (1)
Alcoholic disorder	1 (1)
Epilepsy	1 (1)
Diagnosis unknown	9 (11)

A total of 48 patients had previously diagnosed psychiatric disorder(s)
Some patients had more than one diagnoses: One patient had depressive disorder and/or depressive symptoms and epilepsy; one patient had depressive disorder and/or depressive symptoms and personality disorder; one patient had depressive disorder and/or depressive symptoms and eating disorder; and one patient had bipolar disorder and alcoholic disorder

used in 10 cases (12% of total). Methods of attempted suicide/suicide and types of drugs used to attempt or die by suicide did not differ by gender or by type of institution (data not shown).

The outcomes of suicidal patients and referral rates to a psychiatrist are shown in Table 6. About a half was admitted to medical or surgical service; 6% were admitted to psychiatric departments; and 33% were discharged home. After excluding seven suicide cases who died and one case missing information on referral, overall referral rate to a psychiatrist was 53%. Overall referral rate was significantly lower among patients at secondary EDs compared to tertiary EDs (38% vs. 67%, respectively; $p = 0.02$). Of the cases that were not referred to a psychiatrist ($n = 34$), the ED physicians felt the need to refer the patient to a psychiatrist 53% of the time ($n = 18$; data not shown in table). The main reasons why those patients were not referred to a psychiatrist were because patient or family refused it (33%), psychiatrists were unavailable (28%), or the patient was in coma (22%; data now shown in table). Referral rate was much lower for patients who visited facilities without a psychiatrist compared to patients who visited facilities with a psychiatrist (28% vs. 70%, respectively; $p < .001$). Most of the facilities without a psychiatrist were secondary EDs (Table 1). The outcomes of patients or referral rates did not differ significantly by gender (data not shown).

Table 4 Average number of suicidal patients by day of week and holiday ($N = 81$)

	Average number of cases per day			*p*-value[a]
	Overall	Male	Female	
Day of the week				0.02
Monday	4.0	1.8	2.3	
Tuesday	2.8	1.2	1.6	
Wednesday	2.8	1.6	1.2	
Thursday	1.5	1.0	0.5	
Friday	2.0	0.8	1.3	
Saturday	2.5	0.8	1.8	
Sunday	2.8	1.0	1.8	
Holiday				<.001
Holidays or weekends	2.5	0.8	1.7	
Weekdays	2.7	1.4	1.3	
Day before or after a holiday				
Day before a holiday	2.0	0.8	1.3	NS
Day after a holiday	4.3	2.3	2.0	NS

Two patients were missing information on the day they attempted/died by suicide
[a]Chi-Square Tests, weighted by number of days in each category

Table 5 Methods of suicide and drug types used to attempt or die by suicide ($N = 81$)

	n (% of all patients)
Method of Suicide (not mutually exclusive categories)[a]	
Drug overdose	46 (57)
Stabbing	14 (17)
Hanging	6 (7)
Jumping from height	6 (7)
Pesticide poisoning	5 (6)
Immolation	3 (4)
Carbon monoxide poisoning	2 (3)
Other	1 (1)
Type of drug used to attempt or die by suicide	
Prescription drugs only	39 (48)
Over the counter drugs only	6 (7)
Both prescription and over the counter drugs	1 (1)
Type of prescription drugs used to attempt or die by suicide (not mutually exclusive categories)[b]	
Minor tranquilizer	34 (42)
Major tranquilizer	7 (9)
Other psychoactive drug	15 (19)
Other drug	10 (12)

Methods used by patients who died by suicide ($n = 7$) included: hanging ($n = 2$), immolation ($n = 2$), pesticide poisoning ($n = 2$), and drug overdose ($n = 1$)
[a]Two patients used two methods (both drug overdose and stabbing)
[b]Of the 40 patients who used prescription drugs to attempt suicide, 31 patients used a combination of prescription drug types listed

Discussion

To our knowledge, this was the first published population-based study that examined the characteristics of suicidal patients presenting to secondary and tertiary EDs and that reported the referral rates to a psychiatrist overall and by type of facility. Despite the fact that guidelines recommend ED clinicians to consult the suicidal

Table 6 Outcome of suicidal patients and referral to a psychiatrist ($N = 81$)

	Overall	Secondary EDs	Tertiary EDs	*P*-value [a]
	n (%)	n (%)	n (%)	
Outcome of suicidal patients ($n = 81$)	[$n = 81$]	[$n = 36$]	[$n = 45$]	
Discharged home	27 (33)	12 (33)	15 (33)	NS
Died	7 (9)	1 (3)	6 (13)	0.09
Admitted to medical/surgery department of the institution	38 (47)	18 (50)	20 (44)	NS
Admitted to medical/surgery department of other institution	3 (4)	2 (6)	1 (2)	NS
Admitted to psychiatric department of the institution	3 (4)	1 (3)	2 (4)	NS
Admitted to psychiatric department of other institution	3 (4)	2 (6)	1 (2)	NS
Any referral to a psychiatrist ($n = 73$) [b]	[$n = 73$]	[$n = 34$]	[$n = 39$]	0.02
Any referral to a psychiatrist	39 (53)	13 (38)	26 (67)	
Not referred to a psychiatrist	34 (47)	21 (62)	13 (33)	
Referral to a psychiatrist ($n = 73$) [b]				0.03
Confirmed to have seen a psychiatrist	29 (40)	8 (24)	21 (54)	
Referred but not confirmed if the patient saw a psychiatrist	10 (14)	5 (15)	5 (13)	
Not referred to a psychiatrist	34 (47)	21 (61)	13 (33)	

Percentages may not add up to 100% because of rounding
Abbreviation: *ED* emergency department, *NS* not significant
[a]Chi-Square Tests or Fisher's Exact Tests
[b]Excludes seven cases who died by suicide and one case missing information on referral

patients to a psychiatrist [26–28], in our study, 47% of those alive were not referred to a psychiatrist. Of the cases that were not referred to a psychiatrist, the ED physicians felt the need to refer the patient to a psychiatrist 53% of the time. Referral rate was especially low for cases seen at secondary EDs even though characteristics of suicidal patients were similar between secondary and tertiary EDs. These results are concerning because psychiatrists play a major role in treating the mental illnesses that suicidal patients may have in Japan [41]. Appropriate treatment of medical conditions (especially depression) is associated with reduced likelihood of suicide [42]. If suicidal patients are never referred to a psychiatrist or other mental health professionals after a suicide attempt, opportunities for suicide prevention may be missed [29].

In our study, the top reason for not referring the patient to a psychiatrist was patient and/or family refusal. The reasons for patient and family refusal were not studied, but one possible explanation is the stigma associated with mental health conditions and psychiatric treatment in Japan [43]. Another possible explanation is lack of knowledge about treatment effectiveness among patients and families. One study has shown that the general public in Japan lacks the knowledge that treatments are effective for mental health conditions such as schizophrenia and depression [44]. The same study also showed that the general public in Japan has a strong belief in counsellors, but a psychiatrist was not typically thought as most helpful for mental illnesses. Further research is needed to examine how stigma, knowledge, and beliefs around mental health diagnosis, treatment, and mental health professionals affect patient and family behaviors.

Another major reason why the patients were not referred to a psychiatrist was unavailability of a psychiatrist. There is chronic shortage of psychiatrists in Japan. In 2010, it was estimated that there were 10,844 full-time equivalent psychiatrists in Japan, but the Japanese Ministry of Health, Labour, and Welfare estimated that the number needed to increase to 12,045 to meet the needs [45]. In 2010, for Tochigi prefecture, there were 191 full-time equivalent psychiatrists while the estimated number needed was 207 [45]. The current study showed that there were only a total of 51 full-time equivalent psychiatrists within all the secondary and tertiary emergency hospitals in Tochigi prefecture in 2009, which cover about two million population. Japanese Ministry of Health, Labour, and Welfare does not estimate the number of psychiatrists that need to be available at secondary and/or tertiary EDs, but this number also likely needs to be increased. Nonetheless, there were a total of 191 psychiatrists in Tochigi prefecture at the time of the study [45]. The fact that referral rate was lower at facilities without a psychiatrist (mostly secondary) compared to facilities with a psychiatrist (28% vs. 70%, respectively) indicate that there may be a linkage problem between the EDs and psychiatrists in the community. Psychiatrists who do not work at the facilities with an ED may work at facilities without an ED, stand-alone clinics or stand-alone psychiatric hospitals. The possibility of linking EDs and psychiatrists in the community needs to be explored.

Basic demographic features in our study were similar to those reported in an unpublished study by Tokyo Metropolitan Government involving 422 suicidal patients presenting to 199 EDs in Tokyo Metropolis in the month of December, 2007 [32, 46]. There were 4.1 suicidal patients per 1000 ED visits in Tochigi, which are equivalent to the rates reported in Tokyo Metropolis. In our study, the in-hospital mortality rate was 9% among suicidal patients presenting to secondary/tertiary EDs while this rate was 12% for Tokyo Metropolis [46]. Another study by Ichimura et al. [16] also showed a similar in-hospital mortality rate of 9% among suicidal patients presenting to a single tertiary ED in Japan. Although large scale national studies on suicidal patients presenting to EDs in Japan have not been conducted, our data are consistent with past research in Japan and are likely representative of the situation in Japan.

In our study, at least a quarter of cases had a history of previous suicide attempt, and 60% of them had a recent episode within a year, according to the healthcare providers who completed the survey. These numbers may be an underestimate since the information was not collected directly from the patients. Studies on completed suicides in Japan using police data have shown that 13.4% to 15.9% of suicide cases had previous suicide attempt [4, 32]. According to a study by Inoue et al. [4], visiting a physician for an outpatient treatment was associated with previous suicide attempts in suicide cases. These results stress the importance of referring suicidal patients to proper healthcare when they are presented to EDs. Our study also showed that the majority (71%) had seen a psychiatrist for a psychiatric disorder. Medical professionals, including primary care physicians, ED physicians, and psychiatrists are regarded as one of the key players in preventing future suicides among suicide attempters [41], because medical professionals encounter these patients multiple times as shown in this study and prior studies. Suicide is a preventable event [47], and these results suggest that there clearly are opportunities for intervention by medical professionals, including ED physicians, primary care physicians, and psychiatrists [47]. The types of interventions that should occur between suicidal patients and medical professionals may be difficult to assess because treatment and follow-up need to be tailored to the broad needs of individual patients, most of whom have complex mental illness [47]. Nonetheless, this is the current gap in the literature that needs to be filled by future studies. For example, the interventions at the psychiatric visits such as counseling and medications must be re-evaluated since the visit itself has not been shown to be effective in preventing suicide attempt in this population.

Our study showed that 90% of cases were living with a family member(s). A study by Inoue et al. [4] also showed that living with a family member was associated with previous suicide attempts in suicide cases. It has been reported that conflicts among family members was the third common reason for suicide in Tochigi [32]. Further study is needed to examine if and how family factors can be a risk or protective factors for suicide attempt in Japan.

While suicide rate is higher for men, presentation of suicidal patients at healthcare facilities has been reported to be more common in women in Western countries [48]. Similar trends have been observed in Japan. In 2010, suicide rate for men was 2.6 times greater than that for women (34.1 per 100,000 for men and 13.1 per 100,000 for women) [1]. In our study, the proportion of female cases presenting to EDs was 56%, which is equivalent to what has been reported in Japan (between 56% and 63%) [17–19]. However, our study also showed that age distribution of men presenting to EDs is quite different from that of Western countries. While WHO/EURO study showed that men aged 25 to 34 and women aged 14 to 24 comprised the highest proportion of suicidal patients presenting to hospitals [48], our study showed that middle-aged and elderly men as well as young women (aged 15 to 29 years) comprised the highest proportions. A study from Akita prefecture among patients who present to healthcare facilities showed that attempted suicide was prevalent among men in their 20s and men aged 40 to 59 years while suicide death was most prevalent among men aged 40 to 69 years [49]. Although some claim that completed and attempted suicide population may be different in nature [40, 49, 50], there may be some overlap especially among men because the age distribution between attempted suicide cases and suicide cases overlap. These issues need to be examined in future studies.

In our study, the average numbers of cases were the highest on Mondays and the day after a holiday(s). Men had the highest number of cases earlier in the week (Mondays, Tuesdays, and Wednesdays). These findings are similar to the studies of completed suicide cases reported in Japan [32, 51]. A study by Nakamura et al. [32] on all cases of completed suicides in Tochigi prefecture in 2007 and 2008 also showed that the number of completed suicide cases were the highest on Mondays, Tuesdays, and Wednesdays. Furthermore, a study by Nishi et al. [51] investigated the relationship between suicide and holidays using vital statistics, and found that the highest rate of suicide was found for Mondays and the day after a holiday(s) for both men and women. Our results suggest that attempted suicide and suicide cases presenting to EDs share the similar traits to completed suicide cases (who may or may not present to the ED) in terms of the day of the week they tend to die by suicide. Mondays and the days after a holiday are when most people go back to work or school after a holiday. The people at high risk for suicide should not be left alone on those days. Private community organizations and local government may be able to make arrangements to visit previous suicidal patients on such days [41]. In addition, it is important to educate the family members and the general public on the risk of suicide and suicide attempt on Mondays, on the days after a holiday, and earlier in the week in general.

In our study, the majority of cases had a history of one or more psychiatric disorders. A total of 38% of cases had depressive disorders or had seen a psychiatrist for depressive symptoms. We did not investigate whether these patients were prescribed antidepressants, but only 12% of them used antidepressants to attempt or die by suicide while 42% used benzodiazepines to attempt or die by suicide. It is known that psychiatric disorders are present in the majority of suicide cases, and most of them are undertreated [52, 53]. Depression is undertreated even among patients who previously attempted suicide [54]. Suicidal patients need be referred to psychiatrists in order to receive appropriate psychiatric assessment for mood disorders so that they be diagnosed and be treated with antidepressants appropriately. This may decrease future suicide rates [55, 56]. On the other hand, appropriate use of benzodiazepines is in question because 42% of the cases used benzodiazepines to attempt or die by suicide. A study by Fukuhara et al. [57] showed that internists in Japan overprescribe benzodiazepines to patients with depressive symptoms without the use of antidepressants, which may increase the risk of future suicide and mortality. Benzodiazepines are prescribed more in Japan than anywhere else in the world [58]. Studies have shown that psychiatrists are 1.5 to 2 times more likely to prescribe benzodiazepines in Japan although the appropriateness of prescription by specialty is unknown [59]. Future studies need to examine if patients are prescribed benzodiazepines appropriately in Japan, and whether these patients may benefit from taking antidepressants or receiving (additional) psychotherapy instead.

There are some limitations in our study. Data on suicidal patients were collected only for the month of September. As a result, the sample size was small, and there was inadequate power to conduct multivariable analyses or show statistical significance in sub-analyses. In addition, we were not able to investigate the seasonal variation that may have occurred over the course of a year, which is known to occur among the suicidal population [51, 60]. We had to limit the data collection period to one month because Tochigi has several medically underserved areas. We felt that the study could not be conducted for a longer period of time due to the burden on ED physicians in Tochigi. EDs in Tochigi are already overcrowded, and ED physicians are overworked due to physician shortage [45], which is experienced in various parts of Japan. Nonetheless, we successfully investigated the state of the problem at current EDs.

Another limitation is that we relied solely on reports by administrative and/or clinical staff of each ED about information on cases, which may not have been accurate. Since we did not verify the numbers of attempted suicide and suicide cases by chart review, there is a possibility of underreporting of cases, especially at secondary EDs, where they may be understaffed to collect the information prospectively. Another source of bias associated with the data collection method is that, although this study used a broad definition of attempted suicide and suicide with or without the intention to die, it is possible that ED physicians did not report the cases involving less lethal methods, which will result in overrepresentation of severe cases in our sample. These biases may have affected our results, but the extent of bias is unknown.

In addition, because the questionnaires on each case were filled out exclusively by ED clinicians, no information was obtained directly from the patient, family members, or psychiatrists. Reports on psychiatric diagnosis by ED physicians may not be accurate especially if the patient had been diagnosed at a psychiatric department of another institution. No detailed information about the patient history related to mental illness (e.g., treatment received) was available. Personal information of the patient such as occupational status may not be accurate as well. Nevertheless, the strengths of the study are that it is population-based, covering both secondary and tertiary EDs, and the 100% response rate from eligible EDs.

In Japan, Basic Law on Suicide Countermeasures, which was passed into law in 2006 and revised by the Diet in 2016, specifically states that national government and local public entities should implement necessary policies to secure "effective coordination among psychiatrists and medical doctors who provide emergency medical care" [61]. Low referral rates to a psychiatrist especially at secondary EDs demonstrated in this study suggests that service coordination between secondary EDs and psychiatric departments/hospitals may be a pressing issue. Secondary EDs often do not have psychiatric departments in their facility as shown in this study, and they may not have the resources to link the patients to psychiatric services. Local governments should take initiatives in connecting the EDs to psychiatric hospitals and community resources. Because the number of psychiatrists is limited and not likely to increase soon, the role of other mental health professionals such as nurses, psychologists, and social workers in following up these patients needs to be examined. Recently, a multicenter randomized controlled trial examined the feasibility and effectiveness of assertive case management at 17 hospital EDs in Japan [62]. The study showed that assertive case management reduced the incidence of recurrent suicide attempt up to 6 months, but long term effectiveness was not shown. Similarly, a meta-analysis showed that active contact and follow-up type interventions for suicidal patients who visit EDs were effective for 12 months, but not at 24 months [63]. Nonetheless, these studies are promising that adverse outcomes could be delayed for 6 to 12 months. This is very relevant for clinical practice in Japan since this study showed that more than half (60%) of suicidal patients who previously attempted suicide had the recent episode within a year. Additional interventions are likely needed to improve long-term outcomes beyond 12 months for these patients.

Because this study only investigated the referral rates to a psychiatrist, future studies need to investigate whether suicidal patients presenting to EDs actually receive appropriate psychiatric assessment/evaluation and follow-up after discharge, and whether long term outcomes can be improved (e.g., recurrent suicide attempt and suicide mortality). Furthermore, studies need to examine further what components of interventions are effective in preventing future suicides in the ED settings and in psychiatric settings, taking into consideration the real-world situation and cultural context of Japan.

Conclusions

The study investigated the characteristics and outcomes of suicidal patients presenting to secondary and tertiary EDs in Japan, and the referral rates to a psychiatrist. Findings from our study suggest that psychiatric referral rates were low among suicidal patients presenting to secondary and tertiary EDs in Japan. The study also showed that referral rates were lower in secondary EDs compared to tertiary EDs even though the characteristics of suicidal patients presenting to secondary and tertiary EDs were similar. Future studies should examine the outcomes of patients who are not referred to a psychiatrist at the EDs, and should examine what components of interventions are effective in preventing future suicides among suicidal patients who present to EDs.

Abbreviations

ED: Emergency departments

Acknowledgements

The authors thank all the secondary and tertiary EDs in Tochigi prefecture that participated in the questionnaire survey. This study was supported by the Research Grant from Tochigi Prefectural Local Government.

Funding

This study was supported by the Research Grant from Tochigi Prefectural Local Government. The sponsor played no role in the study design, data collection, analysis, and interpretation or manuscript drafting.

Authors' contributions

Study concept and design: IC, YK, RU, YN; data acquisition: IC, YK, RU, YN; data analysis and interpretation: IC, RA, NM, YM, TS, YA; manuscript preparation: IC, RA, YM, TS, KK, YN; study supervision: RU, NM, YA, KK, YN; final approval: KK, YN. All authors have reviewed and approved the manuscript for submission.

Competing interests

The authors declare that they have no competing interests.

Author details

[1]Division of Public Health, Center for Community Medicine, Jichi Medical University, 3311-1 Yakushiji, Shimotsuke, Tochigi 329-0498, Japan. [2]Department of Neuropsychiatry, Keio University School of Medicine, 35 Shinanomachi, Shinjuku-ku, Tokyo 160-8582, Japan.

References

1. Statistics and Information Department, Minister's Secretariat, Ministry of Health, Labour and Welfare. Vital Statistics of Japan, vol. 1; 2016. Health and Welfare Statistics Association (in Japanese)
2. Suicide Prevention White Paper. Ministry of health, labour and welfare. 2016 http://www.mhlw.go.jp/wp/hakusyo/jisatsu/16/. Accessed 29 July 2017.
3. Hawton K, Zahl D, Weatherall R. Suicide following deliberate self-harm: long-term follow-up of patients who presented to a general hospital. Br J Psychiatry. 2003;182:537–42.
4. Inoue K, Tanii H, Fukunaga T, et al. The importance of the frequency of suicide attempts as a risk factor of suicide. J Forensic Legal Med. 2008;15:24–6.
5. Nordentoft M, Mortensen PB, Pedersen CB. Absolute risk of suicide after first hospital contact in mental disorder. Arch Gen Psychiatry. 2011;68(10):1058–64.
6. Rygnestad T. Mortality after deliberate self-poisoning. A prospective follow-up study of 587 persons observed for 5279 person years: risk factors and causes of death. Soc Psychiatry Psychiatr Epidemiol. 1997;32:443–50.
7. Hawton K, Fagg J. Suicide, and other causes of death, following attempted suicide. Br J Psychiatry. 1988;152:359–66.
8. Hawton K, van Heeringen K. Suicide. Lancet. 2009;373:1372–81.
9. Foster T, Gillespie K, McClelland R. Mental disorders and suicide in Northern Ireland. Br J Psychiatry. 1997;170:447–52.
10. Suokas J, Lonnqvist J. Outcome of attempted suicide and psychiatric consultation: risk factors and suicide mortality during a five-year follow-up. Acta Psychiatr Scand. 1991;84:545–9.
11. Asarnow JR, Baraff LJ, Berk M, et al. An emergency department intervention for linking pediatric suicidal patients to follow-up mental health treatment. Psychiatr Serv. 2011;62(11):1303–9.
12. Stewart SE, Manion IG, Davidson S, Cloutier P. Suicidal children and adolescents with first emergency room presentations: predictors of six-month outcome. J Am Acad Child Adolesc Psychiatry. 2001;40(5):580–7.
13. Owens D, Horrocks J, House A. Fatal and non-fatal repetition of self-harm. Systematic review. Br J Psychiatry. 2002;181:193–9.
14. Perhats C, Valdez AM. Suicide prevention in the emergency department. J Emerg Nurs. 2008;34(3):251–3.
15. Ting SA, Sullivan AF, Boudreaux ED, Miller I, Camargo CA Jr. Trends in US emergency department visits for attempted suicide and self-inflicted injury, 1993-2008. Gen Hosp Psychiatry. 2012;34(5):557–65.
16. Ichimura A, Matsumoto H, Kimura T, et al. Changes in mental disorder distribution among suicide attempters in mid-west area of Kanagawa. Psychiatry Clin Neurosci. 2005;59:113–8.
17. Nakagawa M, Kawanishi C, Yamada T, et al. Characteristics of suicide attempters with family history of suicide attempt: a retrospective chart review. BMC Psychiatry. 2009;9:32.
18. Yamada T, Kawanishi C, Hasegawa H, et al. Psychiatric assessment of suicide attempters in Japan: a pilot study at a critical emergency unit in an urban area. BMC Psychiatry. 2007;7:64.
19. Asukai N. Mental disorder as a risk factor of suicide; a clinical study of failed suicides. Seishin Shinkeigaku Zasshi. 1994;96:415–43.

20. Doihara C, Kawanishi C, Yamada T, et al. Trait aggression in suicide attempters: a pilot study. Psychiatry Clin Neurosci. 2008;62:352–4.
21. Kudo K, Otsuka K, Endo J, et al. Study of the outcome of suicide attempts: characteristics of hospitalization in a psychiatric ward group, critical care center group, and non-hospitalized group. BMC Psychiatry. 2010;10:4.
22. Murase S, Ochiai S, Ueyama M, Honjo S, Ohta T. Psychiatric features of seriously life-threatening suicide attempters: a clinical study from a general hospital in Japan. J Psychosom Res. 2003;55:379–83.
23. Narishige R, Kawashima Y, Otaka Y, Saito T, Okubo Y. Gender differences in suicide attempters: a retrospective study of precipitating factors for suicide attempts at a critical emergency unit in Japan. BMC Psychiatry. 2014;14:144.
24. Hori S. Emergency medicine in Japan. Keio J Med. 2010;59(4):131–9.
25. Ezaki T, Yamada T, Yasuda M, Kannna T, Shiraishi K, Hashizume M. Current status of Japanese emergency medicine based on a cross-sectional survey of one prefecture. Emerg Med Australas. 2007;19(6):523–7.
26. Japanese Society for Emergency Medicine, Providing care for suicide attempters, Guide for emergency department staff (in Japanese). 2009. http://www.mhlw.go.jp/bunya/shougaihoken/jisatsu/dl/07.pdf. Accessed 29 July 2017.
27. The Japanese Association for Emergency Psychiatry, Guidelines for Psychiatric Emergency Treatment (3) Management after Suicide Attempt Version 2009 (in Japanese). 2009. http://www.mhlw.go.jp/bunya/shougaihoken/jisatsu/dl/11.pdf. Accessed 29 July 2017.
28. The Japanese Association for Emergency Psychiatry. Guidelines for Psychiatric Emergency Treatment (in Japanese). 2015. http://www.jaep.jp/gl/2015_all.pdf. Accessed 22 Dec 2017.
29. Ronquillo L, Minassian A, Vilke GM, Wilson MP. Literature-based recommendations for suicide assessment in the emergency department: a review. J Emerg Med. 2012;43(5):836–42.
30. Grupp-Phelan J, Mahajan P, Foltin GL, Jacobs E, Tunik M, Sonnett M, Miller S, Dayan P. Pediatric emergency care applied research network. Referral and resource use patterns for psychiatric-related visits to pediatric emergency departments. Pediatr Emerg Care. 2009;25(4):217–20.
31. Baraff LJ, Janowicz N, Asarnow JR. Survey of California emergency departments about practices for management of suicidal patients and resources available for their care. Ann Emerg Med. 2006;48(4):452–8.
32. Nakamura Y, Ito T, Chihara I, et al. Suicides in Tochigi prefecture in 2007-2008: epidemiologic features based on police data. Nippon Koshu Eisei Zasshi. 2010;57:807–15.
33. Skegg K. Self-harm. Lancet. 2005;366:1471–83.
34. Suominen K, Isometsa E, Suokas J, et al. Completed suicide after a suicide attempt: a 37-year follow-up study. Am J Psychiatry. 2004;161(3):562.
35. Zahl DL. Repetition of deliberate self-harm and subsequent suicide risk: long-term follow-up study of 11583 patients. Br J Psychiatry. 2004;185:70–5.
36. Klonsky ED, May AM, Glenn CR. The relationship between nonsuicidal self-injury and attempted suicide: converging evidence from four samples. J Abnorm Psychol. 2013;122:231–7.
37. Morgan C, Webb RT, Carr MJ, Kontopantelis E, Green J, Chew-Graham CA, Kapur N, Ashcroft DM. Incidence, clinical management, and mortality risk following self harm among children and adolescents: cohort study in primary care. BMJ. 2017;359:j4351.
38. Linehan MM. Suicidal people. One population or two? Ann N Y Acad Sci. 1986;487:16–33.
39. Klonsky ED, May AM, Saffer BY. Suicide, Suicide Attempts, and Suicidal Ideation. Annu Rev Clin Psychol. 2016;12:307–30.
40. Beautrais AL. Suicides and serious suicide attempts: two populations or one? Psychol Med. 2001;31:837–45.
41. Japan Support Center for Suicide Countermeasures. The general principle of suicide prevention policy. Suicide Policy Res. 2017;1:16–45.
42. Zalsman G, Hawton K, Wasserman D, et al. Suicide prevention strategies revisited: 10-year systematic review. Lancet Psychiatry. 2016;3(7):646–59.
43. Ando S, Yamaguchi S, Aoki Y, Thornicroft G. Review of mental-health-related stigma in Japan. Psychiatry Clin Neurosci. 2013;67(7):471–82.
44. Jorm AF, Nakane Y, Christensen H, et al. Public beliefs about treatment and outcome of mental disorders: a comparison of Australia and Japan. BMC Med. 2005;3:12.
45. Ministry of Health, Labour, and Welfare, Estimation of Demand and Supply of Physicians (in Japanese). 2010. http://www.mhlw.go.jp/bunya/iryou/other/iryou01.html. Accessed 29 July 2017.
46. Tokyo Metropolitan Government. Report on Suicide Attempters Presenting to Emergency Departments (in Japanese). 2008. http://www.fukushihoken.metro.tokyo.jp/iryo/tokyokaigi/torikumi/kaigi/kaigi/kaigishiryou200715.files/shiryou6_200715.pdf. Accessed 29 July 2017.
47. Reid WH. Preventing suicide. J Psychiatr Pract. 2010;16(2):120–4.
48. Schmidtke A, Bille-Brahe U, DeLeo D, et al. Attempted suicide in Europe: rates, trends and sociodemographic characteristics of suicide attempters during the period 1989-1992. Results of the WHO/EURO multicentre study on Parasuicide. Acta Psychiatr Scand. 1996;93:327–38.
49. Fushimi M, Sugawara J, Saito S. Comparison of completed and attempted suicide in Akita, Japan. Psychiatry Clin Neurosci. 2006;60:289–95.
50. Kessel N. Self-poisoning. I BMJ. 1965;2:1265–70.
51. Nishi M, Miyake H, Okamoto H, Goto Y, Sakai T. Relationship between suicide and holidays. J Epidemiol. 2000;10:317–20.
52. Henriksson S, Boethius G, Isacsson G. Suicides are seldom prescribed antidepressants: findings from a prospective prescription database in Jamtland county, Sweden, 1985-95. Acta Psychiatr Scand. 2001;103:301–6.
53. Lonnqvist JK, Henriksson MM, Isometsa ET, et al. Mental disorders and suicide prevention. Psychiatry Clin Neurosci. 1995;49(Suppl 1):S111–6.
54. Oquendo MA, Kamali M, Ellis SP, et al. Adequacy of antidepressant treatment after discharge and the occurrence of suicidal acts in major depression: a prospective study. Am J Psychiatry. 2002;159:1746–51.
55. Gibbons RD, Brown CH, Hur K, et al. Early evidence on the effects of regulators' suicidality warnings on SSRI prescriptions and suicide in children and adolescents. Am J Psychiatry. 2007;164(9):1356–63.
56. Gusmão R, Quintão S, McDaid D, et al. Antidepressant utilization and suicide in Europe: an ecological multi-National Study. PLoS One. 2013;8(6):e66455.
57. Fukuhara S, Green J, Albert J, et al. Symptoms of depression, prescription of benzodiazepines, and the risk of death in hemodialysis patients in Japan. Kidney Int. 2006;70:1866–72.
58. Nakao M, Takeuchi T, Yano E. Prescription of benzodiazepines and antidepressants to outpatients attending a Japanese university hospital. Int J Clin Pharmacol Ther. 2007;45:30–5.
59. Nomura K, Nakao M, Sato M, Yano E. Regular prescriptions for benzodiazepines: a cross-sectional study of outpatients at a university hospital. Intern Med. 2006;45(22):1279–83.
60. Christodoulou C, Douzenis A, Papadopoulos FC, et al. Suicide and seasonality. Acta Psychiatr Scand. 2012;125(2):127–46.
61. Research Project Team on Suicide Prevention Policy. Basic law on suicide countermeasures. Suicide Policy Res. 2017;1:1–7.
62. Kawanishi C, Aruga T, Ishizuka N, et al. Assertive case management versus enhanced usual care for people with mental health problems who had attempted suicide and were admitted to hospital emergency departments in Japan (ACTION-J): a multicentre, randomised controlled trial. Lancet Psychiatry. 2014;1(3):193–201.
63. Inagaki M, Kawashima Y, Kawanishi C, et al. Interventions to prevent repeat suicidal behavior in patients admitted to an emergency department for a suicide attempt: a meta-analysis. J Affect Disord. 2015;175:66–7.

5

The association between electrodermal activity (EDA), depression and suicidal behaviour

Marco Sarchiapone[1,2*], Carla Gramaglia[3], Miriam Iosue[4], Vladimir Carli[5], Laura Mandelli[6], Alessandro Serretti[7], Debora Marangon[8] and Patrizia Zeppegno[3,8]

Abstract

Background: Electrodermal activity (EDA) and other peripheral autonomic electrical parameters have been used as indicators of emotional states, including depressive states and suicidal state. We aimed to review EDA research systematically, focusing on EDA's usefulness as a biomarker for depression and suicidal behaviour.

Methods: We searched MEDLINE, Scopus, Cochrane Library, and Web of Science databases, following PRISMA guidelines. The initial screening of articles was based on titles and abstracts; then the full text was reviewed. A preliminary synthesis of findings was developed using tables, thematic analysis and quality ratings.

Results: 1287 articles were screened and 77 relevant studies were identified and included in the systematic review. The studies were fairly consistent in maintaining that hypoactive electrodermal response is an established feature of patients affected by depression. There is also preliminary evidence that monitoring EDA may help to differentiate the phases of mood disorders. A few studies provided evidence that EDA can be used to differentiate acutely suicidal subjects from depressed patients who are not severely suicidal. Although EDA has been shown to be a valid, sensitive marker of suicidal ideation, suicide attempts and violent suicidal behaviour, it also seems to be influenced to some extent by antidepressant treatment.

Conclusions: Most of the studies summarised in this review are quite outdated and employed a variety of designs and methods to evaluate EDA. This limits the generalisability of the results and makes it difficult to draw clear conclusions about the role of EDA in real-world settings. Electrodermal hypoactivity seems to be a reliable feature of depression and a valid marker of suicidal risk. Nevertheless, the potential utility of EDA in diagnosis, prevention, and treatment planning for depression and suicidal behaviour, should be thoroughly studied.

Keywords: Electrodermal activity, Skin conductance, Depression, Suicidal behaviour

* Correspondence: marco.sarchiapone@gmail.com
[1]Department of Health Sciences, University of Molise, Via Francesco De Sanctis, 1, 86100 Campobasso, Italy
[2]National Institute for Health, Migration and Poverty, Via di S. Gallicano 25/a, 00153 Rome, Italy
Full list of author information is available at the end of the article

Background

Rationale

Biological abnormalities may be risk factors for depression, suicidal behaviour or completed suicide; a recent review has identified the following major categories of potential biological predictors of suicide attempt behaviour: (1) results of structural and functional brain imaging and (2) biochemical and genomic findings relating to the major neurotransmitters (serotonin, catecholamines, GABA and glutamate), the hypothalamic pituitary adrenal (HPA) axis, the inflammasome, lipids and neuroplasticity [1]. Nevertheless, there is currently a lack of biomarkers for the psychiatric field, in particular for suicidal behaviour. The prediction of suicidal risk and identification of suicidal patients will only be possible when we have an accurate picture of the interplay between biological and psychosocial factors. The use of the autonomic responses as markers of emotion, attention, decision-making, motor preparation, anticipation of reward or punishment and unconscious detection has grown considerably since the 1980s [2]. The most basic indicators of the state of the autonomic nervous system are heart rate and electrodermal activity (EDA); the former is influenced by the sympathetic and parasympathetic systems, whereas the latter is under sympathetic control only. Since a useful biomarker should be measurable in a non-invasive manner [3], the features of EDA suggest that its potential utility as a biomarker warrants careful consideration.

EDA is now the preferred term for changes in the electrical conductance of the skin, which depend on the quantity of sweat secreted by eccrine sweat glands in the hypodermis of the palmar and plantar regions [4]. Sympathetic nervous activity and variations in the sweating of the skin are regulated by environmental temperature (thermoregulatory sweating) and by central nervous activity related to affective and cognitive states (palmar, mental or emotional sweating) [5, 6]. EDA has been used as an index of emotional stimulation in several experimental studies [7].

EDA has a tonic and a phasic component. The tonic component is related to the slower components and background characteristics of the signal (skin conductance level; SCL). The phasic components are the faster-changing elements of the signal that can be associated with a stimulus (skin conductance response; SCR) or "spontaneous" or "nonspecific" (non-specific skin conductance response; NS.SCR) [8, 9].

It has been hypothesised that the central component of EDA originates in the left hemisphere, but this lateralisation remains controversial [10]. EDA may be modulated by two different pathways: ipsilateral modulation within the limbic system, via the hypothalamus and thermoregulatory pathways and, to a lesser degree, contralateral modulation by the premotor cortex and basal ganglia [8, 11, 12].

In subjects exposed to emotional stimuli the amplitude of electrodermal response increases linearly with perceived arousal [13–16], whilst repeated presentation of identical, non-significant stimuli elicits progressively smaller reactions, a phenomenon known as habituation [8]. Individual trait differences in EDA have been observed and labelled as EDA lability. Some individuals show a high rate of nonspecific EDA and slow habituation to specific stimuli (labile individuals), whereas others show less non-specific EDA and more rapid specific EDA habituation (stable individuals) [16, 17]. EDA lability is influenced by both genetic and environmental factors [18] and is often considered dependent on trait anxiety at the individual level. It has also been proposed as an endophenotype of individual disposition towards emotional expression, self-control and inhibition of contrasting impulses [19, 20]. EDA-labiles people may be described as calm, deliberative, restrained, more good-natured, cooperative, and responsible, whereas EDA--stable people tend to be active, emotionally expressive, animated, assertive, more irritable, more antagonistic, more impulsive and more irresponsible [21, 22]. Both depression and suicide have been extensively investigated from a physiological point of view, and the extant research has consistently demonstrated that depressed and suicidal patients show electrodermal hypoactivity and can therefore be described as EDA-stable [23–26].

To the best of our knowledge the first review of EDA in depression was published by Straub et al. in the early 1990s [25]. It acknowledged that electrodermal hypoactivity had been repeatedly associated with affective disorders, but raised doubts about whether EDA could be considered a marker of depression, pointing to conflicting results and differences in laboratory conditions and suggesting that the impact of person-situation-environment dynamics on EDA had been underestimated. A more recent review of galvanic skin response (GSR) confirmed that patients with mood disorders show low or flat EDA profiles, but the authors pointed out several limitations in the evidence, including that many of the EDA studies are quite old and were conducted using outdated methods and technology [26]. The Vahey & Becerra review [26] anyway focused specifically on mood disorders and yielded a smaller number of eligible studies (41 vs. 77).

A summary of the current knowledge about the relationships between EDA and depression and between EDA and suicidal behaviour is timely, given the lack of recent comprehensive reviews [24] and the recent publication of the study protocol for a multi-centre, naturalistic, clinical study of electrodermal orienting reactivity in a large sample of adult depressed patients [27].

Objectives

Our objective was to carry out a systematic review of studies investigating:

1. The association between EDA and depression (research comparing depressed patients and controls, depression subgroups, depressed patients and other psychiatric patients, elicitation methods and EDA, EDA and hormones, EDA and antidepressants and other studies of EDA characteristics).
2. The association between EDA and suicidal behaviour (including research on suicidal risk, suicidal ideation only, completed/attempted suicide, violent/non-violent suicidal behaviour, impulsive/non-impulsive suicidal behaviour and suicide prevention) in depressed patients.

Methods

Selection of studies

The inclusion criteria were the following:

- EDA was measured.
- Design: randomised controlled trial (RCTs), quasi-experimental (e.g. non-randomised controlled studies and before-and-after studies), observational or meta-analytical.
- Participants of any age or gender in a community or clinical setting.
- The following types of study were eligible for inclusion:
  - studies involving participants with a primary diagnosis of mood disorder (unipolar depression, bipolar disorder, dysthymia, cyclothymia) who were in a depressive phase;
  - studies investigating the effects of an antidepressant compound on EDA;
  - studies involving participants with suicidal ideation or suicidal behaviour (suicide attempts, completed suicide).

Exclusion criteria were:

- Primary focus on psychiatric disorders other than mood disorders.
- Investigation of the effects of EDA on medication other than antidepressants.
- Case report, letter to the editor, conference paper, dissertation, personal opinion or commentary.
- Papers not written in English.

Data sources and search strategy

We carried out an electronic literature search to identify relevant studies. PubMed, Scopus, Cochrane Library and Web of Science were searched from the inception of the databases up to 12th April 2017. The search strings used in each search engine are reported in the Appendix 1. Articles were selected in accordance with the Preferred Reporting Items for Systematic Reviews and Meta-Analyses (PRISMA) diagram [28, 29]. The selection was done by three reviewers (M.S., M.I., V.C.) who independently selected titles, abstracts and full-text publications according to the inclusion and exclusion criteria described above. In the first stage of the selection process titles were screened to exclude those that were clearly not relevant to the review and then each reviewer read the abstract and full text of the remain articles and selected the relevant ones. Disagreements between reviewers were resolved through group discussion.

The following information was extracted from all publications: country, design, characteristics of study participants (number of subjects, diagnosis, mean age, % women), EDA variables and summary of main study findings. Regrettably, availability of information on several issues - sample and diagnosis; study design and protocol; type of EDA assessment; type of data presented in the results etc. - was very uneven and this meant that neither meta-analysis nor quantitative synthesis was possible, nor was it possible to adhere completely to the "Guidance on the conduct of narrative synthesis in systematic reviews"; nonetheless the guidance on data analysis and presentation was followed as closely as possible [30]. Study quality was appraised, where applicable, using the Newcastle-Ottawa Scale (NOS) [31].

Results

The electronic searches identified 1278 studies; once duplicates removed 823 records remained of which 606 were excluded because the title clearly had no relevance to the review; 109 records were excluded based on the Abstract; a further 68 studies were excluded because they were not written in English and 41 studies because the full text was not available. We assessed the full text of 108 articles and excluded 31 studies at this stage. The main reasons for exclusion were: study population did not match inclusion criteria (no primary clinical diagnosis of depression), focus on psychophysiological variables other than EDA (e.g. heart rate), basic, non-clinical research on EDA and wrong type of publication (conference session; letter to the editor; case report). Seventy-seven studies met all the inclusion criteria and were included in this review. The selection process is represented in Fig. 1.

Summaries of all the studies are presented in Tables 1 and 2 (EDA and depression) and 2 (EDA and suicidal behaviour).

Association between EDA and depression

Although low EDA in depressed patients was first described in 1890 [32], interest in this physiological variable as a marker of depressive disorders occurred mainly between the late 1970s and the 1990s.

The studies included in this section are very varied, both regarding sample and EDA variables. For clarity they have been grouped under the following headings: Depressed patients vs. controls; Depression subgroups; Depressed patients vs. other psychiatric patients; Elicitation methods and EDA; Other studies of EDA characteristics; EDA and hormones; EDA and antidepressants.

Depressed patients vs. controls

Nine studies, with a NOS score ranging from 2 (2 studies) to 5 (3 studies), mean NOS score 3.8, reported lower SCL, increased SCR latency and lower SCR amplitude in depressed subjects compared with healthy controls [33–41]. Thorell et al. reported a lower level of EDA in depressed patients than in healthy subjects, reflected in lower central values for SCL, SCR amplitude, SCR rate and an index of non-response during neutral tone stimulation [42].

The overall efficiency of SCR as a means of discriminating between depressed and healthy subjects has been estimated to be about 80% [43]. It has also

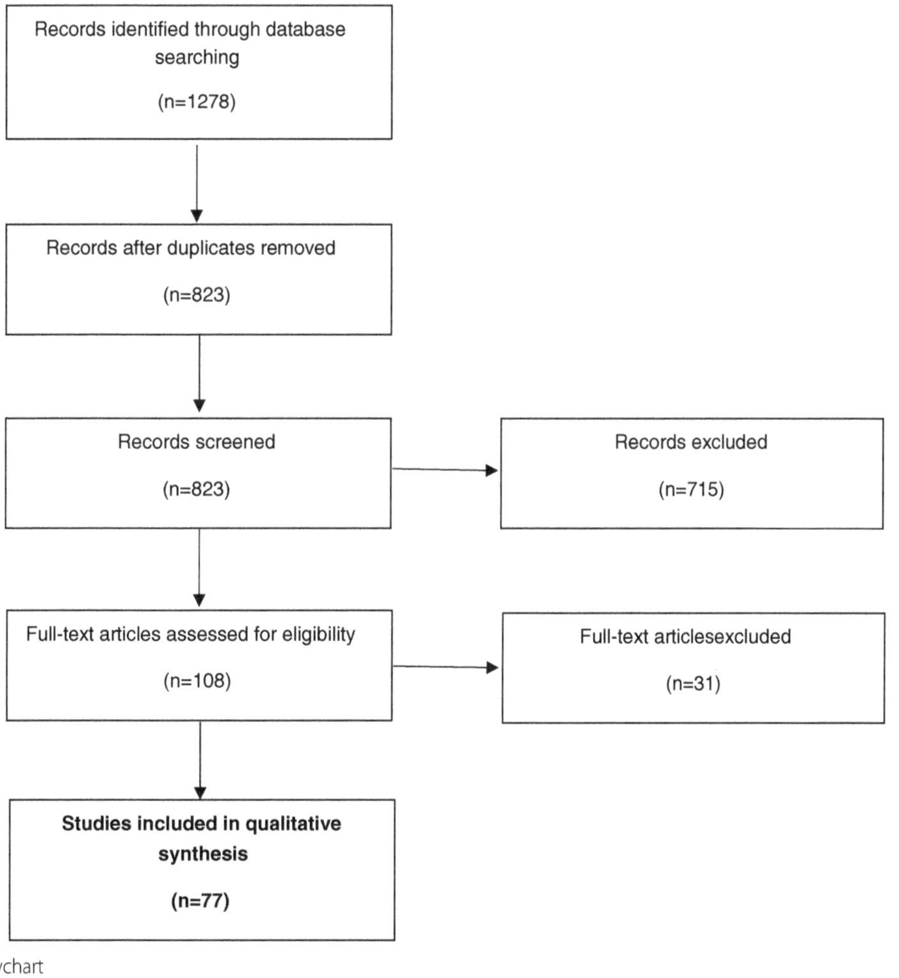

Fig. 1 PRISMA Flowchart

Table 1 Summary of selected studies – Electrodermal activity (EDA) and suicidal behavior

AUTHORS (COUNTRY AND YEAR)	SUBJECTS (DIAGNOSIS; AGE; MALE/FEMALE) AND CONTROLS (AGE; MALE/FEMALE)	MEASURES	MAIN STUDY FINDINGS	STUDY DESIGN (QUALITY[1])
Crowell et al. (USA, 2005)	– 23 parasuicidal adolescent girls, age 14–18, – 23 age-matched controls.	EDA recordings during the last minute of a 10-min resting baseline and for 10 min of recovery following the end of a sad movie.	No significant differences on measures of EDR between parasuicidal girls and healthy controls.	Case-control(3)
Edman et al. (1986)	35 drug-free, suicidal inpatients (mean age 41 years; 63% females): – 24 inpatients after a suicide attempt; – 11 patients with suicidal ideation.	SCL and habituation of the SCR.	No differences in the SCL. Tendency to lower figures in NS.SCR in patients who used violent suicide methods. All violent attempters (at baseline and follow-up) were fast habituators. Lowest frequency of fast habituators in patients with suicidal ideation.	Cross-sectional
Jandl et al. (Germany, 2009)	MDD inpatients divided in 3 groups: – 16 with history of 'hard attempted suicide' (e.g., hanging, stabbing) (47.3±11.9 years; 56% females); – 16 with a history of 'soft attempted suicide' (e.g. poisoning) (49.8±8 years; 69% females); – 18 no attempted suicide (47.9 ±11.6 years; 67% females).	NS.SCR frequency, SCR amplitude and EDA Habituation Rate measured during an auditory habituation paradigm.	Significantly lower EDA habituation rate in both suicide attempters groups. No difference among the 3 groups in SCR amplitude or NS.SCR frequency. Women showed faster habituation.	Cross sectional
Keller et al. (Germany, 1991)	– 23 patients with suicide attempt divided into violent and non-violent method (violent, N=14, 41.4±9.5 years, 64% females; non-violent, N= 9, 37.2±9.7 years, 66.6% females). – Age and sex matched groups (non-suicidal depressed patients/ patients with suicidal thoughts.	Number of stimuli until habituation, nonspecific SC reactions, height of first amplitude and SCL measured during an habituation experiment.	All patients who had used a violent method and patients who committed suicide in the year following the experiment were fast habituators. No difference in EDA between non-suicidal patients, those with suicidal thoughts or suicide attempts.	Case-control (4)
Sarchiapone et al. (Europe, 2017)	-1573 patients with a primary clinical diagnosis of depression, either currently depressed or in remission.	– ElectroDermal Orienting Reactivity (EDOR Test)	It is hypothesized that the EDOR Test will identify electrodermal hyporeactive depressed patients with a high suicidal proneness. Patients who reveal strong death intent are expected to be hyporeactive at the EDOR test, in most cases; non-hyporeactive patients are expected to have suicide attempts with strong death intent in a minority of cases.	Multicentric/ Study protocol
Spiegel (US, 1969)	Inpatients including: - 16 controls with no history of suicide threats or attempts and denying current suicidal thoughts; - 15 inpatients with suicide threats or preoccupations but no history of attempts; - 13 attempters with a history of one or more suicide attempts.	GSR First two sessions: word association. 4 days later, a series of words at irregular intervals, recording skin resistance changes.	Relatively low reactivity of threateners might be a function of depression. Threateners were the least reactive in terms of GSR to the word "suicide" Significant positive association between magnitude of GSR and intensity of affective meaning assigned to the concept "suicide" in all patients.	Crossover
Thorell (Sweden, 1987) Thorell et al. (1987a) Thorell et al. (1987b)	– 59 in- and out-patients with major depressive episode and dysthymic disorders (42±13.2 years; 54% females);	SCL at the onset of the first stimulus, mean SC fluctuation rate (SCFr) per minute, SCR magnitude (SCRm) to the first stimulus, SCR	Significantly lower central SCL, SCRm, SCRr, and SCRi, but not SCFr and habituation values in patients than in controls.	Case-control (5)

Table 1 Summary of selected studies – Electrodermal activity (EDA) and suicidal behavior *(Continued)*

AUTHORS (COUNTRY AND YEAR)	SUBJECTS (DIAGNOSIS; AGE; MALE/FEMALE) AND CONTROLS (AGE; MALE/FEMALE)	MEASURES	MAIN STUDY FINDINGS	STUDY DESIGN (QUALITY[1])
	– 59 mentally and somatically healthy subjects (42.4±13.3 years; 54% females)	rate (SCRr), and index of SC nonresponding (SCRi).	Considering medications, no statistically significant difference in any EDA variable. No significant difference in any EDA variable among dysthymic disorder vs major depressive episode and melancholic vs non-melancholic major depressive episode. Patients with endogenous depression had significantly lower SCL, SCRr, and SCRi. Patients with a high level of inhibition showed significantly lower SCL and SCRi. Suicidal behavior related to low electrodermal responsivity (EDR) and low stimulus-unrelated phasic activity, but unrelated to tonic EDA. Extreme hyporesponsivity in the suicide attempters was observed irrespective of whether the attempt had been made previously or during the current depression.	
Thorell et al. (2009)	– 279 depressed patients – 59 healthy subjects	Habituation of the electrodermal response	Sensitivity 96.6% and specificity 92.9% of electrodermal hyporeactivity for suicide and 83.3% and 92.7%, respectively, for suicide and/or violent attempts	Meta-analysis
Thorell et al. (Germany, 2013)[2]	783 depressive patients (126 bipolar patients; 539 unipolar patients; 118 with other diagnoses) (42.9±11.5; 58% females): – 32 violent suicide; – 4 nonviolent suicide; – 84 violent suicide attempt; – 103 nonviolent suicide attempt; – 560 other or no suicidal behavior.	Habituation of electrodermal responses measured during an auditory habituation paradigm.	Prevalence of electrodermal hyporeactivity was high and highest (80%) among bipolar patients and was independent of severity of depression, trait anxiety, gender and age. Sensitivity and specificity for suicide, and for suicide and violent suicide attempt were 83%, 98% and 74%, 88%, respectively. Hyporeactivity was stable, while reactivity changed into hyporeactivity in a later depressive episode.	Cohort (7)
Wolfersdorf et al. (Germany, 1996)	– 11 patients with personality disorders who attempted suicide (23±4 years; 100% females); – Depressed non-suicidal patients (100% females); – Depressed suicide attempters (100% females); – Schizophrenic non-suicidal patients (100% females); – Schizophrenic suicide attempters (100% females).	SCL, number of NS.SCR, habituation of the SCR	Significant differences in EDA values between women with personality disorders who attempted suicide and non-suicidal women suffering from depression. No difference between personality disorder and depressive patients who attempted suicide . No significant differences in EDA values in a habituation study between personality disorder patients and schizophrenic women with or without histories of suicide attempts.	Cross-sectional

Table 1 Summary of selected studies – Electrodermal activity (EDA) and suicidal behavior *(Continued)*

AUTHORS (COUNTRY AND YEAR)	SUBJECTS (DIAGNOSIS; AGE; MALE/FEMALE) AND CONTROLS (AGE; MALE/FEMALE)	MEASURES	MAIN STUDY FINDINGS	STUDY DESIGN (QUALITY[1])
Wolfersdorf et al. (Germany, 1999)	– 30 depressed violent suicide completers (mean age 43.8 years; 57% females); – Age and sex matched non-suicidal depressed patients; – Age and sex matched depressed patients with suicidal ideations; – Age and sex matched depressed patients with suicide attempts.	Number of stimuli up to habituation (habituation score, HS), SCL and amplitude of SCR after the first stimulus measured during a habituation experiment using auditory stimuli.	Depressed patients who died by suicide showed significantly lower HS, first amplitude of the SCR and SCL than non-suicidal depressed patients. Suicides showed a significant lower HS than non-suicidal patients or depressive patients with suicidal ideation. No significant difference between suicide and suicide attempters groups.	Case-control (5)

Legend:
[1]The "Newcastle-Ottawa Scale (NOS) for assessing the quality of case-control and cohort studies" was used to evaluate the case-control (scores 0-10) and cohort studies (scores 0-12)
[2]The sample comprises patients treated on the Depression Ward of the Centre for Psychiatry, Weissenau in southern Germany between 1985 and 2002. The studies of Keller et al. (1991), Wolfersdorf et al. (1996) and Wolfersdorf et al. (1999) were conducted in the same centre
EDA = Electrodermal Activity; EDOR = ElectroDermal Orienting Response; HS = Habituation Score; MDD = Major Depressive Disorder; NS.SCR = Nonspecific Skin Conductance Response; SCL = Skin Conductance Level; SCF = Skin Conductance Fluctuation; SCR = Skin Conductance Response

been reported that depressed patients show marginally faster habituation of the skin resistance orienting response than healthy controls [44, 45], although one study [35] with a lower NOS score than the others (2 vs. 3 and 5) did not find this.

Some researchers looked at age- and gender-related EDA variability. In adolescents [46] the results were consistent with the notion that EDA is lower in major depressive disorder (MDD) patients than in control subjects. In contrast SCL was similar in patients with dementia, depressed patients (mean age 75.9 ± 7 years) and healthy controls, probably due to a decline in the number of active sweat glands and sweat production in the elderly. As far as gender is concerned, SCLs were lower in women than in men in both depressed patients and healthy controls [47].

A study of GSRfound that patients were hyporesponsive because of depressive inhibition in an experimental condition, but failed to find any difference in GSR variables between patients and controls in two rest periods and in a no-response experimental condition [48].

Unlike most studies in this field Lapierre and Butter reported a higher SCL and higher basal skin resistance in depressed patients than in controls. The amplitude of SCR and number of non-specific SCRs were similar in depressed patients and controls [49]. Other studies reported higher SCLs in depressed subjects than in healthy controls [50, 51] and psychiatric controls [50]. A couple of studies [52, 53] failed to find any difference between depressed patients and healthy controls with respect to SCL [52] and SCR [53] variables.

It should be noted that the Lapierre and Butter study scored 0 on the NOS because of the lack of information about the study design, whereas the other studies [50–52] described above had higher NOS scores (5,4, and 4, respectively).

Briefly, lower EDA, especially lower SCL and SCR, in depressed patients than in healthy controls was the most consistently reported result.

Depression subgroups

It has been suggested that in depressed patients level of EDA may be a function of the type of depression. A recent, cross-sectional study offered preliminary evidence that EDA levels may differentiate the phases (depressive vs. mixed vs. euthymic) of bipolar disorder [54].

Lower EDA levels were found in patients with psychomotor retardation or symptoms of inhibition than in agitated depressed patients ([55, 56, 58], mean NOS score 4.3; [57, 59] cross-sectional studies), except for the study by Lapierre and Butter, which was the least robust in terms of NOS score [49; NOS score 0]. Patients classified as suffering from "psychotic" (rather than "neurotic") [60] and "endogenous" (rather than "non-endogenous") [61, 62] depression had lower EDA levels, although this finding was not consistent across all studies. Moreover, the published research on this issue [40, 58, 59, 63] is highly heterogeneous with respect to NOS score (2, 5, not applicable, and 1, respectively).

The absence of a SCR was observed in depressed patients with predominance of anxiety symptoms [40].

Table 2 Summary of selected studies – Association between EDA and depression

AUTHORS (COUNTRY AND YEAR)	SUBJECTS (DIAGNOSIS; AGE; MALE/FEMALE) AND CONTROLS (MEAN AGE; MALE/FEMALE)	MEASURES	MAIN STUDY FINDINGS	STUDY DESIGN (QUALITY[1])
Barg et al. (Germany, 1996)	– 16 depressed patients (36.1±1.9 years; 50% females), no medication; – 16 depressed patients (45.8±10.2 years; 50% females) treated with paroxetine; – 16 depressed patients (45.4±9.9 years; 50% females) treated with imipramine.	SCL, non-specific SCR, SCR	Patients treated with imipramine showed a higher heart rate and lower EDA than the other two groups.	Case-Control (5)
Bernstein et al. (US, 1988)	– 50 schizophrenic patients (34.8±9.5; 30% females); – 50 depressive patients (32.5±9.7 years; 66% females); – 50 controls (27.3±7.6 years; 58% females).	SCR recorded during auditory stimuli presentation. A subsample of each group was told they needed do nothing during tone presentations (habituation series); other subsamples had to press a pedal for each designated target signal, ignoring all nontarget tones.	No differences between hands in SCR for any diagnostic group Compared to normal controls, schizophrenic patients showed higher nonresponding in the habituation series, but no difference when target tones were presented. Depressives were equally nonresponsive during the habituation series, but they did not show a decrease in SCR nonresponding to the target tone.	Case-control (4)
Bernstein et al. (US, 1995)	– 69 schizophrenic patients (34.9±8.5 years; 42% females); – 45 mood disorder patients (36.6±10.1 years; 62% females); – 67 normal controls (31.2±10.1 years; 49% females).	SCR recorded during exposure to tones.	Schizophrenic and depressed patients were significantly more often classified as non-responders. The proportion of non-responders did not vary with neuroleptic or antidepressant medication.	Case-control (4)
Bob et al. (2011)	– 44 unipolar depressed outpatients, (37.06±8.72); – 35 healthy controls (35.12±8.10; 57% females).	EDA measured bilaterally.	Absence of differences between EDA in relapse and in remissions as well as between pharmacotherapy response and EDA.	Case-control (4)
Bonnet et al. (France, 2004)	– 9 non-depressed Chronic Low Back Pain (CLBP) patients, (43 years; 55% females); – 9 depressed CLBP patients, (46.1 years; 55% females); – 9 depressed controls free of pain (DCs), (44.1 years; 55% females); – 9 healthy controls free of pain and depression, (45.3 years; 55% females).	EDA recorded during a 3-min rest period and during a subsequent stimulation period. Stimuli were 3 identical pure tones.	Non-depressed patients presented an increased EDA, especially a higher frequency of non-specific fluctuations, than the 3 other groups. SCL was lower in the 2 groups of depressed participants than in the healthy control group.	Case-control (4)
Brankovic (Serbia, 2008)	– 57 patients with major depressive disorder and currently in depressive episode (43.1±10.9 years; 56% females); – 52 healthy controls (39.8±8.1 years; 60% females).	5 parameters of the SCR recorded when reading emotional eliciting stories.	Initial SCR was larger in controls than depressed patients. Positive feedback loop was greater in depressed patients than controls. Negative feedback loop was stronger in depressed patients than controls. Length of time needed for the magnitude of SCRs to decrease to half of the original response magnitude was longer in	Case-control (3)

Table 2 Summary of selected studies – Association between EDA and depression *(Continued)*

AUTHORS (COUNTRY AND YEAR)	SUBJECTS (DIAGNOSIS; AGE; MALE/FEMALE) AND CONTROLS (MEAN AGE; MALE/FEMALE)	MEASURES	MAIN STUDY FINDINGS	STUDY DESIGN (QUALITY[1])
			depressed patients than controls.	
Breyer-Pfaff et al. (1982)	37 patients with primary depressive disorders (22 endogenous and 15 non endogenous) (81% females) treated with amitriptyline.	SCLs, SF, habituation and amplitude of the SCR recorded during the exposure to tones and during active and passive situations. Measures repeated on the day before treatment began and again after 14 and 28 days of treatment.	Compared to baseline levels, EDA state at day 14 can be considered inhibited and labile (larger phasic and tonic reaction amplitudes). After 4 weeks of treatment, lability had returned to baseline, but inhibition was unchanged. No significant correlation between EDA measures and plasma drug levels.	Case-series
Byrne (Australia, 1975)	– 18 acute depressive inpatients (20-60 years; 50% females): – 10 "neurotic depressive"; – 8 "psychotic depressive"; – 11 normal controls (24-45 years; 45% females).	SCR amplitude, NS.SCR, habituation rate.	Higher mean SCR, higher frequency of NS.SCRs, and slower skin response habituation rata in the neurotic depressive sample. Higher mean SCR amplitude in the control sample. No significant difference between skin response habituation rates of either the control and neurotic depressive, or control and psychotic depressive samples.	Case-control (1)
Carney et al. (US, 1981)	– 15 inpatients with primary affective disorder (32±6.9 years; 100% females) – 15 age-and race-matched controls (31.5±7.5; 100% females)	SCL	Significantly lower SCL in depressed subjects. No significant correlation between SCL and measures of anxiety or depression for patients with primary affective disorder. Significant correlations between a measure of depression and SCL in normal controls.	Case-control (5)
Dawson et al. (US, 1977) Dawson et al. (1985)	– 20 hospitalized depressed patients (63.8±7.8 years; 80% females); – 20 non-depressed controls (62.2±7.6 years; 80% females).	SCL and SCR recorded at rest and during a variety of tasks before and after a series of electroconvulsive shock treatments (ECTs)	Depressed patients, compared to non-depressed controls during the pre-ECT test, exhibited lower SCLs, smaller phasic SCRs with longer latencies. Little EDA changes following ECT. Overall efficiency of SCL was of 70% and of SCR was 80%.	Case-control (4)
Donat & McCollough (US, 1983)	– 10 chronically depressed subjects (18-25 years; 100% females); – 10 controls (18-25 years; 100% females).	SCL	SCL correctly identified 9 of the 10 depressed group subjects and 7 of the 10 control group members under resting conditions. No difference between depressed subjects and controls under conditions of laboratory stress and of imaginal-role stress.	Case-control (4)

Table 2 Summary of selected studies – Association between EDA and depression *(Continued)*

AUTHORS (COUNTRY AND YEAR)	SUBJECTS (DIAGNOSIS; AGE; MALE/FEMALE) AND CONTROLS (MEAN AGE; MALE/FEMALE)	MEASURES	MAIN STUDY FINDINGS	STUDY DESIGN (QUALITY[1])
			SCL reliably identified group membership, with lower levels in the depressed group.	
Falkenberg et al. (Germany, 2012)	– 16 patients with MDD (37±15 years; 50% females); – 16 healthy controls (35±14 years; 50% females).	SCR recorded during standardized mood induction using happy and neutral pictures and funny and neutral cartoons.	MDD patients had higher SCRs in the cartoon condition than controls. Women revealed lower overall SCRs compared to men.	Case-control (5)
Fraguas et al. (US, 2007)	8 unmedicated patients diagnosed with MDD (35±12 years; 62,5% females) treated with fluoxetine 20 mg per day for 8 weeks.	SCL and SCR measured at basal condition and during four induced emotional states: happy, angry, sad and neutral.	Significant positive correlations between the percentage reduction in depression scores and increases in SCR only during the neutral emotion condition.	Case-series
Giedke et al. (Germany, 1980)	– 18 patients with primary depression (15 unipolar, 3 bipolar) (46.2±13.1 years; 83% females); – 27 age-matched healthy controls (45.1±15.4 years; 70.4% females).	GSR/SRR (Skin Resistance Responses). Response condition: participants were asked to react to the second of two identical tone stimuli.	In the experimental response condition controls increased their number and amplitude of SRRs to tone-stimuli more than patients. No significant correlation between GSR and both self-rated and physician-rated psychopathology.	Case-control (5)
Giedke & Heimann (1987)	– 59 drug free patients with primary MDD (47±11 years; 69% females) assigned to a double-blind treatment with amitriptyline or oxaprotiline; – 30 healthy controls matched for age and sex.	SR and habituation of SR orienting response.	Patients with primary MDD exhibited significantly fewer spontaneous fluctuations of SR and a faster habituation rate of SR orienting response. SR level did not differ between groups. Most patient/control differences remained unaffected irrespective of the drug applied.	Case-control + RCT (5)
Greco et al. (Italy, 2014)	– 10 patients affected by bipolar disorder I or II; – 10 healthy subjects (20-32 years; 50% females).	Tonic and phasic features of EDA measured during an emotional elicitation protocol.	Phasic features well discriminated among depression, mixed state, and euthymia. Mixed-state shows a strong tonic hypoactivity compared to euthymic state. Healthy subjects showed no statistical difference on each of the EDA feature patterns.	Cross-sectional
Hattangadi et al. (Canada, 1968)	- 263 psychiatric inpatients, including 51 depressed patients (27 neurotic and 24 psychotic depression); - 58 healthy controls.	GSR	Patients responded less than controls to the indifferent stimuli. No significant difference in response frequency between patient categories. No significant difference in latency, either between normal subjects and	Case-control (4)

Table 2 Summary of selected studies – Association between EDA and depression *(Continued)*

AUTHORS (COUNTRY AND YEAR)	SUBJECTS (DIAGNOSIS; AGE; MALE/FEMALE) AND CONTROLS (MEAN AGE; MALE/FEMALE)	MEASURES	MAIN STUDY FINDINGS	STUDY DESIGN (QUALITY[1])
			patients, or between any two diagnostic categories. All psychiatric patients in all categories gave lower amplitude responses than the normal group. No significant difference between medicated and non-medicated patients in any diagnostic group as far as GSR frequency and latency. Patients receiving antidepressant medication had higher amplitudes than those receiving anti-psychotic medications.	
Have et al. (Iceland, 1991)	– 21 patients with Alzheimer dementia (80.6 ± 9.8 years); – patients with depression (75.9 ± 7 years); – 19 healthy volunteers (79 ± 11.4 years).	SCL	No difference in SCL among patients' groups. Very low SCL in the overall sample, likely due to a decline in the number of active sweat glands in old people and diminished sweat production.	Case-control (3)
Heimann (Germany, 1978)	– 95 depressive and depressive-anxious patients; – 18 of these 95 treated with amytriptylin for 4 weeks; – 27 of these 95 retested at a 1-year follow-up.	SRR, SRL (Skin Resistance Level). Orienting reaction and habituation tested after two minutes of rest, with a series of tones and of flashes. Assessment of changes in the dimension of activation after 14 and 28 days of treatment with amytriptylin, and 1-year follow up after the first examination during a depressive state.	Patients in the activated and inhibited cluster showed the smallest changes at follow-up, whereas all four patients of the labile-activated cluster change to another group. Preponderance of cases with lower activation after treatment with amitriptylin.	Cross-sectional
Iacono et al. (1983) Iacono & Tuason (1983)	– 26 unipolar depressed patients (37.8±12.7 years; 23% females); – 24 with bipolar affective disorder (36±12 years; 33% females); – 46 healthy control patients (35±11.9 years; 17.4% females).	SCL.	The EDA of affective disorder patients was uniformly depressed across all tasks and conditions. No consistent bilateral asymmetries in EDA were observed.	Case-control (5)
Iacono et al. (1984)[2]	– 22 unipolar outpatients in remission (41±12.7 years; 77% females); – 22 bipolar outpatients in remission (38.5±14.4 years; 68% females); – 26 controls (41.3±12.2 years; 88% females).	SCLs and SCRs recorded during blowing up a balloon until it burst and during the exposure to tones, and eight familiar sounds.	Compared to the control subjects, the affective disorder patients (especially the unipolar patients) responded significantly less to the balloon task, the highest tones, and the familiar sounds, had lower tonic levels and a larger proportion of them failed to respond to the stimuli. Several measures of EDA displayed moderately high one-year retest stability.	Case-control (3)

Table 2 Summary of selected studies – Association between EDA and depression *(Continued)*

AUTHORS (COUNTRY AND YEAR)	SUBJECTS (DIAGNOSIS; AGE; MALE/FEMALE) AND CONTROLS (MEAN AGE; MALE/FEMALE)	MEASURES	MAIN STUDY FINDINGS	STUDY DESIGN (QUALITY[1])
Ikeda et al. (Japan, 1982)	20 healthy volunteers (23.1 years; 0% females): – Amitriptyline 30 mg/day, 3 times, for 3 days; – Nomifensine 100 mg/day, 2 times, for 3 days; – Placebo 3 times, for 3 days.	SCR recorded before the experiment and 8 hours after the final dose.	In the amitriptyline group, the NS.SCR decreased. In the nomifensine group, NS.SCR tended to increase.	
Kamenskaya & Mikhailova (Russia, 1985)	– 50 manic-depressive patients in the depressive phase prior to treatment (20-45 years), divided into 3 groups according to the nature of the principal affect (anguish, anxiety, or apathy); – 25 healthy individuals (20-45 years).	SCR in the background and during the presentation of indifferent stimuli (opening the eyes, light flashes) and in a stress situation.	Depressed patients had an increased latency and lower amplitude of the SCR than healthy subjects. The absence of a SCR was observed in 20% of patients, more often with a dominant anxiety affect.	Case-control (2)
Lader & Wing (UK, 1969)	– 35 inpatients with a primary diagnosis of moderate or severe depression: – 17 Predominantly agitated (45.8 years; 59% females); – 13 Predominantly retarded (42.3 years; 69% females); – 5 Uncomplicated depressives (30.2 years); – 35 age and sex matched controls.	SCLs, SCRs, NS.SCRs and habituation rate recorded during exposure to tones.	Agitated patients and retarded patients had, respectively, significantly higher and lower mean SCL than controls. Agitated depressives had the highest conductance levels at the end of the recording session than at the start. Healthy subjects were the most reactive ones, and habituated significantly more rapidly than did the agitated depressives. Retarded patients gave a significant lower number of SCRs than agitated patients. The agitated patients had significantly more and the retarded patients had significantly less fluctuations than the normal subjects.	Case-control (4)
Lapierre & Butter (Canada, 1978)	– 20 agitated depressed patients (mean age 38 years and 2 months; 75% females); – 20 retarded depressed patients (mean age 37 years and 8 months; 70% females).	Spontaneous GSR was monitored for 5 minutes. The patient was then given a series of 6 randomized visual and/or auditory stimuli, and the latency period for a EDA response and the magnitude of the response was assessed. Then: Maprotiline and imipramine administration, double-blind. Measurement were repeated after 3 hours, 4, 7, 14 and 28 days.	Basal skin resistance was significantly lower for the agitated depressive. The GSR response was consistently greater in the agitated depressives than in the retarded. Gradual but nonsignificant increase in skin resistance and reduction in the magnitude of the GSR response as treatment progressed in both drug groups. Still the agitated depressives maintained more reactivity on this parameter. No major difference in GSR was found between imipramine and maprotiline.	Double blind controlled study

Table 2 Summary of selected studies – Association between EDA and depression *(Continued)*

AUTHORS (COUNTRY AND YEAR)	SUBJECTS (DIAGNOSIS; AGE; MALE/FEMALE) AND CONTROLS (MEAN AGE; MALE/FEMALE)	MEASURES	MAIN STUDY FINDINGS	STUDY DESIGN (QUALITY[1])
Lapierre & Butter (Canada, 1980)	– 20 agitated depressed patients (mean age 38 years; 75% females); – 20 retarded depressed patients (mean age 38 years; 70% females); – 20 volunteer controls (mean age 24 years; 75% females).	SCL and SCR recorded prior, during and after visual and auditory non-signal sensory stimulations and a reaction time stimulation.	SCLs significantly higher for both depressed groups. Depressed patients had longer latency time of onset of an EDA response than in volunteers.	Case-control (0)
Lemaire et al. (France, 2015)	– 45 bipolar outpatients: – 15 remitted (41.67±10.19 years; 47% females); – 15 moderately depressed (43.4±11.65 years; 80% females); – 15 moderately manic (41.53±8.13 years; 73% females); – 101 healthy controls (43.86±11.96 years; 49% females).	Maximum SCR amplitude recorded following the presentation of affective and neutral pictures during passive viewing and during experiential suppression.	Negative and positive pictures elicited SCRs of similar maximum amplitudes, greater than those elicited by neutral pictures. The maximum SCR amplitude was reduced during experiential suppression in all groups but this effect was more pronounced in depressed patients.	Case-control (4)
Levinson (US, 1991)	– 36 schizophrenic patients (31.4±6.9 years; 36% females); – 17 patients schizoaffective disorder (30.3±9 years; 59% females); – 24 inpatients with MDD (psychotic or nonpsychotic), or the mainly affective subtype schizoaffective disorder (36.9±12.4 years; 54% females); – 25 control subjects (30.6±9 years; 44% females).	SCL, SCR, NS.SCR, SC non-response, habituation score, reaction time recorded during four paradigms: – a series of tones in a no-task habituation paradigm; – a similar series of higher tones; – a series of tones with a button-press (reaction time) task; – a loud white noise stimulus (without task).	Schizoaffective subjects were more likely to be non-responders, and had lower (faster) mean habituation scores than other groups. Schizophrenic, depressed and controls subjects had similar mean habituation scores and proportions of non-responders. Depressed subjects showed some evidence of autonomic hyperarousal (higher tonic SC level, trend toward more NS.SCRs).	Case-control (4)
Lewinsohn et. al (USA,1973)	Two studies on the same sample composed by – -12 depressed patients; – -12 psychiatric control patients; – -12 healthy control subjects.	Autonomic response (skin resistance) to aversive stimulation and adaptation over repeated presentations of the same aversive situation.	In both studies, the depressed group was found to be more responsive to the aversive stimulus and the overall SCL was highest for the depressed subjects.	Case-control (5)
Lindsey et al. (US, 2011)	- 24 currently depressed Seasonal Affective Disorder (SAD) participants (41.58±11.72 years; 92% females); - 24 demographically-matched controls with no depression (41.83±12.75; 92% females).	SCL, surface facial electromyography and self-reported emotional responses to light- and season-relevant stimuli Task: 30 digital photographs of 5 scenes presented under 6 conditions (light intensity – 2 conditions; seasonal cues – 3 conditions).	SAD participants displayed more frequent SCR, greater SCR magnitude, and more self-reported depressed mood in response to overcast stimuli and lower SCR magnitude, and less self-reported depressed mood in response to sunny stimuli.	Case-control (5)
Mardaga & Hansenne (Belgium, 2009)	– 20 subjects with MDD (22-59 years; 55% females); – 20 healthy controls (24-59 years; 55% females).	SCR recorded following the presentation of neutral, pleasant, and unpleasant pictures.	Pleasant pictures elicited more and larger responses than unpleasant ones in control but not in depressed subjects. Depressed subjects showed generally faster half-recovery times.	Case-control (6)

Table 2 Summary of selected studies – Association between EDA and depression *(Continued)*

AUTHORS (COUNTRY AND YEAR)	SUBJECTS (DIAGNOSIS; AGE; MALE/FEMALE) AND CONTROLS (MEAN AGE; MALE/FEMALE)	MEASURES	MAIN STUDY FINDINGS	STUDY DESIGN (QUALITY[1])
Mestanikova et al. (Slovak Republic, 2015)	– 25 depressed adolescents (14.6± 0.4 years; 52% females); – 25 age/gender matched healthy controls.	EDA measured in sitting and supine position, at rest.	EDA diminished in the supine resting position in MDD patients compared to healthy controls.	Case-control (4)
Miquel et al. (Spain, 1999)	– 27 depressed outpatients (4 bipolar disorder in the depressive cycle; 17 MDD; 5 depressive neurosis; 1 subject non-specified depressive disorder) (34.63±10.05 years; 19; 70% females); – 27 normal subjects (33.44±10.27 years; 63% females).	SCL and SCR recorded during a series of tones.	Depressive patients displayed lower basal SCLs and lower conductance amplitudes to the first stimulus and to stimulus change. A trend towards habituation was detected in both groups, but neither difference between them, nor differences in habituation speed were found between depressive and healthy subjects.	Case-control (2)
Mirkin & Coppen (1980	– 13 depressive inpatients (58.6±1.9 years; 72% females). – 15 normal controls (54.2±1.7 years; 60% females).	SCL and SCR recorded during exposure to tones.	Higher proportion of electrodermal non-responders in patients than controls. Endogenous depressive patients had significantly lower SCLs than either the non-endogenous patients or controls.	Case-control (1)
Myslobodsky & Horesh (Israel, 1971)	– 10 endogenous depressive patients (51±6.79 years; 70% females); – 9 reactive depression patients (43±6.29 years; 89% females); – 14 normal subjects (48±17.59 years; 57% females).	EDA recorded at rest and during three experimental conditions: a visual-imagery task, a verbal task, a neutral tone habituation sequence.	In endogenous depression EDA was higher on the left hand compared with the right under all the conditions studied. In reactive depression EDA was higher on the left side during the verbal task and tone habituation sequence and on the right side in the visual task.	Case-control (3)
Nissen et al. (2010)	– 23 patients with MDD; 35 healthy control matched for sex, age, and IQ.	SCR recorded during the presentation of Conditioned (CS+) and non-Conditioned (CS-) Stimuli.	MDD patients responded stronger to the CS+ than to the CS-.	Case-control (4)
Noble & Lader (UK, 1971)	– 34 inpatients with a primary diagnosis of depression (12 males, 44.3±13.6 years; 22 females, 35.7±11.4 years); – Subgroups of 10 agitated and 10 retarded depression patients.	SCLs, SCRs, NS.SCRs recorded at rest and during mental arithmetic, before and after ECT.	The stress of mental arithmetic was associated with increase in skin conductance. The difference between the basal and stress recordings (reactivity) was highly significant. Reactivity was reduced after ECT. Low skin conductance correlated significantly with severity of depression. A reduction in NS.SCR correlated with high scores for depressed mood and retardation. Before ECT the agitated patients had significantly	Cross-sectional

Table 2 Summary of selected studies – Association between EDA and depression *(Continued)*

AUTHORS (COUNTRY AND YEAR)	SUBJECTS (DIAGNOSIS; AGE; MALE/FEMALE) AND CONTROLS (MEAN AGE; MALE/FEMALE)	MEASURES	MAIN STUDY FINDINGS	STUDY DESIGN (QUALITY[1])
			more fluctuations than the retarded group. No significant overall change in EDA measures after ECT.	
O'Kearney & Parry (Australia, 2014)	– 24 depressive episode (39.6±16.98 years; 67% females); – 24 PTSD (31.7±16.49 years; 50% females); – 24 healthy controls (35.8±15.73 years; 50% females).	SCR.	PTSD showed higher SCR during trauma recall compared with recall of other events and compared with depressed controls. No significant difference in reactivity between depressed and non-disordered participants.	Case-control (4)
Pazderka-Robinson et al. (2004)	– 43 patients with chronic fatigue syndrome (46.3±9.6 years; 100% females); – 25 depressed patients (35.3±10.5 years; 100% females); – 44 controls (27.8±9.3; 100% females).	SCL and SCR recorded during an orienting task.	SCLs were markedly lower for the chronic fatigue syndrome group, with no difference between controls and depressives.	Case-control (4)
Perez-Reyes & Cochrane (US, 1967)	– 108 neurotic depressed inpatients; – 82 psychotic depressed inpatients; – 69 healthy volunteers.	SCL and mean number of SCRs per minute.	No difference in initial SCL or SCR frequency, but significant differences in SCR susceptibility among the three groups.	Case-control (1)
Pruneti et al. (Italy, 2010)	– Outpatients (38.4±9.7 years; 52% females) with the following diagnoses: – Generalized Anxiety Disorder (GAD, n = 24); – Major Depression Episode (MDE, n = 14); – Panic Disorder (PAD, n = 12); – Obsessive-Compulsive Disorder (OCD, n = 10).	SCR registered in three consecutive phases: baseline (registration at rest), stress presentation, and recovery.	SCR mean values are much higher for GAD and PAD patients than for MDE and OCD. The amplitude of the SCR was also significantly different among groups.	Cross-sectional
Rohde et. al (Germany, 2014)	– 43 currently depressed patients (36.34±11.36 years; 60% female); – 36 controls (32.19±12.26 years; 66% female); – physiological data of 32 currently depressed participants and 23 controls.	SCR, EMG corrugator activity at baseline and during a Mindful Breathing Exercise. Mindful episode: the patient mindfully observed his/her breathing. Drifted episode: the patients had his/her mind wandering, not focused on the task.	SCR: no significant differences were found between currently depressed patients and controls. In both groups, greater SCRs recorded during drifted episodes, while weaker SCRs were elicited within mindful episodes.	Case-control (4)
Rottenberg et al. (2002, USA)	– 71 depressed persons (mean age 33.4 years; 66% females); – 33 non-depressed healthy controls (mean age 32.3 years; 70% females).	SCL and SCR recorded at baseline and after stimuli (neutral film and cry-inducing film).	During the sad film, non-depressed criers had greater number of SCR than non-depressed non-criers. Non-depressed non-criers exhibited significant decreases in SCL from the neutral to the sad film. Depressed criers exhibited significantly smaller increases in SCL and SCR rate to the sad film than did non-depressed criers.	Case-control (5)

Table 2 Summary of selected studies – Association between EDA and depression *(Continued)*

AUTHORS (COUNTRY AND YEAR)	SUBJECTS (DIAGNOSIS; AGE; MALE/FEMALE) AND CONTROLS (MEAN AGE; MALE/FEMALE)	MEASURES	MAIN STUDY FINDINGS	STUDY DESIGN (QUALITY[1])
Schneider (US, 1983)	– 10 depressed inpatients (9 with unipolar and 1 with bipolar disorder) (mean age 43.1 years; 0% females); – 23 schizophrenic inpatients (13 who underwent drug 'washout' and 10 who didn't) (mean age 45.2 years; 0% females); – 10 healthy controls (mean age 40.9 years; 0% females).	SCL, SCR and NS.SCR recorded during exposure to tones.	SCLs were higher in the normal and schizophrenic groups than in the other two groups. The depressives' mean laterality index, unlike that of the controls, reflected lower SCLs and SCRs from the right hand than from the left. The indices from the other two patient groups did not significantly differ from controls' ones. The patient groups generally had a lower proportion of 'responders' than did the health controls group, a lower number of SFs and a lower SF amplitude.	Case-control (2)
Schneider D. et al. (Germany, 2012)	– 28 in- and out-patients with unipolar MDD (age range 21–54 years; 43% females); – 28 age- and education-matched control participants.	Galvanic skin conductance (GSC), galvanic skin responses (GSR). Stimuli: 96 short video-clips conveying one of 4 emotion categories (happy, sad, fear, disgust) or no emotion (neutral).	Patients displayed more GSRs than healthy controls in all emotion categories. In patients, the number of GSRs did not differ between emotion categories, and neutral video clips evoked less GSRs than happy, sad, fearful and disgusted clips.	Case-control (4)
Siepmann et al. (Germany, 2001)	12 healthy volunteers (mean age 25 years; 0% females): – Reboxetine 4 mg, twice a day, for 13 days; – Placebo, twice a day, for 13 days.	SCL and SCR recorded following a single deep inspiration.	SCR was decreased after multiple dosing with reboxetine.	Crossover
Siepmann et al. (Germany, 2003)	12 healthy volunteers (mean age 34 years; 0% females): – Sertraline 50 mg, once a day, for 14 days; – Placebo, once a day, for 14 days.	SCL and SCR recorded following a single deep inspiration	Sertraline caused a significant reduction of SCL, whereas SCR was not changed.	Crossover
Siepmann et al. (Germany, 2004b)	12 healthy volunteers (mean age 27 years; 0% females): – Moclobemide 150 mg, twice a day, for 14 days; – Placebo, twice a day, for 14 days.	SCL and SCR recorded following a single deep inspiration	SCRs did not change after treatment with moclobemide.	Crossover
Siepmann et al. (Germany, 2004a)	12 healthy volunteers (25±3 years; 0% females): – Amitriptyline 25 mg, 3 times daily for 13 days; – St. John's wort extract, 3 times daily for 13 days; – Placebo, 3 times daily for 13 days.	- SCR recorded following a single deep inspiration.	St. John's wort extract had no effect on SCR. SCR significantly decreased during treatment with amitriptyline at all time points of measurement.	Crossover
Sigmon et al. (USA, 2007)	-15 MDD patients, Recurrent, with Seasonal Pattern (MDD-SAD; 80% females); -15 MDD patients (MDD; 66.7% females); -15 controls (80% females). Mean age 38.93 years.	Baseline SCL recordings obtained for a 5-min baseline period and average SCL collected across the baseline period. SCR at baseline and after presentation of winter and summer scenes were recorded.	MDD-SAD patients exhibited a greater number of SCR and greater SCR amplitude in reaction to the winter scenes, than individuals in the MDD and control groups. Individuals in the control and MDD groups did not significantly differ on frequency of SCR or strength of SCR amplitude	Case-control (5)

Table 2 Summary of selected studies – Association between EDA and depression *(Continued)*

AUTHORS (COUNTRY AND YEAR)	SUBJECTS (DIAGNOSIS; AGE; MALE/FEMALE) AND CONTROLS (MEAN AGE; MALE/FEMALE)	MEASURES	MAIN STUDY FINDINGS	STUDY DESIGN (QUALITY[1])
			in response to winter scenes. Individuals in the three groups did not significantly differ on SCR amplitude, in reaction to the summer scenes.	
Silva et al. (Brazil, 2000)	-29 adult healthy volunteers (86% females) received - 100 mg Nefazodone (NF) (mean age 25 years); - 200 mg NF (mean age 26.6 years); - placebo (mean age 24.9 years). (Double-blind condition).	Test 1: (1) amplitude of SCR - fluctuations that occurred within 5 s from a sound stimulus; (2) number of spontaneous fluctuations – those occurring be yond the above mentioned 5-s window; (3) SCL – average level of conductance during the intervals between fluctuations.	Conditioned fear. NF decreased the number of spontaneous fluctuations of skin conductance in a dose-dependent way, although the drug did not affect the amplitude of the SCR to the tone.	Crossover Double-blind
Storrie et al. (US, 1981)	– 10 inpatients with Primary Affective Disorder, free from psychoactive medications for at least 3 days prior the initial testing (48±4 years; 0% females); – 10 healthy subjects without history of depressive dysfunction or psychosis (49±5 years; 0% females).	SCL and SCR recorded during Valsalva maneuvers. Measures repeated three weeks after initiation of therapy with tricyclic antidepressants or antipsychotic medication.	Laterality hypothesis not confirmed. Mean SCL and SCR significantly higher in the control group than in depressed patients. No significant difference in SCL and SCR between treated and untreated patients.	Case-control (5)
Thorell & D'Elia (Sweden, 1988)[3]	– 28 in- and out-patients with major depressive episode and dysthymic disorders (42.5; 50% females); – 59 mentally and somatically healthy subjects.	SCL at the onset of the first stimulus, mean SC fluctuation rate (SCFr) per minute, SCR magnitude (SCRm) to the first stimulus, the SCR rate (SCRr), and the index of SC nonresponding (SCRi).	Significantly higher EDA during remission than during depression according to all 5 EDA variables. No significant difference in EDA between patients in remission and healthy subjects. Among suicide attempters, EDA at follow-up did not change significantly, but was not significantly lower than in healthy subjects. However, SCRm and SCRi in suicide attempters were significantly lower at follow-up than in the healthy group. The extremely hyporesponsive patients, including suicide attempters, when in remission, did not reach the levels of the healthy subjects except for SCFr. The patient with recurrent major depressive episodes when in remission did not reach the electrodermal responsivity levels found in the healthy subjects.	Case-control (5)

Table 2 Summary of selected studies – Association between EDA and depression *(Continued)*

AUTHORS (COUNTRY AND YEAR)	SUBJECTS (DIAGNOSIS; AGE; MALE/FEMALE) AND CONTROLS (MEAN AGE; MALE/FEMALE)	MEASURES	MAIN STUDY FINDINGS	STUDY DESIGN (QUALITY[1])
Thorell et al. (1988, Sweden)	– 59 depressed patients; – 59 healthy controls.	After 5 min without stimulation, 37 tones were presented. SCL at onset of the first stimulus; stimulus-unrelated SC fluctuation rate (SCFr) during the whole stimulation session except for 10 s after onset of each stimulus; SC response magnitude (SCRm) to the first stimulus; SCR rate (SCRr); index of SC nonresponding (SCRi). Cortisol in plasma and in urine were dosed, dexamethasone suppression test (DST) was performed.	No significant correlation between EDA and cortisol in patients' plasma and urine. No relationship between EDA and the outcome of DST, neither any simple relationship between EDA and cortisol in plasma and in urine. Positive correlation between SCL and morning plasma cortisol and negative correlations between EDR and nocturnal urinary cortisol in the suicide attempters. In the suicide attempters, the already extremely low EDR is additionally suppressed with increased nocturnal urinary cortisol excretion while SCL, and to some extent also EDR, are elevated with increased morning plasma cortisol. This pattern is opposite to that obtained in the healthy subjects and in the non-suicidal patients for SCL and plasma cortisol.	Case-control (5)
Thorell et al. (Sweden, 1993)	– 50 depressive patients (42.2±13.4 years; 52% females); – 50 age and gender-matched healthy subjects (42.6±13.5 years; 48% females).	Blood and urine for the measurement of basal hormone levels were collected at 8 a.m., immediately followed by clinical ratings and EDA measurements.	Positive relationships between SCL and basal levels of thyroid hormones in the healthy subjects were absent or reversed in the depressive patients. No relationships between electrodermal responsivity and thyroid hormones in depressive and healthy subjects. No significant difference between drug-free patients and patients treated with antidepressant medications regarding the EDA variables.	Case-control (4)
Toone et al. (UK, 1981)	– 22 schizophrenic patients (mean age 35.8 years; 64% females); – 11 unipolar depressed patients (mean age 40.6 years; 73% females); – 4 manic patients (mean age 38.7 years; 50% females); – 12 anxiety state patients (mean age 30.1 years; 50% females); – 22 healthy controls (mean age 36.7 in males and 39.3 in females; 36% females).	SCLs, SCRs and SF recorded at rest and during 32 flashes.	No group showed a distinctive pattern of lateral asymmetry; the only significant difference was in the adaptation of SCL during stimulation. Among depressed males the adaptation of SCL during stimulation on the left exceeded the right; among depressed females the trend was reversed. The frequency of SF in EDA was greater in the	Case-control (6)

Table 2 Summary of selected studies – Association between EDA and depression *(Continued)*

AUTHORS (COUNTRY AND YEAR)	SUBJECTS (DIAGNOSIS; AGE; MALE/FEMALE) AND CONTROLS (MEAN AGE; MALE/FEMALE)	MEASURES	MAIN STUDY FINDINGS	STUDY DESIGN (QUALITY[1])
			anxiety state and schizophrenic groups and in those patients who reported auditory hallucinations during recording.	
Tsai et al. (US, 2003)	– 12 Spanish-speaking latinas with major depressive episode (28.28±7.45; 100% females); – 10 non-depressed Spanish-speaking latinas (28.28±7.45; 100% females).	SCL during sad and amusing film clips of human and animal content.	Depressed Latinas demonstrated less electrodermal reactivity across all the film clips than non-depressed Latinas.	Case-control (4)
Ward et al. (USA, 1983)	– 33 depressed patients (mean age 42.58 years; 36% females); – 71 healthy controls (mean age 35.59 years; 46% females).	SCL was examined during 15 minutes during the first week of hospitalization.	Healthy and depressed women had significantly lower SCLs than healthy and depressed men; subjects with recurrent depression had significantly lower SCLs than subjects with a first episode depression. Significant positive correlation between age and SCL in the depressed group but not in the control group. No significant SCL differences between medicated and unmedicated patients. No significant SCL differences between endogenous-nonendogenous, situational-non-situational, primary-secondary, or DST suppressor-DST non-suppressor depression. SCL proved a very sensitive and specific test for distinguishing non-geriatric unipolar depressed adults from physically healthy normal controls.	Case-control (3)
Ward & Doerr (1986)	– 37 in- and out- patients with major affective disorder (mean age 35.3 years; 59% females); – 71 controls (control group 1) (mean age 35.5 years; 46% females); – 334 "stressed" normal controls (control group 2) who were first parents of newborns (mean age 28.7 years; 51% females).	Resting SCL.	Lowest SCLs in the depression group. No difference between the two control groups. For women, SCL less than 3.0 micronho/cm2 yielded a sensitivity of 95% and a specificity of 91% for Control Group 1. For males, a criterion of SCL less than 4.8 yielded a sensitivity of 93% and a specificity of 89% for Control Group 1. No significant difference in SCL between drug-free and medicated patients. SCL was abnormally low in all depression subtypes.	Case-control (3)

Table 2 Summary of selected studies – Association between EDA and depression *(Continued)*

AUTHORS (COUNTRY AND YEAR)	SUBJECTS (DIAGNOSIS; AGE; MALE/FEMALE) AND CONTROLS (MEAN AGE; MALE/FEMALE)	MEASURES	MAIN STUDY FINDINGS	STUDY DESIGN (QUALITY[1])
Weckowicz et al (Alberta, 1971)	– 212 depressed inpatients included; data at follow-up available for 170 (mean age 38 years; 69% females).	Galvanic skin responses (GSR) to a noxious stimulus, obtained one minute after the last basal reading. Patients were tested after admission and before starting therapy. Second assessment after 3 weeks of therapy.	GSR was not a predictor for ECT, it was a near-significant predictor for psychotherapy and for drug therapy.	Cross-Sectional
Williams et al. (1985)	36 primary depressive patients: – 27 unipolar (37.4±12.5 years; 74% females); – 9 bipolar (46.2±10.1 years; 55% females).	SCL and SCR recorded for two experimental conditions: – auditory stimuli during relaxation; – a task requiring responding to specific tones pressing a foot pedal.	No differences in tonic or phasic EDA in unipolar or bipolar subtype, response to the dexamethasone suppression test, severity of depression, medication status, or gender. Patients with psychomotor retardation had significantly lower levels of tonic EDA than non-retarded ones.	Cross-sectional
Zullino et al. (Switzerland, 2015)	– 58 patients randomly assigned to 8-week Venlafaxine treatment (44.9±8 years; 36.7% females) or applied relaxation (45.6±11.3 years; 46.4% females).	Skin conductance.	Patients treated with Venlafaxine had significantly lower EDA than the other group, both at week 4 and 8.	Randomized comparative

Legend:
[1]The "Newcastle-Ottawa Scale (NOS) for assessing the quality of case-control and cohort studies" was used to evaluate the case-control (scores 0-10) and cohort studies (scores 0-12)
[2]Follow-up study of Iacono et al. (1983)
[3]Follow-up study of Thorell et al. 1987
CLBP= Chronic Low Back Pain; CS = Conditioned Stimuli; ECT=Electroconvulsive therapy; EDA = Electrodermal Activity; EDR = Electrodermal Response; GSC = Galvanic skin conductance; GSR = Galvanic skin response; MDD = Major Depressive Disorder; MDE = Major Depressive Episode; NS.SCR = Nonspecific Skin Conductance Response; OCD = Obsessive-Compulsive Disorder PTSD = Post-traumatic Stress Disorder; SAD = Seasonal Affective Disorder; SCL = Skin Conductance Level; SCFr = Skin Conductance Fluctuation rate; SCR = Skin Conductance Response; SF= Spontaneous Fluctuation; SR = Skin Resistance; SRR = Skin Resistance Response

In brief, patients classified as suffering from "psychotic" and "endogenous" depression had lower EDA levels compared to "neurotic" and "non-endogenous" depression. However, in view of the significant differences in the methodology and design of the relevant studies and their inconsistent results, the utility of EDA as a means of discrimination between subgroups of depressive patients remains to be demonstrated.

Depressed patients vs. other psychiatric patients

Comparisons of EDA in depressed patients and patients with other psychiatric disorders have been performed to ascertain whether EDA can be used as a marker of depressive states.

EDA abnormalities have been described in schizophrenic patients [64]. Compared with normal controls, both schizophrenic and depressed patients showed high levels of non-response in the habituation series, but schizophrenics - unlike the depressed patients - showed a decrease in SCR non-response to the target tone [55, 65]. In contrast Levinson [51] found no substantial differences between schizophrenic and depressed patients and normal controls with respect to SCR.

Pruneti et al. [66] found that patients with generalised anxiety disorder or panic disorder had higher SCRs than patients with major depression or obsessive-compulsive disorder.

Have et al. [67] reported that depressed patients, patients with degenerative dementia of the Alzheimer type and healthy controls had similar SCLs.

In summary, there have been only six studies comparing depressed patients to other psychiatric patients, and they deal with different disorders, making it hard to draw clear conclusions.

Elicitation methods and EDA

The published research using emotional elicitation protocols and other tasks to investigate EDA is highly heterogeneous with respect to sample, EDA variables, task and NOS score (range: 3 - 6), making it very hard to compare studies and to draw unequivocal conclusions.

Lower EDA, lower SCRs and higher SCL/SCRs were found in depressed subjects compared with controls in response to various emotional elicitation protocols (including exposure to pleasant and unpleasant pictures, exposure to sad and amusing film clips, and suppression of emotional reaction to pictures) [68–71]. Other studies found contrasting or mixed results depending on the type of task [72–75, 50]. For instance, in a standardised mood induction experiment, MDD patients had higher SCRs than controls in the cartoon condition, but not when mood was induced through happy and neutral pictures [73]. Schneider et al. [75] found that depressed subjects showed increased reactivity and autonomic arousal (elevated GSRs) in response to affective stimuli, compared to healthy controls [75]. Rohde and coworkers [76] studied depressed patients and healthy controls performing a Mindful Breathing Exercise task and found no difference in SCR between the two groups.

A couple of studies including elicitation protocols compared depressed patients with a seasonal pattern (seasonal affective disorder) and healthy controls. When exposed to overcast stimuli [77] or winter scenes [78] patients with seasonal affective disorder displayed more frequent SCRs and SCRs of greater magnitude, whereas the opposite pattern was found for sunny stimuli [77] and there was no disease by stimulus interaction for SCLs [77].

In short, the heterogeneity of study designs does not allow to draw clear conclusions in this field.

EDA and hormones

Only two studies dealt with this topic and they concerned different hormones, so it is not possible to generalise from the results. Based on the dexamethasone suppression test EDA in depressive patients does not appear to be related to dysfunctions of the hypothalamic-pituitary-adrenal axis. On the other hand, suicide attempters exhibited opposite correlations between EDA and cortisol in plasma and in urine, suggesting that there may be a complex relationship between EDA and cortisol production [79].

The positive correlations found between basal levels of thyroid hormones and SCL in healthy subjects were absent or reversed in depressed patients [80].

EDA and antidepressants

A cross-sectional study by Weckowicz [81] found GSR was a near-significant predictor of psychotherapy and drug therapy in depressed patients.

Several studies [37, 43, 55, 59, 82] failed to find any difference in EDA levels in depressed patients in response to antidepressant treatment or other medication, but it is hard to draw clear conclusions from these studies, many of which assessed non-specified antidepressants and/or antipsychotic medication.

Other studies investigating the effects of antidepressant compounds on EDA have found different results, but they cover a range of drugs and the results are mixed. Of the studies selected for this review, 6 assessed the effects of tricyclic antidepressants (imipramine [83, 84], amitriptyline [85–88]); 1 a tetracyclic antidepressant (maprotiline; [83]); 1 a serotonin antagonist and reuptake inhibitor (nefazodone; [89]); 3 selective serotonin reuptake inhibitors (paroxetine; [84], sertraline; [90], fluoxetine; [91]); 1 a noradrenaline reuptake inhibitor (reboxetine; [92]); 1 a serotonin-noradrenaline reuptake inhibitor (venlafaxine; [93]); 1 a reversible inhibitor of monoamine oxidase A (moclobemide; [94]); and 1 an unspecified antidepressant [95].

Imipramine-treated patients showed lower EDA than controls [84]. Regarding amitriptyline, findings were not consistent across studies, spanning from no correlation between the drug plasma level and EDA measures [86], to lower activation and decreased NS.SCRs and SCR in patients treated with amitriptyline [78, 87, 88]. Reboxetine reduced SCR after multiple dosing [92], while sertraline, moclobemide and nefazodone-treated patients showed no change in SCR [90, 94, 89]. On the other hand, sertraline-treated patients had lower SCL compared to controls [90]. Venlafaxine caused a reduction of EDA measures [93]. See Tables 1 and 2 for further details.

Very briefly, studies of EDA and antidepressants, either found no correlation between drugs and EDA measures, or a reduction of EDA measures (NS.SCRs, SCR, SCL) in subjects taking medications.

Other studies of EDA characteristics

A couple of follow-up studies investigated the temporal stability of EDA. In the studies of Iacono and coworkers [42, 45] the EDA variables were moderately stable at the one-year follow-up, whereas in the study of Thorell and d'Elia [43, 61] patients' EDA was elevated in the remission phase and similar to that of the matched healthy subjects. It should be noted, however, that the mean follow-up period in this study was 2 years, which suggests that the recovery of tonic EDA in patients with affective disorders is probably a very slow process. Thorell and d'Elia's study had a more robust design than the Iacono studies (NOS 5 vs. NOS 3).

A one-year cross-sectional follow-up study of depressive and depressive-anxious patients found mixed results with respect to the temporal stability of EDA: changes were smallest in stable patients, and greatest in all four labile-activated patients [85].

The laterality of EDA has also been explored and it has been hypothesised that there is right-hemisphere hyperexcitability in depressive conditions. After the original 1978 study by Myslobodsky and Horesh [96] others reported that EDA levels were lower on the right hand than the left under various experimental conditions, including rest [97]. Nevertheless, contrasting results were obtained both at rest and during stimulation [65, 98], and during different phases of illness, including remission [37, 99]. Notably, the first two studies cited in this paragraph had lower NOS scores (3 and 2) than the last four (respectively 4, 6, 5, 5); the existence of lateral differences in EDA remains to be confirmed.

EDA and suicidal behaviour

It has been suggested that differences in EDA may be specific to suicidality rather than depression [100]. Although there has been less research on EDA in individuals exhibiting suicidal behaviour than in people with depression, there is consistent evidence of electrodermal hypoactivity in depressed suicide attempters compared with non-suicidal depressed patients and healthy controls [61, 58, 101, 102].

Correlations between EDA and the type and level of suicide risk have been suggested. For instance, one study compared patients recently admitted to the hospital because of suicide threats or preoccupations, but with no history of attempts, controls with no history of suicide threats or attempts and no reported suicidal thoughts at the time of data collection and suicide attempters with a history of one or more suicide attempts. The first group showed the smallest GSR to the word 'suicide', suggesting generally lower reactivity [103].

Other studies have assessed SCR habituation in individuals with different patterns of suicidal behaviour. Violent suicide attempters and suicide completers were both found to be fast habituators [101, 104, 105]. The findings on non-violent suicide attempters, patients with suicidal ideation and non-suicidal depressed patients are less clear: one study found that non-violent suicide attempters showed either fast or slow habituation [101] but another found no differences among these groups (violent and non-violent suicide attempters, patients with suicidal ideation, non suicidal patients) [104]. Jandl et al. found no difference in the habituation of violent and non-violent suicide attempters, but corroborated the general finding of hyporeactivity in suicide attempters compared with non-attempters [106]. A study comparing parasuicidal adolescent girls with healthy controls found no differences in EDA variables [107].

Thorell et al. [24] carried out a meta-analysis of earlier research covering a total of 297 depressed patients and 59 healthy subjects. Electrodermal hyporeactivity was strongly associated with high suicide risk. Extremely low electrodermal reactivity had a sensitivity of 96.6% and a specificity of 92.9% for suicide and a sensitivity of 83.3% and specificity of 92.7% for suicide and/or violent suicide attempt.

A further analysis of data from 783 depressive patients by Thorell et al. [108] confirmed that electrodermal hyporeactivity is a marker of suicidal tendency in both unipolar and bipolar depression, independently of severity of depression, trait anxiety, gender and age.

Recently the protocol for a study involving 1573 patients with a primary diagnosis of depression recruited from 15 centres in nine European countries that will test the predictive value of electrodermal hyporeactivity (measured with the electrodermal orienting reactivity EDOR test) for suicide and suicide attempt has been published. The extant literature suggests that suicide attempt with intent to die and completed suicide will be associated with electrodermal hyporeactivity [27].

Discussion

The aim of this review is to offer a comprehensive overview of the EDA literature with a view to assessing its potential utility as a biomarker of depressive states and risk of suicidal behaviour, and its potential role in advanced, integrated physiological evaluation systems.

Overall, our review of the literature supports the hypothesis that electrodermal hypoactivity is a feature of depression. Nevertheless, considering the number and robustness of studies, EDA seems to be more useful in discriminating depressive patients from healthy controls than from other psychiatric patients. Moreover, specific EDA features (e.g., SCL, SCR, NS.SCR, habituation rate, etc.) seem to be differently affected, and the extremely contrasting nature of studies and of the variables used cannot be overlooked. Briefly, specific patterns of electrodermal hypoactivity may be a reliable marker of a depressive state at population level, but they should be carefully combined with other physiological and non-physiological indicators when used for preventive and diagnostic purposes.

Another area that deserves further investigation is the potential use of EDA to distinguish between subtypes of depression. At present the evidence suggests that patients with psychomotor retardation, endogenous and psychotic depression show lower EDA values than patients with agitation, non-endogenous and neurotic depression, respectively.

It has been hypothesised that electrodermal hypoactivity is a rather stable trait of patients affected by depression, although increases in EDA may indicate euthymia or remission [61, 54]. It should be noted that extremely hyporesponsive depressive patients, including suicide attempters and patients with recurrent major depression, may fail to reach the EDA levels of healthy subjects even when in remission [54].

There is even more debate about the effects of antidepressants on EDA and research has yielded mixed results. In the context of experimental anxiety conditioning tasks some antidepressants blunt EDA in healthy subjects, but the data from depressed patients are not consistent and there is no clear correlation between EDA and clinical improvement. As Thorell hypothesised, electrodermal hypoactivity may be a rather stable trait of depressed patients; EDA appears to be only marginally affected by treatment and clinical improvement, and normalisation may not occur until several months - or even years - after clinical recovery [61]. Moreover, there is only limited evidence in relation to each drug and for most drugs it comes from just one study.

As far as suicidal behaviour is concerned, extreme hyporeactivity has been consistently reported in both suicide attempters and at baseline in subjects who eventually committed suicide during a follow-up period; moreover, hyporeactivity seems to be related to the choice of a violent method for attempted or completed suicide [101, 104, 105]. On this basis it has been hypothesised that extreme electrodermal hypoactivity is a marker of suicidal tendencies in depressed patients, and it appears to be independent of severity of depression [61, 102]. Recent studies [24, 108] showed that EDA discriminates well between patients who will subsequently commit suicide, make a non-violent suicide attempt or make a violent suicide attempt, but it is less clear that EDA can be used to distinguish individuals with current suicidal ideation from depressed patients who are not currently suicidal. Nevertheless, it has been suggested that the evidence is sufficient to warrant strict monitoring of both euthymic and depressed patients who are show extreme electrodermal hyporeactivity, even in the absence of suicidal ideation. Obviously close monitoring and adequate antidepressant therapy are even more necessary in hyporeactive patients with suicidal ideation [24].

Assessment of the robustness of the synthesis and limitations

We adhered to the PRISMA statement [28, 29], which requires the use of defined inclusion/exclusion criteria, a rigorous search strategy and assessment of the quality assessment of included studies. Nevertheless, several limitations of this review should be acknowledged. First, as shown by the NOS scores, the quality of several of the included studies is questionable and most are quite old. The criteria for 'depression' vary somewhat between studies. Most of studies used the Diagnostic and Statistical Manual of Mental Disorders (DSM-III and DSM-IV) criteria [109, 110], but some used the International Classification of Diseases (ICD-9 and ICD-10) [111, 112], the Research Diagnostic Criteria [113], the Feighner Research Criteria or multiple classification systems [114]. Definitional inconsistency is also a problem in comparisons of subtypes of depression as there are no standard criteria for distinguishing between, for example, retarded and agitated depression, endogenous and non-endogenous depression or psychotic and neurotic depression. Furthermore, most studies included patients with various mood disorder diagnoses (e.g., unipolar depression, bipolar depression, dysthymia), without specifying the illness phase or the treatment patients were receiving. Finally, comorbidity was not always accounted for in comparisons between depression and other pathological conditions.

Besides diagnostic issues, over time the EDA assessment methods have changed, leading to inconsistencies. Not all the studies have assessed the same EDA parameters, and despite improvements in measuring equipment since the discovery of electrodermal phenomena more than 100 years ago [32], much of the research reviewed in the present article is limited to observational measurements performed over short periods of time, in laboratory settings or artificial clinical environments.

Conclusions

This review offers a more comprehensive assessment of the extant EDA literature than previous ones [25, 26] and it corroborates their findings, namely that there are associations between electrodermal hypoactivity and depression and suicidal behaviour. EDA appears to be a reliable marker, with high sensitivity and specificity, of depressive states, suicidal tendencies and suicidal behaviour [24, 39, 43, 108]. Nevertheless, further studies are required to validate EDA as an indicator of other clinical features, such as depression subtypes, response to treatment and acute suicide risk.

Appendix 1

Table 3 Search strings

Search Engine	Search String
PubMed (advanced search, All fields)	*((electrodermal activity) OR (electrodermal response) OR (skin conductance response) OR (skin conductance level)) AND ((depression) OR (depressive disorder) OR (mood disorder) OR (affective disorder) OR (suicide) OR (suicide attempt) OR (suicidal behavior) OR (suicidal ideation) OR (antidepressant))*
Scopus	*((TITLE-ABS-KEY (("electrodermal activity" OR "electrodermal response" OR "skin conductance response" OR "skin conductance level")) AND TITLE-ABS-KEY (("depression" OR "depressive disorder" OR "mood disorder" OR "affective disorder" OR "suicide" OR "suicide attempt" OR "suicidal behavior" OR "suicidal ideation" OR "antidepressant")))*
Cochrane Library	("electrodermal activity" OR "electrodermal response" OR "skin conductance response" OR "skin conductance level") AND ("depression" OR "depressive disorder" OR "mood disorder" OR "affective disorder" OR "suicide" OR "suicide attempt" OR "suicidal behavior" OR "suicidal ideation" OR "antidepressant")
Web of Science	*((TITLE-ABS-KEY (("electrodermal activity" OR "electrodermal response" OR "skin conductance response" OR "skin conductance level")) AND TITLE-ABS-KEY (("depression" OR "depressive disorder" OR "mood disorder" OR "affective disorder" OR "suicide" OR "suicide attempt" OR "suicidal behavior" OR "suicidal ideation" OR "antidepressant")))*

Abbreviations

EDA: Electrodermal activity; GSR: Galvanic skin response; MDD: Major depressive disorder; NS.SCR: Non-specific skin conductance response; PRISMA: Preferred reporting items for systematic reviews and meta-analyses; SCL: Skin conductance level; SCR: Skin conductance response; SRR: Skin resistance response

Acknowledgements

Not applicable.

Funding

This study received no specific grant from any funding agency in the public, commercial, or not-for-profit sectors.

Authors' contributions

VC, AS, MS and PZ contributed to planning, supervision, writing, and analysis of the study; MS, MI, VC independently selected titles, abstract and full text; CG, MI, LM and DM each contributed to data collection, writing the manuscript and review of the literature. All authors have read and approved the final manuscript.

Consent for publication

Not applicable.

Competing interests

The authors declare that they have no conflict of interests.

Author details

[1]Department of Health Sciences, University of Molise, Via Francesco De Sanctis, 1, 86100 Campobasso, Italy. [2]National Institute for Health, Migration and Poverty, Via di S. Gallicano 25/a, 00153 Rome, Italy. [3]Department of Translational Medicine, Azienda Ospedaliero Universitaria Maggiore della Carità, University of Piemonte Orientale, Via Solaroli 17, 28100 Novara, Italy. [4]Department of Health Sciences, University of Molise, Via Francesco De Sanctis, 1, 86100 Campobasso, Italy. [5]National Centre for Suicide Research and Prevention of Mental Ill-Health (NASP), Karolinska Institute, -171 77 Stockholm, SE, Sweden. [6]Department of Biomedical and Neuromotor Sciences, Institute of Psychiatry, University of Bologna, Via Altura 3, 40139 Bologna, Italy. [7]Department of Biomedical and Neuromotor Sciences, Institute of Psychiatry, University of Bologna, Via Altura 3, 40139 Bologna, Italy. [8]Institute of Psychiatry, Maggiore della Carità Hospital of Novara, C.so Mazzini 18, 28100 Novara, Italy.

References

1. Sudol K, Mann JJ. Biomarkers of suicide attempt behavior: towards a biological model of risk. Curr Psychiatry Rep. 2017;19(6):31. https://doi.org/10.1007/s11920-017-0781-y. Review. PubMed PMID: 28470485
2. Öhman A, Hamm A, Hugdahl K. Cognition and the autonomic nervous system: orienting, anticipation, and conditioning. In Cacioppo JT, Tassinary LG & Berntson GG (Eds.), Handbook of psychophysiology (2nd ed.). New York, NY: US: Cambridge University Press; 2000. pp. 533–575.
3. Pandey GN, Dwivedy Y. The neurobiological basis of suicide. Boca Raton (FL): CRC Press, Taylor & Francis, Chapter 20 Peripheral biomarkers for suicide, 2012.
4. Groscurth P. Anatomy of sweat glands. Curr Probl Dermatol. 2002;30:1–9.
5. Gunnar Wallin B, Fagius J. The sympathetic nervous system in man — aspects derived from microelectrode recordings. Trends Neurosci. 1986;9: 63–7. https://doi.org/10.1016/0166-2236(86)90024-X.
6. Asahina M, Suzuki A, Mori M, Kanesaka T, Hattori T. Emotional sweating response in a patient with bilateral amygdala damage. Int J Psychophysiol. 2003;47(1):87–93.
7. Bradley MM, Lang PJ. Measuring emotion: behavior, feeling and physiology. In Cognitive Neuroscience of Emotion. Eds. R.D. Lane and L. Nadel. New York: Oxford University Press. 2000.
8. Boucsein, W. Electrodermal activity (2nd ed.). New York: Springer Science & Business Media; 2012.
9. Braithwaite JJ, Watson DG, Jones R, Rowe M. A guide for analysing electrodermal activity (EDA) & skin conductance responses (SCRs) for psychological experiments. Psychophysiology. 2013;49:1017–34.
10. Yoon JH, Ko CM, Ahn YS, Park KS, Choe KH, Yoo KJ, et al. Mechanism of decrease in heart rate by peripheral dopaminergic D2-receptors. Yonsei Med J. 1994;35(4):411–9.
11. Lee GP, Arena JG, Meador KJ, Smith JR, Loring DW, Flanigin HF. Changes in autonomic responsiveness following bilateral amygdalectomy in humans. Neuropsychiatry, Neuropsychol Behav Neurol. 1988;1(2):119–29.
12. Mangina CA, Beuzeron-Mangina JH. Direct electrical stimulation of specific human brain structures and bilateral electrodermal activity. Int J Psychophysiol. 1996;22(1-2):1–8. https://doi.org/10.1016/0167-8760(96)00022-0.
13. Lang PJ, Greenwald MK, Bradley MM, Hamm AO. Looking at pictures: affective, facial, visceral, and behavioral reactions. Psychophysiology. 1993; 30(3):261–73. https://doi.org/10.1111/j.1469-8986.1993.tb03352.x.
14. Manning SK, Melchiori MP. Words that upset Urban College students: measured with GSRs and rating scales. J Soc Psychol. 1974;94(2):305–6. https://doi.org/10.1080/00224545.1974.9923225.

15. Winton WM, Putnam LE, Krauss RM. Facial and autonomic manifestations of the dimensional structure of emotion. J Exp Soc Psychol. 1984;20(3):195–216. https://doi.org/10.1016/0022-1031(84)90047-7.
16. Lacey JI, Lacey BC. The relationship of resting autonomic activity to motor impulsivity. Res Publ Assoc Res Nerv Ment Dis. 1958;36:144–209.
17. Mundy-Castle AC, McKiever BL. The psychophysiological significance of the galvanic skin response. J Exp Psychol. 1953;46(1):15–24. https://doi.org/10.1037/h0060100.
18. Crider A, Kremen WS, Xian H, Jacobson KC, Waterman B, Eisen SA, et al. Stability, consistency, and heritability of electrodermal response lability in middle-aged male twins. Psychophysiology. 2004;41(4):501–9. https://doi.org/10.1111/j.1469-8986.2004.00189.x.
19. Gottesman II, Hanson DR. Human development: biological and genetic processes. Annu Rev Psychol. 2005;56(1):263–86. https://doi.org/10.1146/annurev.psych.56.091103.070208.
20. Iacono WG. Identifying psychophysiological risk for psychopathology: examples from substance abuse and schizophrenia research. Psychophysiology. 1998;35(06):621–37.
21. Crider A. Electrodermal response Lability-stability: individual difference correlates. In J.-C. Roy, W. Boucsein, D. C. Fowles, & J. H. Gruzelier (Eds.), Progress in Electrodermal Research Springer US; 1993. New York: Plenum. 1993:173–186.
22. Crider A. Personality and Electrodermal response Lability: an interpretation. Applied Psychophysiology and Biofeedback. 2008;33(3):141–8. https://doi.org/10.1007/s10484-008-9057-y.
23. Straub R, Jandl M, Wolfersdorf M. Depressive state and Electrodermal activity of depressed inpatients during an acute suicidal state. Psychiatr Prax. 2003;30(Suppl 2):183–6. https://doi.org/10.1055/s-2003-39762.
24. Thorell LH. Valid electrodermal hyporeactivity for depressive suicidal propensity offers links to cognitive theory. Acta Psychiatr Scand. 2009;119(5):338–49. https://doi.org/10.1111/j.1600-0447.2009.01364.x.
25. Straub R, Hole G, Wolfersdorf M. Electrodermal hypoactivity in depression: psychobiological marker or differential psychophysiologic disposition? Schweiz Arch Neurol Und Psychiatrie (1985). 1992;143(1):41–59.
26. Vahey, R., Becerra, R. (2015). Galvanic Skin Response in Mood Disorders: A Critical Review. 2015. http://www.redalyc.org/articulo.oa?id=56041176008. Accessed 15 Dec 2016.
27. Sarchiapone M, Iosue M, Carli V, Amore M, Baca Garcia E, Batra A, et al. EUDORA multicentre research program: a naturalistic, European multicentre clinical study of EDOR test in adult patients with primary depression. BMC Psychiatry. 2017;17(1):108. https://doi.org/10.1186/s128880171246x.
28. Moher D, Shamseer L, Clarke M, Ghersi D, Liberati A, Petticrew M, et al. Preferred reporting items for systematic review and meta-analysis protocols (PRISMA-P) 2015 statement. Syst Rev. 2015;4(1):1. https://doi.org/10.1186/2046-4053-4-1.
29. Shamseer L, Moher D, Clarke M, Ghersi D, Liberati A, Petticrew M, et al. Preferred reporting items for systematic review and meta-analysis protocols (PRISMA-P) 2015: elaboration and explanation. The BMJ. 2015;349:g7647. https://doi.org/10.1136/bmj.g7647.
30. Popay J, Roberts H, Sowden A, Petticrew M, Arai L, Rodgers M, et al. Guidance on the conduct of narrative synthesis in systematic reviews. A Product from the ESRC Methods Programme. Version, 1. 2006 http://www.lancaster.ac.uk/shm/research/nssr/research/dissemination/publications/NS_Synthesis_Guidance_v1.pdf. Accessed 15 Dec 2016.
31. Wells GA, Shea B, O'connell D, Peterson JEA, Welch V, Losos M, et al. The Newcastle-Ottawa scale (NOS) for assessing the quality of nonrandomised studies in meta-analyses. 2000. http://www.medicine.mcgill.ca/rtamblyn/Readings/The%20Newcastle%20-%20Scale%20for%20assessing%20the%20quality%20of%20nonrandomised%20studies%20in%20meta-analyses.pdf. Accessed 15 Dec 2016.
32. Vigouroux A. Etude sur la résistance électrique chez les mélancoliques. Paris: Méd; 1890.
33. Carney RM, Hong BA, Kulkarni S, Kapila A. A comparison of EMG and SCL in normal and depressed subjects. Pavlov J Biol Scie. 1981;16(4):212–6.
34. Dawson ME, Schell AM, Catania JJ. Autonomic correlates of depression and clinical improvement following electroconvulsive shock therapy. Psychophysiology. 1977;14(6):569–78. https://doi.org/10.1111/j.1469-8986.1977.tb01201.x.
35. Miquel M, Fuentes I, Garcia-Merita M, Rojo L. Habituation and sensitization processes in depressive disorders. Psychopathology. 1999;32(1):35–42. https://doi.org/10.1159/000029064.
36. Storrie MC, Doerr HO, Johnson MH. Skin conductance characteristics of depressed subjects before and after therapeutic intervention. J Nerv. 1981;169(3):176–9.
37. Bonnet A, Naveteur J. Electrodermal activity in low back pain patients with and without comorbid depression. Int J Psychophysiol. 2004;53(1):37–44. https://doi.org/10.1016/j.ijpsycho.2004.01.004.
38. Donat DC, McCullough JP. Psychophysiological discriminants of depression at rest and in response to stress. J Clin Psychol. 1983;39(3):315–20. https://doi.org/10.1002/1097-4679(198305)39:3&lt 315:AID-JCLP2270390303&gt 3.0.CO 2-H.
39. Ward NG, Doerr HO. Skin conductance: a potentially sensitive and specific marker for depression. J Nerv Ment Dis. 1986;174(9):553–9. https://doi.org/10.1097/00005053-198609000-00008.
40. Kamenskaya VM, Mikhailova FS. Ratios of electroencephalographic and autonomic indexes in a stress situation in patients with different types of depression. Neurosci Behav Physiol. 1985;15(6):483–7. https://doi.org/10.1007/BF01184258.
41. Iacono WG, Lykken DT, Peloquin LJ, Lumry AE, Valentine RH, Tuason VB. Electrodermal activity in euthymic unipolar and bipolar affective disorders. A possible marker for depression. Arch Gen Psychiatry. 1983;40(5):557–65.
42. Thorell LH, Kjellman BF, d'Elia G. Electrodermal activity in antidepressant medicated and unmedicated depressive patients and in matched healthy subjects. Acta Psychiatr Scand. 1987;76(6):684–92. https://doi.org/10.1111/j.1600-0447.1987.tb02940.x.
43. Dawson ME, Schell AM, Braaten JR, Catania JJ. Diagnostic utility of autonomic measures for major depressive disorders. Psychiatry Res. 1985;15(4):261–70. https://doi.org/10.1016/0165-1781(85)90063-0.
44. Iacono WG, Peloquin LJ, Lykken DT, Haroian KP, Valentine RH, Tuason VB. Electrodermal activity in euthymic patients with affective disorders: one-year retest stability and the effects of stimulus intensity and significance. J Abnorm Psychol. 1984;93(3):304–11. https://doi.org/10.1037/0021-843X.93.3.304.
45. Giedke H, Heimann H. Psychophysiological aspects of depressive syndromes. Pharmacopsychiatry. 1987;20(5):177–80. https://doi.org/10.1055/s-2007-1017098.
46. Mestanikova A, Ondrejka I, Mestanik M, Hrtanek I, Snircova E, Tonhajzerova I. Electrodermal activity in adolescent depression. Adv Exp Med Biol. 2016;935(26):83–8. https://doi.org/10.1007/5584_2016_40.
47. Ward NG, Doerr HO, Storrie MC. Skin conductance: a potentially sensitive test for depression. Psychiatry Res. 1983;10:295–302.
48. Giedke H, Bolz J, Heimann H. Evoked potentials, expectancy wave, and skin resistance in depressed patients and healthy controls. Pharmakopsychiatr Neuropsychopharmakol. 1980;13(3):91–101.
49. Lapierre YD, Butter HJ. Agitated and retarded depression. Neuropsychobiology. 1980;6(4):217–23. https://doi.org/10.1159/000117755.
50. Lewinsohn PM, Lobitz WC, Wilson S. "Sensitivity" of depressed individuals to aversive stimuli. J Abnorm Psychol. 1973;81(3):259–63.
51. Levinson DF. Skin conductance orienting response in unmedicated RDC schizophrenic, schizoaffective, depressed, and control subjects. Biol Psychiatry. 1991;30(7):663–83. https://doi.org/10.1016/0006-3223(91)90012-B.
52. Pazderka-Robinson H, Morrison JW, Flor-Henry P. Electrodermal dissociation of chronic fatigue and depression: evidence for distinct physiological mechanisms. Int J Psychophysiol. 2004;53(3):171–82. https://doi.org/10.1016/j.ijpsycho.2004.03.004.
53. O'Kearney R, Parry L. Comparative physiological reactivity during script-driven recall in depression and posttraumatic stress disorder. J Abnorm Psychol. 2014;123(3):523–32. https://doi.org/10.1037/a0037326.
54. Greco A, Valenza G, Lanata A, Rota G, Scilingo EP. Electrodermal activity in bipolar patients during affective elicitation. IEEE J Biomed Health Inform. 2014;18(6):1865–73. https://doi.org/10.1109/JBHI.2014.2300940.
55. Bernstein AS, Schnur DB, Bernstein P, Yeager A, Wrable J, Smith S. Differing patterns of electrodermal and finger pulse responsivity in schizophrenia and depression. Psychol Med. 1995;25(01):51–62. https://doi.org/10.1017/S0033291700028087.
56. Lader MH, Wing L. Physiological measures in agitated and retarded depressed patients. J Psychiatr Res. 1969;7(2):89–100. https://doi.org/10.1016/0022-3956(69)90014-4.
57. Noble P, Lader M. The symptomatic correlates of the skin conductance changes in depression. J Psychiatr Res. 1971;9(1):61–9. https://doi.org/10.1016/0022-3956(71)90008-2.
58. Thorell LH, Kjellman BF, d'Elia G. Electrodermal activity in relation to diagnostic subgroups and symptoms of depressive patients. Acta

Psychiatr Scand. 1987;76(6):693–701. https://doi.org/10.1111/j.1600-0447.1987.tb02941.x.

59. Williams KM, Iacono WG, Remick RA. Electrodermal activity among subtypes of depression. Biol Psychiatry. 1985;20(2):158–62. https://doi.org/10.1016/0006-3223(85)90075-7.
60. Byrne DG. A psychophysiological distinction between types of depressive states. Aust N Z J Psychiatry. 1975;9(3):181–5.
61. Thorell LH, d'Elia G. Electrodermal activity in depressive patients in remission and in matched healthy subjects. Acta Psychiatr Scand. 1988;78(2):247–53. https://doi.org/10.1111/j.1600-0447.1988.tb06332.x.
62. Mirkin AM, Coppen A. Electrodermal activity in depression: clinical and biochemical correlates. Br J Psychiatry. 1980;137(1):93–7. https://doi.org/10.1192/bjp.137.1.93.
63. Perez-Reyes M, Cochrane C. Differences in sodium thiopental susceptibility of depressed patients as evidenced by the galvanic skin reflex inhibition threshold. J Psychiatr Res. 1967;5(4):335–47.
64. Dawson ME, Schell AM. What does electrodermal activity tell us about prognosis in the schizophrenia spectrum? Schizophr Res. 2002;54(1):87–93.
65. Bernstein AS, Riedel JA, Graae F, Seidman D, Steele H, Connolly J, et al. Schizophrenia is associated with altered orienting activity: depression with electrodermal (cholinergic?) deficit and normal orienting response. J Abnorm Psychol. 1988;97(1):3–12. https://doi.org/10.1037/0021-843X.97.1.3.
66. Pruneti CA, Lento RM, Fante C, Carrozzo E, Fontana F. Autonomic arousal and differential diagnosis in clinical psychology and psychopathology. J Psychopathology. 2010;16:43–52.
67. Have G, Kolbeinsson H, Pétursson H. Dementia and depression in old age: psychophysiological aspects. Acta Psychiatr Scand. 1991;83(5):329–33. https://doi.org/10.1111/j.1600-0447.1991.tb05550.x.
68. Mardaga S, Hansenne M. Autonomic aspect of emotional response in depressed patients: relationships with personality. Neurophysiol Clin. 2009; 39(4-5):209–16. https://doi.org/10.1016/j.neucli.2009.06.002.
69. Lemaire M, El-Hage W, Frangou S. Increased affective reactivity to neutral stimuli and decreased maintenance of affective responses in bipolar disorder. European Psychiatry. 2015;30(7):852–60. https://doi.org/10.1016/j.eurpsy.2015.07.008.
70. Tsai JL, Pole N, Levenson RW, Muñoz RF. The effects of depression on the emotional responses of Spanish-speaking Latinas. Cult Divers Ethn Minor Psychol. 2003;9(1):49–63. https://doi.org/10.1037/1099-9809.9.1.49.
71. Rottenberg J, Gross JJ, Wilhelm FH, Najmi S, Gotlib IH. Crying threshold and intensity in major depressive disorder. J Abnorm Psychol. 2002;111(2):302–12.
72. Branković SB. System identification of skin conductance response in depression–an attempt to probe the neurochemistry of limbic system. Psychiatr Danub. 2008;20(3):310–22.
73. Falkenberg I, Kohn N, Schoepker R, Habel U. (2012). Mood induction in depressive patients: a comparative multidimensional approach. PLoS ONE. 2012; 7(1) e30016; doi:https://doi.org/10.1371/journal.pone.0030016.
74. Nissen C, Holz J, Blechert J, Feige B, Riemann D, Voderholzer U, et al. Learning as a model for neural plasticity in major depression. Biol Psychiatry. 2010;68(6):544–52. https://doi.org/10.1016/j.biopsych.2010.05.026.
75. Schneider D, Regenbogen C, Kellermann T, Finkelmeyer A, Kohn N, Derntl B, et al. Empathic behavioral and physiological responses to dynamic stimuli in depression. Psychiatry Res. 2012;200(23):294–305. https://doi.org/10.1016/j.psychres.2012.03.054.
76. Rohde K, Adolph D, Dietrich DE, Michalak J. Mindful attention regulation and non-judgmental orientation in depression: a multi-method approach. Biol Psychol. 2014;101:36–43.
77. Lindsey KT, Rohan KJ, Roecklein KA, Mahon JN. Surface facial electromyography, skin conductance, and self-reported emotional responses to light- and season-relevant stimuli in seasonal affective disorder. J Affect Disord. 2011;133(1-2):311–9. https://doi.org/10.1016/j.jad.2011.04.016.
78. Sigmon ST, Whitcomb-Smith S, Boulard NE, Pells JJ, Hermann BA, Edenfield TM, et al. Seasonal reactivity: Attentional bias and Psychophysiological arousal in seasonal and nonseasonal depression. Cogn Ther Res. 2007;31:619–38.
79. Thorell LH, Kjellman BF, d'Elia G, Kagedal B. Electrodermal activity in relation to cortisol dysregulation in depressive patients. Acta Psychiatr Scand. 1988; 78:743–53.
80. Thorell LH, Kjellman BF, d'Elia G. Electrodermal activity in relation to basal and post-dexamethasone of thyroid stimulating hormone and basal levels of thyroid hormones in major depressive patients and healthy subjects. Psychiatry Res. 1993;47(1):23–36. https://doi.org/10.1016/01651781(93)90052I.
81. Weckowicz TE, Yonge KA, Cropley AJ, Muir W. Objective therapy predictors in depression: a multivariate approach. J Clin Psychol. 1971;27(1):4–29.
82. Bob P, Jasova D, Raboch J. Subclinical Epileptiform process in patients with Unipolar depression and its indirect Psychophysiological manifestations. PLoS One. 2011;6(11):e28041. https://doi.org/10.1371/journal.pone.0028041.
83. Lapierre YD, Butter HI. Imipramine and maprotiline in agitated and retarded depression: a controlled psychiatric and psychiphysical assessment. Prog Neuro-Psychopharmacology. 1978;2:207–16.
84. Barg T, Wolfersdorf M, Ruppe A. The influence of various antidepressants on heart rate and Electrodermal activity during Psychophysiological examinations. Pharmacopsychiar. 1996;29:216–9.
85. Heimann H. Changes of psychophysiological reactivity in affective disorders. Arch Psychiatr Nervenkr. 1978;225(3):223–31. https://doi.org/10.1007/BF00344009.
86. Breyer-Pfaff U, Gaertner HJ, Giedke H. Plasma levels, psychophysiological variables, and clinical response to amitriptyline. Psychiatry Res. 1982;6(2): 223–34. https://doi.org/10.1016/0165-1781(82)90010-5.
87. Ikeda Y, Nomura S, Sawa Y, Nakazawa T. The effects of antidepressants on the autonomic nervous system-a current investigation. J Neural Transm. 1982;54(1-2):65–73. https://doi.org/10.1007/BF01249279.
88. Siepmann M, Kirch W, Krause S, Joraschky P, Mueck-Weymann M. The effects of St. John's wort extract and amitriptyline on autonomic responses of blood vessels and sweat glands in healthy volunteers. J Clin Psychopharmacol. 2004(a);24(1):79–82. https://doi.org/10.1097/01.jcp.0000104911.75206.f0.
89. Silva M, Hetem LAB, Guimaraes FS, Graeff FG. Opposite effects of nefazodone in two human models of anxiety. Psychopharmacology. 2001; 156:454–60.
90. Siepmann M, Grossmann J, Mück-Weymann M, Kirch W. Effects of sertraline on autonomic and cognitive functions in healthy volunteers. Psychopharmacology. 2003;168(3):293–8. https://doi.org/10.1007/s00213-003-1448-4.
91. Fraguas R, Marci C, Fava M, Iosifescu DV, Bankier B, Loh R, et al. Autonomic reactivity to induced emotion as potential predictor of response to antidepressant treatment. Psychiatry Res. 2007;151(1-2):169–72. https://doi.org/10.1016/j.psychres.2006.08.008.
92. Siepmann M, Mück-Weymann M, Joraschky P, Kirch W. The effects of reboxetine on autonomic and cognitive functions in healthy volunteers. Psychopharmacology. 2001;157(2):202–7.
93. Zullino D, Chatton A, Fresard E, Stankovic M, Bondolfi G, Borgeat F, et al. Venlafaxine versus applied relaxation for generalized anxiety disorder: a randomized controlled study on clinical and electrophysiological outcomes. Psychiatr Q. 2015;86(1):69–82. https://doi.org/10.1007/s11126-014-9334-2.
94. Siepmann M, Handel J, Mueck-Weymann M, Kirch W. The effects of moclobemide on autonomic and cognitive functions in healthy volunteers. Pharmacopsychiatry. 2004(b);37(2):81–7. https://doi.org/10.1055/s-2004-815530.
95. Hattangadi S, Lidsky A, Lee H, Ban TA. Orienting-reflex behavior and clinical psychopathology. Cond reflex. 1968;3(1):29–33. https://doi.org/10.1007/BF03001134.
96. Myslobodsky MS, Horesh N. Bilateral electrodermal activity depressive patients. Biol Psychol. 1978;6(2):111–20. https://doi.org/10.1016/0301-0511(78)90050-9.
97. Schneider SJ. (1983). Multiple measures of hemispheric dysfunction in schizophrenia and depression. Psychol Med. 1983;13(02):287–97. https://doi.org/10.1017/S003329170005090X.
98. Toone BK, Cooke E, Lader MH. Electrodermal activity in the affective disorders and schizophrenia. Psychol Med. 1981;11(03):497–508. https://doi.org/10.1017/S0033291700052818.
99. Iacono WG, Tuason VB. Bilateral electrodermal asymmetry in euthymic patients with unipolar and bipolar affective disorders. Biol Psychiatry. 1983; 18(3):303–15.
100. Wolfersdorf M, Straub R, Barg T. Electrodermal activity (EDA) and suicidal behavior. Crisis. 1996;17(2):69–77.
101. Edman G, Åsberg M, Levander S, Schalling D. Skin conductance habituation and cerebrospinal fluid 5-hydroxyindoleacetic acid in suicidal patients. Arch Gen Psychiatry. 1986;43(6):586–92. https://doi.org/10.1001/archpsyc.1986.01800060080010.

102. Thorell LH. Electrodermal activity in suicidal and nonsuicidal depressive patients and in matched healthy subjects. Acta Psychiatr Scand. 1987;76(4): 420–30.
103. Spiegel D. Autonomic reactivity in relation to the affective meaning of suicide. J Clin Psychol. 1969;25(4):359–62.
104. Keller F, Wolfersdorf M, Straub R, Hole G. Suicidal behaviour and electrodermal activity in depressive inpatients. Acta Psychiatr Scand. 1991; 83(5):324–8. https://doi.org/10.1111/j.1600-0447.1991.tb05549.x.
105. Wolfersdorf M, Straub R, Barg T, Keller F, Kaschka WP. Depressed inpatients, electrodermal reactivity, and suicide - a study about psychophysiology of suicidal behavior. Arch Suicide Res. 1999;5(1):1–10. https://doi.org/10.1080/13811119908258311.
106. Jandl M, Steyer J, Kaschka WP. Suicide risk markers in major depressive disorder: a study of Electrodermal activity and event-related potentials. J Affect Disord. 2010;123(1-3):138–49. https://doi.org/10.1016/j.jad.2009.09.011.
107. Crowell SE, Beauchaine TP, McCauley E, Smith CJ, Stevens AL, Sylvers P. Psychological, autonomic, and serotonergic correlates of parasuicide among adolescent girls. Dev Psychopathol. 2005;17:1105–27.
108. Thorell LH, Wolfersdorf M, Straub R, Steyer J, Hodgkinson S, Kaschka WP, et al. Electrodermal hyporeactivity as a trait marker for suicidal propensity in uni- and bipolar depression. J Psychiatr Res. 2013;47(12):1925–31. https://doi.org/10.1016/j.jpsychires.2013.08.017.
109. American Psychiatric Association, APA. Diagnostic and statistical manual of mental disorders, fourth edition: DSM-IV-TR®: American Psychiatric Association; 2000.
110. American Psychiatric Association, APA. Diagnostic and statistical manual of mental disorders. 3rd ed. DSM-III: American Psychiatric Association; 1980.
111. ICD-9-CM: International Classification of Diseases, 9th Revision, Clinical Modification. Salt Lake City, Utah: Medicode, 1996. Print.
112. The ICD-10 Classification of Mental and Behavioural Disorders: Clinical Descriptions and Diagnostic Guidelines. Geneva: World Health Organization, 1992. Print.
113. Spitzer RL, Endicott J, Robins E. Research diagnostic criteria: rationale and reliability. Arch Gen Psychiatry. 1978;35(6):773–82. https://doi.org/10.1001/archpsyc.1978.01770300115013.
114. Feighner JP, Robins E, Guze SB, Woodruff RA, Winokur G, Munoz R. Diagnostic criteria for use in psychiatric research. Arch Gen Psychiatry. 1972; 26(1):57–63.

Evaluation of an electronic consultation service in psychiatry for primary care providers

Douglas Archibald[1,2*], Julia Stratton[3], Clare Liddy[1,2], Rachel E. Grant[4], Douglas Green[3] and Erin J. Keely[5,6]

Abstract

Background: This study explores the effectiveness of an electronic consultation (eConsult) service between primary care providers and psychiatry, and the types and content of the clinical questions that were asked.

Methods: This is a retrospective eConsult review study. All eConsults directed to Psychiatry from July 2011 to January 2015 by Primary care providers were reviewed. Response time and the amount of time reported by the specialist to answer each eConsult was analyzed. Each eConsult was also categorized by clinical topic and question type in predetermined categories. Mandatory post-eConsult surveys for primary care providers were analyzed to determine the number of traditional consults avoided and to gain insight into the perceived value of eConsults.

Results: Of the 5597 eConsults, 169 psychiatry eConsults were completed during the study period. The average response time for a specialist to a primary care provider was 2.3 days. Eighty-seven percent of clinical responses were completed by the psychiatrist in less than 15 min. The primary care providers most commonly asked clinical questions were about depressive and anxiety disorders. 88.7% of PCPs rated the eConsult service a 5 (excellent value) or 4.

Conclusions: This study indicates that an eConsult psychiatry service has tremendous potential to improve access to psychiatric advice and expand the capacity to treat mental illness in primary care. Future research may include follow-up with PCPs regarding the implementation of specialist advice.

Keywords: Electronic consultation, eConsult, Primary health care, Psychiatry

Background

Wait times to access mental healthcare services remains a concern in Canada, where the average wait time for psychiatric service is 20.8 weeks [1]. Wait times vary drastically between provinces, with the shortest wait times being in British Columbia (16.3 weeks) and the longest in Newfoundland & Labrador (83.0 weeks). Canadians living in rural and remote communities also face a unique set of challenges. The Canadian Mental Health Association suggests the rates of Major Depressive Disorder (MDD) are higher amongst those living within rural and remote regions, yet these individuals face a number of barriers to receiving psychiatric care within their own communities, such as geographical barriers, limited health resources and services, and challenges in recruiting and retaining healthcare professionals [2].

In an effort to improve access to psychiatric care, curbside consultations are an important component of patient care. Informal consultations can occur as spontaneous, face-to-face chats with medical professional colleagues. Several methods to facilitate formal curbside consultation have been developed over the years for psychiatric care [3]. Bergus et al. [4] report on an electronic e-mail service for consultations between primary healthcare physicians and specialists. Carr et al. [5] present details on a consultation liaison service as a way for family physicians to consult with an onsite trainee psychiatrist who provides expert knowledge to family physicians. More recently, alternatives such as telepsychiatry and electronic consultations (eConsults) have been explored. Telepsychiatry uses

* Correspondence: douglas.archibald@uottawa.ca
[1]Department of Family Medicine, University of Ottawa, Ottawa, ON, Canada
[2]Bruyère Research Institute, 85 Primrose Avenue, Ottawa, ON K1R 6M1, Canada
Full list of author information is available at the end of the article

videoconferencing to conduct psychiatric consultations in real-time (synchronous), or primary care providers (PCP) can record patient information and electronically send to the psychiatrist to review at a later time (asynchronous) [6, 7]. A limitation of synchronous telepsychiatry is that it requires access to high-quality video conferencing software and a strong and consistently reliable internet connection [7] which may not be feasible in remote and rural areas of Canada [2]. Additionally, healthcare professionals spend the same amount of time with each patient as if it were face-to-face, and some patients may not want to be videotaped [7].

eConsults are asynchronous systems which allow for secure web-based communication between PCPs and specialists. As they do not require real-time connections or video processing, they do not necessarily have the same potential bandwidth issues as telepsychiatry. By using eConsult, PCPs can submit questions to specialists, who in turn offer recommendations in a timely manner, thus enabling access with the potential of also avoiding a face-to-face consultation.

Evidence suggests that eConsults are associated with improved access to specialty care and high levels of PCP and patient satisfaction [8, 9]. The Champlain BASE ™ (Building Access to Specialists through eConsultation) eConsult service was developed in Ottawa, Ontario to address excessive wait times, which exceeded 9 months in some specialties for non-urgent cases [10]. The system was launched as a proof of concept in 2010 [11], and was piloted between 2011 to 2012 [12]. The program is now a full service funded through the Ontario Ministry of Health [13]. The Champlain BASE ™ eConsult service has since grown to include 1355 registered PCPs (including 1160 family physicians and 195 nurse practitioners) and 102 specialty services. Over 33,000 eConsults have been completed to date.

The purpose of this study was to analyze all psychiatry eConsults that were completed between April 2011 and January 2015. This paper reports on four specific objectives:

1. To determine the most common clinical topics and types of questions asked;
2. To determine the impact of eConsults on PCP's course of action and decision to refer;
3. To estimate the number of psychiatry referrals that were avoided through using the eConsult service;
4. To ascertain the perceived value of eConsults by PCPs.

Methods

Setting

The Champlain BASE™ eConsult service is a secure online application that facilitates asynchronous communication between PCPs and specialists. The service is based in the Champlain health region of Eastern Ontario, Canada, which has a population of 1.3 million individuals, roughly half of whom reside in the city of Ottawa.

Champlain BASE™ eConsult service

A PCP creates an eConsult by logging on to the web portal and filling out an electronic form that includes the patient's medical history and the clinical question being asked to the psychiatrist. PCPs can also attach files, such as laboratory tests, images or videos. A submitted eConsult is then assigned to one of the eConsult psychiatrists based on availability. He or she receives an email alerting them that they have received an eConsult. The specialist then has a week to respond to the PCP within the secure eConsult portal. Specialists can request additional information, provide clinical advice, or advise an in-person consultation. Asynchronous communication can continue between both parties until the PCP decided to close the case within the eConsult service. Following the closing of a case, the PCP is presented with an obligatory close-out survey (Table 1).

Electronic healthcare services, such as the Champlain BASE™ eConsult Service, require that providers are proficient in telespsychiatric competencies [14]. PCPs must be able to present a clear and detailed patient history in order for specialists to confirm and suggest a new management or treatment plan. Over time as specialist advice is implemented and telepsychiatric competencies are applied, entrustment and a working relationship develops [14, 15].

Study design

This retrospective eConsult review examined all psychiatry eConsults submitted from April 2011 to January 2015. Eligible cases were retrospectively categorized by clinical topic using a hybrid framework of the International Classification for Primary Care, version 2 (ICPC-2) [16] and experiences of the Champlain BASE eConsults medical specialists (see Appendix 1 for our classification taxonomy). The DSM5 was used to classify the various clinical topics that were raised by the PCPs. Ely et al.'s taxonomy of generic clinical questions (TGCQ) [17] was used to classify the "type" of question. The TGCQ uses 4 levels of classification and a total of 64 subcategories to identify the type of question being asked for the first 2 levels of classification and examples of questions. The highest overarching level consists of 6 broad areas, including diagnosis, treatment, management, epidemiology, nonclinical, and unclassified questions. This scale was modified to include the most relevant areas for a referral question. The close-out survey for each eConsult was also included in the dataset. This allowed for the quantification of how the eConsult impacted PCPs course of action and decision for referral, as well as the perceived value of eConsults to PCPs. All data were exported into an Excel spreadsheet and examined through descriptive statistics

Table 1 Content of close-out survey for primary care providers

Question	Response Options
Q1. Which of the following best describes the outcome of this eConsultation for your patient:	1. I was able to confirm a course of action that I originally had in mind; 2. I got new advice for a new or additional course of action; 3. I did not find the response very useful; 4. None of the above.
Q2. As a result of the eConsultation would you say that:	1. Referral was originally contemplated but now avoided at this stage; 2. Referral was originally contemplated and is still needed – this eConsult likely leads to a more effective visit; 3. Referral was not originally contemplated and is still not needed – this eConsult provided useful feedback/instruction; 4. Referral was not originally contemplated, but eConsult process resulted in a referral being initiated; 5. There was no particular benefit to using eConsult in this case; 6. Other (please explain).
Q3. Please rate the overall value of the eConsult.	Minimal 1 2 3 4 5 Excellent
Q4. Please rate the overall value of the eConsult service in this case for you as a primary care providers.	Minimal 1 2 3 4 5 Excellent
Q5. We would value any additional feedback you provide:	

including frequencies and content analysis for classification of question type.

Results

Of the 5597 eConsults directed to the service during the study period, 169 were to psychiatry (3.0%). Of these cases, 153 (90.5%) were from family physicians, 150 (88. 8%) were from clinicians in urban practices, and 146 (86%) were from female providers. The average response time was just under 3.2 days (median was less than 2. 1 days), and the fastest response time was less than 5 min. The majority of eConsults (87.6%) took less than 15 min for the psychiatrist to answer. The vast majority of the eConsults (75%) were completed through a single question/response asynchronous interaction. The remaining consults required more back and forth communication due to the specialist requiring question clarification or more information.

Clinical topic

Depressive disorders were the most common clinical topic, accounting for 30.2% of all psychiatry eConsults (Table 2). Depressive disorders included all listed in the DSM-5 Depressive Disorder Section: Disruptive Mood Dysregulation Disorder, MDD, Persistent Depressive Disorder, Premenstrual Dysphoric Disorder, Substance/ Medication induced Depressive Disorder and Depressive Disorder Due to Another Medical Condition (APA,

Table 2 List of content topics in electronic consultation

Content Topic	No. eConsults	% eConsults
Depressive Disorders	51	30.2%
Anxiety Disorders	28	16.6%
Neurodevelopmental Disorders	21	12.4%
Bipolar and Related Disorders	20	11.8%
Schizophrenia Spectrum and Other Psychotic Disorders	18	10.7%
Personality Disorders	5	3.0%
Substance-Related and Addictive Disorders	5	3.0%
Obsessive-Compulsive and Related Disorders	4	2.4%
Disruptive, Impulse-Control, and Conduct Disorders	3	1.8%
Medication-Induced Movement Disorders and Other Adverse Effects of Medication	3	1.8%
Neurocognitive Disorders	3	1.8%
Sleep-Wake Disorders	3	1.8%
Somatic Symptom and Related Disorders	2	1.2%
Feeding and Eating Disorders	1	0.6%
Trauma- and Stressor-Related Disorders	1	0.6%
Unable to classify	1	0.6%

2013). Other common clinical topics included Anxiety Disorders (16.6%), Neurodevelopmental Disorders (12.4%), Bipolar and Related Disorders (11.8%), and Schizophrenia Spectrum and Other Psychotic Disorders (10.7%).

Question type

Questions pertaining to drug treatment were most common (75.7% of consults). Types of drug treatment questions included drug of choice (39.1% of eConsults), adverse effects from medications (16.0%), how to prescribe a particular drug (5.9%), interactions between medications (3.6%), indications / goals of treating a particular condition (2.4%), and other (8.9%). Questions pertaining to management (13.6%) and diagnosis (10.1%) were less common (Table 3).

The questions submitted for the Depressive Disorders – the most common clinical topic– predominately concerned drug treatment (88.2%), particularly *drug of choice* (52.9%). Drug treatment also dominated the other most common clinical areas of Anxiety Disorders (82.1%), Neurodevelopmental Disorders (61.9%), Bipolar and Related Disorders (70%), and Schizophrenia Spectrum and Other Psychotic Disorders (66.7%). *Drug of choice* was the most common drug treatment question across four of these five groups. The exception was the Schizophrenia Spectrum and Other Psychotic Disorders category, where the most common drug treatment questions pertained to *adverse effects of drugs*. Appendix 2 shows de-identified examples of eConsult clinical questions.

Post-eConsult survey

Course of action and decision for referral

PCPs were asked about how the eConsultation affected the course of action for the patient. The majority of the PCPs (62.1%) indicated they received advice for a new or additional course of action, while 32.5% indicated it confirmed a course of action the PCP already had in mind. PCPs were also asked about referrals. In 30.7% of the eConsults, PCPs indicated they no longer needed to refer the patient for a face–to-face appointment based on the information provided by the specialist (Table 4). In 27.8% of eConsults, it was determined that a face-to-face visit was still needed.

Overall value

PCPs were asked to rank the overall value in using the eConsultation service for this patient using a Likert scale ranging from 1 (minimal value) to 5 (excellent value). Using this scale, 88.7% of PCPs gave the eConsult service a 4 (27.8%) or a 5 (60.9%) for its value to the patient. One of the reasons PCPs valued the eConsult was that the average response time was much shorter than traditional referrals. A PCP highlighted how one of their patients appreciated the eConsult service:

Table 3 Classification of question type

Question Type	No. eConsults	% eConsults
Drug Treatment		
Drug of choice	66	39.1%
Adverse effects of drugs	27	16.0%
Other	15	8.9%
How to prescribe a particular drug	10	5.9%
Interactions between drugs	6	3.6%
Indications / goals of treating a particular condition	4	2.4%
Drug treatment total	128	75.7%
Clinical Management		
General management question	17	10.1%
Other providers available	6	3.6%
Clinical management total	23	13.6%
Diagnosis		
Interpretation of a clinical finding	11	6.6%
Other	3	1.8%
What test to choose	2	1.2%
Interpretation of a laboratory test	1	0.6%
Diagnosis total	17	10.1%
No specific question	1	0.6%

Table 4 Responses to close-out survey question 2: As a result of the eConsultation would you say that...

Response	No. eConsults	% eConsults
1. Referral was originally contemplated but now avoided at this stage;	52	30.8%
2. Referral was originally contemplated and is still needed – this eConsult likely leads to a more effective visit;	47	27.8%
3. Referral was not originally contemplated and is still not needed – this eConsult provided useful feedback/instruction;	60	35.5%
4. Referral was not originally contemplated, but eConsult process resulted in a referral being initiated;	2	1.2%
5. There was no particular benefit to using eConsult in this case;	5	3.0%
6. Other (please explain).	3	1.8%

> *"It is great to receive such detailed advice. I was able to have a good discussion with my patient about what the next steps are for her and she is happy to have an early contact with the specialist about her case."*

Only one PCP reported minimal value to their patient, in the clinical context of patient urgency and safety concerns that required emergency intervention which could not be addressed by the service.

Using a Likert scale of 1 (minimal) to 5 (excellent), PCPs were asked to rate the overall value of the eConsult service in this case to them as a PCP. The majority (91.1%) rated the value to be a 4 (20.7%) or 5 (70.4%). Many PCPs indicated that they found the advice and/or resources provided by specialists to be helpful and efficient. For example:

> *"Excellent collaboration, very quick response – so glad to have access to this service!"*

> *"Thank you to the specialist for providing effective practical advice and for the research literature information."*

Discussion

Our study found that the eConsult psychiatry service is a useful and valued tool to assist in addressing the significant treatment gap for mental illness in primary care settings. In keeping with the evidence for prevalence of mental illness, this study found that depression was the most common clinic topic for which clinical assistance was requested, followed by anxiety, neurodevelopment, bipolar, and schizophrenia spectrum disorders. MDD is the second leading cause of disability worldwide [18], more than breast, colorectal, lung, and prostate cancers [19]. Thus, timely access to care is paramount.

By far the most common questions asked pertained to pharmacotherapy recommendations around how to choose, augment and switch between commonly used psychotropic medications. These included, but were not limited to, frequently prescribed Selective Serotonin Reuptake Inhibitors, Selective Norepinephrine Reuptake Inhibitors, and First and Second Generation Antipsychotics. Questions regarding dosing and side effect profiles were more often asked about Methylphenidate and Amphetamine based Stimulants, Mood Stabilizers and Anticonvulsants. Polypharmacy concerns and medical monitoring were commonly asked across all classes. A possible explanation why there are more treatment type questions than diagnosis questions is that it is harder to easily diagnose patients in psychiatry as specialists do not have investigations to rely upon. Furthermore, PCPs may be able to diagnose cases more easily but need more assistance with treatment options.

In a similar study by Lowenstein et al. [20], the authors describe the implementation of eConsults specifically for psychiatric services. The authors evaluated 50 psychiatry eConsults, which revealed that PCPs most commonly asked questions about depressive disorders (20/50, 40%). (49/50, 98%) were related to the management of the disease, most often for managing medications. The average response time for specialists reported in the Lowenstein study was 1.4 days, slightly lower than the response time reported here, 2.3 days.

In another specialist classification study using eConsult data, Wren et al. [21] found that 46% of PCP cases were related to treatment compared to almost 76% in our analysis. However, the Wren study included nine specialties but no psychiatry questions. Goberstein et al. [22] recently published a study exploring the effects of electronic psychiatric consultations of mental health care. They found that PCPs reported high levels of confidence in treating depression with medication, through referral. However, there is no indication of how many consults were related to treatment.

Analysis of results indicates that the eConsult service had a significant impact on PCPs course of action, as it provided them with advice and/or information that they anticipated would lead to a more effective visit with their patient in a majority of cases. In the study by Lowenstein et al. [20], 38/50 (76%) of PCPs implements the specialists' recommendation. Although we did not directly ask this question it can be assumed that the vast majority of PCPs implemented the specialist's advice as it was either new or confirming information (95.3%).This transmission of clinical knowledge may have the potential for capacity building when PCPs encounter similar cases in their practice.

Moreover, if eConsults continue to reduce referrals to specialty services, this has important implications for both patients and the health care system. Benefits could include decreased wait times for patients who require face-to-face specialist care, and cost savings as an alternative model for the delivery of specialty services within the health care system. The service proved to be highly valued by PCPs for its high-quality advice and provision of rapid access to specialist knowledge and recommendations.

Although not the only solution to the treatment gap in the provision of mental health care in the primary care setting, eConsult has demonstrated clinical utility in narrowing the gaps for both patients and providers in Eastern Ontario. Therefore, expanding the service to other healthcare regions in Ontario and across Canada, which our group is currently doing, could yield similar success. Future research analyzing and comparing eConsult analysis between different jurisdictions to identify patterns in the healthcare needs of the population would help to identify gaps in healthcare services.

The findings of this study are susceptible to several limitations. First, as a study completed at a single center in Eastern Ontario, Canada, the result may not be generable to other health urban or rural centers with varying infrastructures. However, the results of the study align with similar studies in other health regions [20]. The data were analyzed retrospectively which also poses as a limitation as some of the consults dated back to 2011. The sample analyzed was a convenience sample, and thus might not have been representative of the population being examined.

Conclusions

eConsult can facilitate greater collaboration between PCPs and psychiatrists, and as such aligns with recommendations made in the 2011 position paper *The Evolution of Collaborative Mental Health Care in Canada: A Shared Vision for the Future* [23] which was developed by the Canadian Psychiatric Association and the College of Family Physicians of Canada. This paper highlights the importance of effective communication between providers as well as the need for rapid access to advice. It also supports the need to "explore innovative ways for mental health providers to work more closely with PCPs" (p.6). Certainly eConsult represents an excellent example of such an innovation. The Mental Health Commission of Canada similarly recommends the importance of the "medical home" and the need to support collaboration with mental health providers, in recognition of the fact that most mental health care is provided in the primary care setting. eConsult exemplifies a facet of the Canadian collaborative shared care model, which brings together patients, families, primary care providers and mental health providers with the goal of improving mental health outcomes for patients.

Appendix 1

Table 5 Psychiatry content taxonomy for classifying eConsults

Anxiety Disorders
Bipolar and Related Disorders
Depressive Disorders
Dissociative Disorders
Disruptive, Impulse-Control, and Conduct Disorders
Elimination Disorders
Feeding and Eating Disorders
Gender Dysphoria
Medication-Induced Movement Disorders and Other Adverse Effects of Medication
Neurocognitive Disorders
Neurodevelopmental Disorders
Obsessive-Compulsive and Related Disorders
Paraphilic Disorders
Personality Disorders
Schizophrenia Spectrum and Other Psychotic Disorders
Sexual Dysfunctions
Sleep-Wake Disorders
Substance-Related and Addictive Disorders
Trauma-and Stressor-Related Disorders

Appendix 2

Table 6 Examples of eConsult clinical questions

Depression
35 year old woman with dysthymia. Has been seeing a psychologist for over a year. Symptoms of low mood, decreased motivation and anhedonia. Not suicidal. No alcohol or drug use. No significant anxiety symptoms. Was started on Prozac and dose increased up to 40 mg without effect. She was then switched to Effexor with dose titrated up to 225 mg with little response. Do you have any suggestions?
ADHD
21 year old university student with diagnosis of ADD. Treated with Concerta 54 mg in the morning and Ritalin 30 mg at lunch/early afternoon as he has an evening class. He has asked to increase the dose of Concerta but I am uncomfortable with that as the dose is already high. Otherwise healthy. Takes no other medications. What would you advise?
Anxiety/Insomnia
My question is about insomnia. 42 year old woman is severely anxious and reports episodes of panic attacks. She is currently on sertraline 50 mg which is being titrated up but still has primary and secondary insomnia. She has responded to zopiclone 3.25 mg prn for small periods of time but I do not want to continue this due to the risk of tolerance/dependence. She is unable to tolerate trazodone. Is it reasonable to use zopiclone long term? Otherwise would nortriptyline be safe to use with sertraline? If so at what dose? Do you have other suggestions?

Abbreviations

Champlain BASE ™: Building Access to Specialists through eConsultation; eConsult: electronic consultations; ICPC-2: International Classification for Primary Care, version 2; MDD: Major Depressive Disorder; PCP: primary care provider; TGCQ: Taxonomy of Generic Clinical Questions

Acknowledgements

We thank Lesley Ananny for her administrative and project management support, Amir Afkham for his technical assistance in retrieving data, and Sheena Guglani for helping with manuscript revisions.

Funding

University of Ottawa, Department of Medicine, Education Grant.
Royal College of Physicians and Surgeons of Canada Medical Education Research Grant.
The funders had no role in the design of the study, data collection, analysis, interpretation of data nor writing of the manuscript.

Authors' contributions

DA contributed to study design, data collection, data analysis, and reviewed and contributed to drafts of the manuscript. JS contributed to the data analysis, and reviewed and contributed to drafts of the manuscript. CL co-created the eConsult service including the survey questions, conceived of and contributed to study design, data collection, data analysis and reviewed and contributed to drafts of the manuscript. REG contributed to the data analysis and drafting of the manuscript. DG contributed to the data analysis and contributed to drafts of the manuscript. EJK is one of the co-founders of the BASE eConsult service. She contributed to study design, data collection, data analysis and reviewed and contributed to drafts of the manuscript. All authors have read and approved the final manuscript.

Competing interests

The authors declare that they have no competing interests.

Author details

[1]Department of Family Medicine, University of Ottawa, Ottawa, ON, Canada. [2]Bruyère Research Institute, 85 Primrose Avenue, Ottawa, ON K1R 6M1, Canada. [3]Department of Psychiatry, University of Ottawa, Ottawa, ON, Canada. [4]Faculty of Education, University of Ottawa, Ottawa, ON, Canada. [5]Department of Medicine, University of Ottawa, Ottawa, ON, Canada. [6]Ottawa Hospital Research Institute, Ottawa, ON, Canada.

References

1. Barua B, Ren F. Waiting your turn - wait times for health care in Canada, 2016 report. 2016. https://www.fraserinstitute.org/studies/waiting-your-turn-wait-times-for-health-care-in-canada-2016.
2. Canadian Mental Health Association Ontario. Rural and northern community issues in mental health. 2009. https://ontario.cmha.ca/documents/rural-and-northern-community-issues-in-mental-health/.
3. Manian FA, Janssen DA. A closer look at curbside consultations. JAMA. 1996;275:145–7.
4. Bergus GR, Sinift SD, Randall CS, Rosenthal DM. Use of an E-mail curbside consultation service by family physicians. J Fam Pract. 1998;47:357–64.
5. Carr VJ, Faehrmann C, Lewin TJ, Walton JM, Reid AA. Determining the effect that consultation-liaison psychiatry in primary care has on family physicians' psychiatric knowledge and practice. Psychosomatics. 1997;38:217–29. https://doi.org/10.1016/S0033-3182(97)71458-0.
6. Yellowlees PM, Odor A, Parish MB, Iosif AM, Haught K, Hilty D. A feasibility study of the use of asynchronous telepsychiatry for psychiatric consultations. Psychiatr Serv. 2010;61:838–40.
7. Butler TN, Yellowlees P. Cost analysis of store-and-forward telepsychiatry as a consultation model for primary care. Telemed e-Health. 2012;18:74–7. https://doi.org/10.1089/tmj.2011.0086.
8. Liddy C, Drosinis P, Keely E. Electronic consultation systems: worldwide prevalence and their impact on patient care — a systematic review. Fam Pract. 2016;33:274–85.
9. Vimalananda VG, Gupte G, Seraj SM, Orlander J, Berlowitz D, Fincke BG, et al. Electronic consultations (e-consults) to improve access to specialty care: a systematic review and narrative synthesis. J Telemed Telecare. 2015;21:323–30. https://doi.org/10.1177/1357633X15582108.
10. Liddy C, Afkham A, Drosinis P, Joschko J, Keely E. Impact of and satisfaction with a new eConsult service: a mixed methods study of primary care providers. JABFM. 2015;28:394–403.
11. Liddy C, Rowan MS, Afkham A, Maranger J, Keely E. Building access to specialist care through e-consultation. Open Med. 2013;7:e1–8.
12. Keely E, Liddy C, Afkham A. Utilization, benefits, and impact of an e-consultation service across diverse specialties and primary care providers. Telemed e-Health. 2013;19:733–8.
13. Liddy C, Drosinis P, Deri Armstrong C, McKellips F, Afkham A, Keely E. What are the cost savings associated with providing access to specialist care through the Champlain BASE eConsult service ? A costing evaluation. BMJ Open. 2016;6:1–9.
14. Hilty DM, Crawford A, Teshima J, Chan S, Sunderji N, Yellowlees PM, et al. A framework for telepsychiatric training and e-health: competency-based education, evaluation and implications. Int Rev Psychiatry. 2015;27:569–92.
15. Keely EJ, Archibald D, Tuot DS, Lochnan H, Liddy C. Unique educational opportunities for PCPs and specialists arising from electronic consultation services. Acad Med. 2017;92:45–51.
16. Wood M, Lamberts H, Meijer J, Hofmans-Okkes IM. The conversion between icpc and icd-10. Requirements for a family ofclassification systems in the nextdecade. Fam Pract. 1992;9:340–8.
17. Ely JW, Osheroff JA, Ebell MH, Bergus GR, Barcey T, Chambliss ML, et al. Information in practice patient care, vol. 319; 1999. p. 358–61.
18. Lam RW, Kennedy SH, Grigoriadis S, McIntyre RS, Roumen M, Ramasubbu R, et al. Canadian network for mood and anxiety treatments (CANMAT) clinical guidelines for the management of major depressive disorder in adults. III. Pharmacotherapy. J Affect Disord. 2009; 117:S26–43. https://doi.org/10.1016/j.jad.2009.06.041.
19. Ratnasingham S, Cairney J, Manson H, Rehm J, Lin E, Kurdyak P. The burden of mental illness and addiction in Ontario. Can J Psychiatr. 2013;58:529–37.
20. Lowenstein M, Bamgbose O, Gleason N, Feldman MD. Psychiatric consultation at your fingertips: descriptive analysis of electronic consultation from primary care to psychiatry. J Med Internet Res. 2017;19:e279.
21. Wrenn K, Catschegn S, Cruz M, Gleason N, Gonzales R. Analysis of an electronic consultation program at an academic medical Centre: primary care provider questions, specialist responses, and primary care provider actions. J Telemed Telecare. 2016;23:217–24. https://doi.org/10.1177/1357633X16633553.
22. Golberstein E, Kolvenbach S, Carruthers H, Druss B, Goering P. Effects of electronic psychiatric consultations on primary care provider perceptions of mental health care: survey results from a randomized evaluation. Healthcare. 2016; https://doi.org/10.1016/j.hjdsi.2017.01.002.
23. Kates N, Mazowita G, Lemire F, Jayabarathan A, Bland R, Selby P, et al. The evolution of collaborative mental health Care in Canada: a shared vision for the future. Can J Psychiatr. 2011;56:1–10.

7

High prevalence rates for multiple psychiatric conditions among inmates at French Guiana's correctional facility: diagnostic and demographic factors associated with violent offending and previous incarceration

Mathieu Nacher[1*], Gulen Ayhan[1], Romain Arnal[2], Célia Basurko[1], Florence Huber[3], Agathe Pastre[4], Louis Jehel[5], Bruno Falissard[6] and Vincent About[4]

Abstract

Background: French Guiana has the highest incarceration rate among French territories, it is higher than that of Brazil, Colombia or Venezuela. It is well known that mental health problems are over-represented in correctional facilities. Our objectives were to describe the prevalence of various psychiatric conditions and to study factors associated with violence and repeated offenses among arriving detainees at the sole correctional facility of French Guiana.

Methods: The study was cross-sectional. All consenting new adult prisoners incarcerated between 18/09/2013 and 31/12/2014 at the penitentiary centre of French Guiana were included. The Mini International Neuropsychiatric Interview (MINI) was used to screen for psychiatric diagnoses. In addition sociodemographic data was collected.

Results: Overall 647 men and 60 women were included.

The participation rate was 90%.Overall 72% of patients had at least one psychiatric diagnosis (Fig. 2). Twenty percent had three or more diagnoses. Violent index offences were not more frequent among those with a psychiatric diagnosis (crude odds ratio 1.3 (95%CI = 0.9–2), $P = 0.11$.

Multivariate analysis showed that after adjusting for sex and age, psychosis, suicidality and post-traumatic stress disorder were independently associated with violent offences. Generalized anxiety disorder was less likely to be associated with incarceration for violent offences.

Having a history of a previous incarceration was significantly associated with a psychiatric condition in general (any diagnosis) OR = 3 (95%CI = 2–4.3), $P < 0.0001$.

Calculations of the population attributable risks showed that in the sample 31.4% of repeat incarcerations were attributable to antisocial personality disorder, 28.3% to substance addiction, 17.3% to alcohol addiction, 8.7% to depression and 7% to psychosis.

(Continued on next page)

* Correspondence: mathieu.nacher66@gmail.com
[1]Centre d'Investigation Clinique CIC INSERM 1424, Centre Hospitalier de Cayenne, 97300 Cayenne, French Guiana
Full list of author information is available at the end of the article

(Continued from previous page)
Conclusions: The very high prevalence of psychiatric disorders observed in our sample, and the relative lack of psychiatric facilities, suggest that part of the problem of very high incarceration rate may be explained by transinstitutionalization. Improving psychiatric care in prison and coordination with psychiatric care in the community after release is likely to be important.

Background

French Guiana is a French overseas territory located between Brazil and Suriname, and thus a part of the European Union. It has the highest GDP per capita on the Latin American continent and therefore attracts numerous immigrants in search of a better life (https://www.insee.fr/fr/statistiques/2011101?geo=DEP-973). However, unemployment is high and much of the population lives in precarious social conditions. The soil is rich in gold and attracts large numbers of illegal gold miners [1]. French Guiana is also a hub for cocaine trafficking towards France and Europe. Drugs are relatively cheap and there are high rates of substance use, impacting on HIV rates [2]. A quarter of families are single parent families, and one in five families includes four children or more, demographic conditions that further increase social vulnerability (https://www.insee.fr/fr/statistiques/2011101?geo=DEP-973).

The natural population growth in French Guiana is 2.45% per year, the second highest in Latin America on a par with Guatemala [3]. This very rapid growth compounds social problems and challenges the French social system, which struggles to keep up in terms of education, health infrastructure, and appropriate housing. These difficult social conditions and the illegal "opportunities to make money" may fuel the high crime rate and lead French Guiana to have the highest incarceration rate (328 per 100,000) among French territories, a rate that is higher than that of Brazil (319 per 100,000), Colombia (231 per 100,000) or Venezuela (173 per 100,000) [4].

As for other government services, the judiciary and penitentiary systems struggle to keep up. The only correctional facility in French Guiana is thus saturated and its overpopulation and poor living conditions have been repeatedly described [5, 6].

It is well known that mental health problems are over-represented in correctional facilities [7, 8]. Psychiatric illnesses often increase the risk of suicide, the risk of death after release from incarceration, and the risk of new offences and reincarceration. Until recently, there had never been any study of the mental health issues of detainees in this particular territory at the crossroad between France and Latin America. A first study showed focused on the risk of suicide and its predictors among arriving detainees [9]. The objective of the present study was to describe the relation between various psychiatric conditions and violence or repeated offenses among arriving detainees at the sole correctional facility of French Guiana.

Methods

The study was cross-sectional. All consenting new adult prisoners incarcerated between 18/09/2013 and 31/12/2014 at the penitentiary centre of French Guiana at Cayenne were included.

This is slightly different from the study on suicide risk factors [9] because the questionnaire and case record form used was modified after a test phase; we only used data collected with the finalized version of the data collection tool.

Inmates with an assigned legal guardian were excluded in order not to compromise the incarceration procedures for our study because the presence of the legal guardian would have been logistically very difficult given the restricted access to the mental health ward [9].

After incarceration, all new arrivals are seen for physical examination by a doctor of the "Unité de consultation et de soins ambulatoires (UCSA)", the ambulatory care unit of the prison and then by a psychiatrist or psychiatric nurse in the "Unité fonctionnelle de psychiatrie intra-carcérale (UFPI)" (the psychiatric ward). Patients had a 15 day window after arrival in which they could be included.

In addition to this normal procedure upon admission for the purpose of our study we added the Mini International Neuropsychiatric Interview (MINI). The MINI is a short diagnostic structured interview (DSI) developed in France and the United States to explore 17 disorders according to the Diagnostic and Statistical Manual (DSM)-V diagnostic criteria. The validity and reliability of the MINI has been confirmed in several studies [10, 11]. The MINI is structured to allow administration by non-specialized interviewers for the research of current disorders. It is currently one of the most used psychiatric diagnostic tools [12]. For each mental illness, one or two screening questions rule out the diagnosis when answered negatively. The MINI is thus adapted for epidemiological studies requiring a short but robust tool. The estimated time for the interview is 15 min. The MINI has been translated and validated in 46 languages, including the main languages found in French Guiana: French, English, Portuguese, Dutch and Spanish.

All psychiatrists and nurses performing the MINI were trained in order to correctly use the questionnaire. Socio-demographic questions were added (age, birthplace, residence, languages, presence of a translator, family status, children, siblings, position among siblings, professional situation), history of detention (reason for detention, previous imprisonment) and psychiatric history. A training period preceded our study in order to test the feasibility of the MINI and to familiarize staff with the protocol and to verify that the staff was proficient with the tool before starting the study. Since there were 2 phases with some changes in the ancillary questionnaire, we only analyzed the data collected with the final questionnaire in order to obtain a homogenous data set.

Inclusion criteria

Incarcerated adults accepting to participate were only included.

Exclusion criteria

Minors, persons with a legal guardian, or persons refusing to participate were not included.

Statistical analysis

Descriptive analysis of qualitative and quantitative variables was followed by bivariate analysis in order to identify significant variables for incarceration for violent index offences. Variables were included in a multivariate model for logistic regression in order to identify independent diagnoses at increased risk for incarceration for violent index offences. The modelling strategy was purely exploratory and the variables were retained in the model except obsessive compulsive disorder, anorexia and bulimia which were too rare to be included in a multivariate model (respectively, 15, 5 and 3 persons). Collinearity was tested using the Collin package (STATA, College Station, Texas) and verifying that variance inflation factors were < 4. The Hosmer-Lemeshow goodness-of-fit test was used to test the model.

A similar procedure was used for bivariate and multivariate analysis of variables associated with repeated incarcerations.

Principal component analysis was performed and a loading plot of the different diagnoses was performed.

Stata13 (College Station, Texas, USA) was used.

Ethical and regulatory aspects

The study was approved by the Ethical committee of Bordeaux (Comité de Protection des Personnes, CPP) (reference number DC 2012/115). The study was also approved by the Ethical committee of INSERM CEEI in 2013 (IRB00003888). Inmates gave informed consent (oral and written) to participate in the study.

Results

General results

Between September 18th 2013 and December 31st 2014, 785 new prisoners were registered. The survey participation rate was 90% (707/785) [9]. Overall 647 men and 60 women were included. The mean age was 30 years (SD = 10.7 years) for men and 27.7 years (SD 10 years) for women. Figure 1 shows the over-representation of younger age groups.

Birth place and spoken language

Overall 47.8% of persons were born in French Guiana, 3% in other French territories, 15.1% were born in neighboring Suriname, 14.3% were born in Guyana, 10.6% in Brazil, 3.1% in Haiti, and the rest were born elsewhere or missing. 57.3% spoke French, 14% spoke English, 9.1% spoke Portuguese, 7.4% spoke Nengue Tongo, and 7% spoke Haitian Creole.

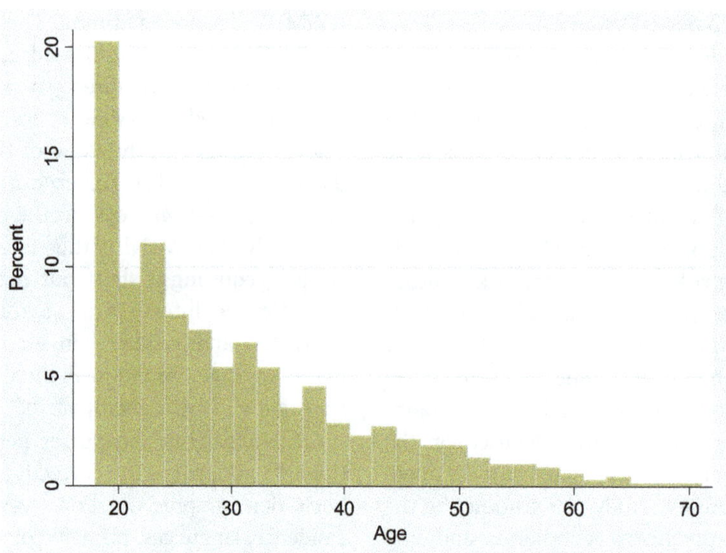

Fig. 1 Age of incarcerated persons included in the study at the sole correctional facility of French Guiana

Marital status

Regarding their marital status 48.4% were single, and 41.02% lived in a couple, 6.3% were married and 1% were divorced or widowed. Sixty percent (368/613 respondents) of inmates had parents who were separated (13.3% of non response).

Work

Among respondents (92%) to the work status question, 22.4% of men and 48% of women were unemployed; 46% of men and 26% of women declared having odd jobs; and 24.6% of men and 10% of women had a work contract.

Trauma

Nearly 2% (11/564 respondents) declared having experienced prior sexual trauma with 18.2% not responding to the question. A third of respondents declared the death of a close family member (233/691 respondents).

Incarceration motives

Incarceration resulted from violent offences in 28% of cases (assault 7.9%, homicide without intent 2.2%, intentional homicide 3.5%, rape 4.5%, violence 9.8%) and drugs in 34.4% of cases.

Psychiatric diagnoses

Overall 72% of patients had at least one psychiatric diagnosis (Fig. 2). Twenty percent had three or more diagnoses. Violent offences were not more frequent among those with a psychiatric diagnosis (crude odds ratio 1.3 (95%CI = 0.9–2), $P = 0.11$, Median 1 in both groups, $p = 0.49$).

Overall 36 of 51 (70.6%) persons with psychosis also had substance addictions. Conversely, 36 of 235 persons with substance addictions (15.3%) were also psychotic. Among the study population, 307 took cannabis (43%), 58 took crack cocaine (8.2%) and 15 cocaine (2.1%).

The individual prevalence for individual diagnoses is shown in Fig. 3.

Overall, 2% reported past sexual trauma (95%CI = 1–3.5%) and 5.9% (95%CI = 4.2–8%) reported a family history of psychiatric problems.

Principal component analysis

Figure 4 shows a loading plot after the principal component analysis of the different diagnoses obtained by the MINI. A cluster of depressive signs is found on the lower right part, the bottom center is mostly linked to a cluster of neurotic manifestations; the top center cluster pertains to addictions, which lie close to antisocial disorder.

Incarceration for violence

Table 1 shows the proportion of patients for listed MINI- diagnoses who had been charged with violent and non-violent crimes. Multivariate analysis showed that after adjusting for sex and age, psychosis, suicidality, and post-traumatic stress disorder were independently associated with violent offences for incarceration. Generalized anxiety disorder was less likely to be associated with incarceration following a violent index offence.

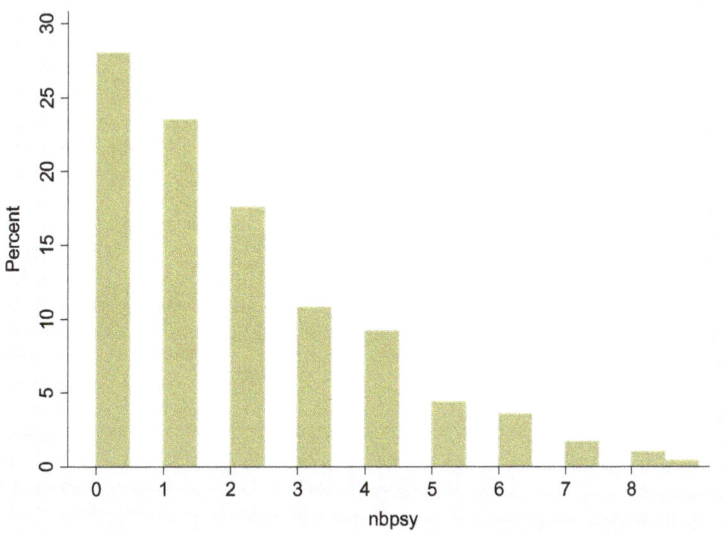

Fig. 2 Number of psychiatric diagnoses among inmates incarcerated in the sole correctional facility of French Guiana

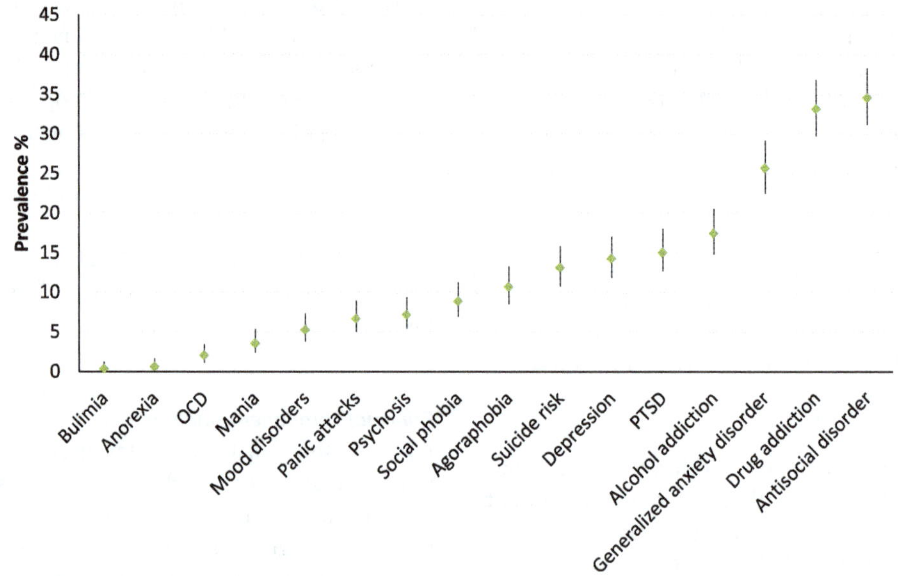

Fig. 3 Prevalence and 95% confidence intervals of different psychiatric conditions in Prisoners in French Guiana using the MINI 5.0 screening tool at the time of incarceration

Repeat offenders

Overall, 48.6% of inmates had already been previously incarcerated. Having a history of a previous incarceration was significantly associated with a psychiatric condition in general (any diagnosis) OR = 3 (95%CI = 2–4.3), $P < 0.0001$. Table 2 shows the detail by psychiatric diagnosis. Calculations of the population attributable risks showed that in the sample 31.4% of repeat incarcerations were attributable to antisocial personality disorder, 28.3% to substance addiction, 17.3% to alcohol addiction, 8.7% to depression and 7% to psychosis.

Discussion

The present study emphasizes the high prevalence of mental illness among detainees in French Guiana [9]. Overall, 512/707 inmates (72%) presented at least 1 psychiatric disorder. The most common diagnoses were antisocial personality disorder (34.6%), substance addiction (33.2%),

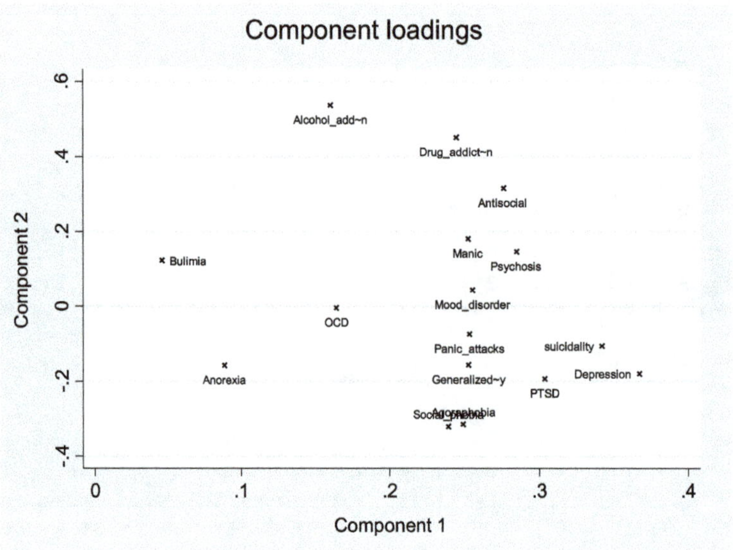

Fig. 4 Principal component analysis of the different psychiatric diagnoses among inmates incarcerated in the sole correctional facility of French Guiana

Table 1 Variables associated with violent and non violent crimes, bivariate and multivariate analysis

	Total	Incarceration linked to violence N(%)	Incarceration not linked to violence N(%)	Crude odds ratio (95% CI)	Adjusted odds ratio (95% CI), *P*
Age in years Mean [SD]	707	29.6 [10.3]	31 [11.2]	1 (0.99–1.02)	1(0.98–1.02), *P* = 0.5
Sex					
Male	647	195 (98.5)	452(88.8)	8.2(2.5–26.5)	8 (2.4–26.4), *P* = 0.001
Female	60	3(1.5)	57(11.2)		
Antisocial disorder					
Yes	245	67(33.8)	178 (35)	0.9 (0.67–1.3)	0.9 (0.6–1.3), *P* = 0.5
No	462	131 (66.2)	331(65)		
Generalized anxiety disorder					
Yes	182	39(19.7)	143(28.1)	0.6 (0.4–0.9)	0.5 (0.3–0.8), *P* = 0.006
No	525	159(80.3)	366(71.9)		
Psychosis					
Yes	51	23(11.6)	28(5.5)	2.2 (1.2–4)	2.4 (1.2–4.6), *P* = 0.01
No	656	175(88.4)	481(94.5)		
Substance addiction					
Yes	235	61(30.8)	174(34.2)	0.8(0.6–1.2)	0.7 (0.4–1), *P* = 0.05
No	230	197 (69.2)	33(65.8)		
Alcohol addiction					
Yes	144	39(19.7)	85(16.7)	1.2 (0.8–1.8)	1.4 (0.86–2.2), *P* = 0.19
No	583	159(80.3)	424(83.3)		
PTSD					
Yes	107	40(20.2)	67(13.1)	1.7(1.1–2.6)	1.8 (1.08–3), *P* = 0.02
No	600	158(79.8)	442(86.8)		
Social phobia					
Yes	63	15(7.6)	48(9.4)	0.8 (0.4–1.44)	0.7 (0.4–1.5), *P* = 0.4
No	644	183(92.4)	461(90.6)		
Agoraphobia					
Yes	76	28(14.1)	48(9.4)	1.6 (0.96–2.6)	1.6 (0.9–2.9), *P* = 0.1
No	631	170(85.9)	461(90.6)		
Panic attacks					
Yes	48	15(7.6)	33(6.5)	1.2 (0.6–2.2)	1 (0.5–2), *P* = 0.9
No	659	183(92.4)	476(93.5)		
Mania					
Yes	26	5(2.5)	21(4.1)	0.6 (0.2–1.6)	0.4 (0.1–1.2), *P* = 0.1
No	681	193(97.5)	488(95.9)		
Mood disorders					
Yes	38	11(5.5)	27(5.3)	1 (0.5–2.1)	0.9 (0.4–2.2), *P* = 0.9
No	669	187(94.5)	482(94.7)		
Suicidality					
Yes	93	35(17.7)	58(11.4)	1.7 (1.05–2.6)	2.1 (1.2–3.8), *P* = 0.009
No	614	163(82.3)	451(88.6)		
Depression					
Yes	101	28(14.1)	73 (14.3)	1 (0.6–1.6)	0.8 (0.4–1.5), *P* = 0.5
No	606	170(85.9)	436(85.7)		

generalized anxiety disorder (25.7%), alcohol addiction (17.5%), post traumatic stress disorder (15.1%), and major depression (14.3%) (Fig. 3).

Prevalence of psychosis was greater in our sample (7.6%) than in large meta-analyses (3.7–4%) [8, 13]. Prevalence of depression was also higher. This may reflect the use of the MINI, rather than the use of other diagnostic instruments in other studies in the literature. Although antisocial personality disorder was the most frequent diagnosis, its prevalence was less frequent than in the largest meta-analysis of

Table 2 Variables associated with previous incarcerations, bivariate and multivariate analysis

	Total	Previously incarcerated N(%)	First incarceration N(%)	Crude odds ratio (95% CI)	Adjusted odds ratio (95% CI), *P*
Age in years Mean [SD]	707	32 [10.5]	28.1 [10.3]	1 (0.99–1.02)	1.04(1.02–1.06), $P < 0.001$
Sex					
Male	647	333(96.8)	314 86.5)	4.7(2.4–9.2)	4.3 (2–9.1), $P < 0.001$
Female	60	11(3.2)	49(13.5)		
Antisocial disorder					
Yes	245	162(47.1)	83 (22.9)	3 (2.2–4.1)	2.6 (1.8–3.7), $P < 0.001$
No	462	182 (52.8)	280(77.1)		
Generalized anxiety disorder					
Yes	182	92(26.7)	90(24.8)	1.1 (0.8–1.5)	0.8 (0.5–1.3), $P = 0.4$
No	525	252(73.3)	273(75.2)		
Psychosis					
Yes	51	37(10.7)	14(3.9)	3 (1.6–5.7)	1.4 (0.7–2.9), $P = 0.01$
No	656	307(89.3)	349(96.1)		
Substance addiction					
Yes	235	153(44.5)	82(22.6)	2.7(2–3.8)	1.9 (1.3–2.7), $P = 0.001$
No	472	191 (55.52)	281(77.4)		
Alcohol addiction					
Yes	124	88(25.6)	36(9.9)	3.1 (2–4.7)	1.7 (1.1–2.8), $P = 0.02$
No	583	256(74.4)	327(90.1)		
PTSD					
Yes	107	64(18.6)	43(11.9)	1.7(1.1–2.6)	1.3 (0.8–2.2), $P = 0.3$
No	600	280(81.4)	320(88.1)		
Social phobia					
Yes	63	34(9.9)	29(8)	1.2 (0.74–2.1)	1.2 (0.6–2.3), $P = 0.6$
No	644	310(90.1)	334(92)		
Agoraphobia					
Yes	76	46(13.4)	30(8.2)	1.7 (1.05–2.8)	1.1 (0.6–2.1), $P = 0.6$
No	631	298(86.4)	333(91.8)		
Panic attacks					
Yes	48	27(7.9)	21(5.8)	1.4 (0.7–2.5)	0.8 (0.4–1.6), $P = 0.5$
No	659	317(92.1)	342(94.2)		
Manic					
Yes	26	18(5.2)	8(2.2)	2.56 (1.05–5.7)	1.3 (0.5–3.6), $P = 0.5$
No	681	326(94.8)	355(97.8)		
Mood disorders					
Yes	38	19(5.5)	19(5.2)	1.1 (0.5–2)	0.5 (0.2–1.2), $P = 0.13$
No	669	325(94.5)	344(94.8)		
Suicidality					
Yes	93	54(15.7)	39(10.7)	1.5 (0.99–2.4)	1.2 (0.7–2), $P = 0.6$
No	614	290(84.3)	324(89.3)		
Depression					
Yes	101	63 (18.3)	38 (10.53)	1.9 (1.2–3)	1.7 (0.96–3), $P = 0.06$
No	606	281(81.7)	325(89.5)		

cross-sectional prevalence rates of mental illness among prisoners internationally [13]. It has been observed that in low to middle income countries the prevalence of psychosis and major depression is higher than in high income countries. French Guiana, despite being a French territory thus has a profile that is closer to low and middle income countries [8]. In low and middle income countries, lower budgets for psychiatric care of psychoses may lead to a shift from mental health care towards incarceration. Another hypothesis pertains to different social and cultural norms regarding mental illness, and possible poor legal representations of mentally ill patients in the justice system [8].

When comparing our results with the study in French prisons, which used the MINI and examination by a psychiatrist, there were some differences between mainland France and the French territory of French Guiana. A striking difference was the weight of addictions in French Guiana (33.2% for drugs and 17.5% for alcohol) relative to mainland France (8.9 and 8.7%, respectively). This level of addictions was comparable to what is observed in neighboring Brazil [14, 15]. PTSD and generalized anxiety seemed more frequent in French Guiana than in mainland France (15.1 and 25.7%, versus 6.6 and 15.4%) whereas depression was less frequent in French Guiana than in mainland France (14.3 versus 22.9%). Some of these differences may be due to methodological differences, but others may be due to the "Latin American socio economic and cultural context" in French Guiana. Thus what applies in mainland France may not apply in French Guiana, and French-trained mental health professionals require some adaptation of their epidemiological assumptions.

After adjusting for age, males, antisocial personality disorder, substance and alcohol addictions, depression and psychoses were significantly associated with repeat offenses as described elsewhere [16, 17]. We did not find any association with bipolar disorder. It may be that our sample size was insufficient to detect any effect because the crude odds ratio, but not the adjusted one, was significantly associated with repeat incarceration. The calculation of population-attributable fractions is arguable in this cross-sectional design. It was meant to estimate, what proportion of repeat offenses could be attributed to the psychiatric conditions, and thus what could theoretically be gained if they were controlled. We believe it emphasizes the importance of enhancing psychiatric and social care in prison.

The variables significantly associated with incarceration for violent crimes were male sex, psychosis, suicide risk. Generalized anxiety disorder on the contrary was associated with a lower probability of incarceration for a violent crime. The direction of causality is not clear with regard to suicide risk: perhaps remorse explained the association, but hetero-aggressive behavior in persons with suicidal thought is also a possible explanation. We have previously described predictive factors for suicide risk for this population [9].

Substance addiction has been reported to be associated with violence [18]. However, here we did not find any significant association perhaps because violence between drug users may be less frequently reported to the police and less frequently prosecuted. Prison is likely to represent an opportunity to initiate addiction treatment and medical services that should aim for a smooth transition with the services outside of prison [19, 20].

The transinstitutionalization hypothesis posits that mentally ill persons without proper care will be over-represented in the criminal justice system. This hypothesis is debated. Some authors argue that this is reductionist and that psychiatric desinstitutionalization does not necessarily lead to a direct increase in the number of prisoners with mental health issues, and that increasing psychiatric facilities will not necessarily reduce numbers of detainees with mental health issues [7, 21–25].

French Guiana has a structural lag in health care personnel, notably in terms of specialized physicians. In terms of the density of psychiatrists French Guiana is six times lower than in mainland France [26]. The number of beds per capita is much lower than in mainland France and even than other French overseas territories [27]. In terms of psychiatric care, the number of beds per 100,000 persons in French Guiana is lower than in other territories (90 in France, in Martinique, 70 in Guadeloupe, and 40 in French Guiana). When we compare the incarceration rate and the psychiatric facilities, the contrast between French territories is even more salient: in France there are 1.12 inmates per psychiatric bed, in Guadeloupe 3, in Martinique 3.3 and in French Guiana 8.2.

It is noteworthy that in early 2017, following a wave of violent crime, French Guiana erupted in mass protests over notably security issues and deficient health infrastructures [28]. When looking at the very high prevalence of psychiatric disorders observed in our sample, and when looking at the relative lack of psychiatric facilities, it is tempting to hypothesize that part of the problem can be explained by transinstitutionalization and the Penrose hypothesis [21, 29]. At least, we hope these data will help fuel strategic debates in French Guiana.

There are several limitations to our study: The cross sectional design and the use of declarative data in a context of incarceration may have led to biased estimates. The MINI scale is a validated screening tool but it may not always be sufficiently sensitive notably for certain borderline personality disorders which are associated with incarceration. Finally the inclusion of study participants directly after incarceration– a stressful period-may have impacted responses to the questions.

Conclusions

Mentally ill detainees should benefit from effective screening, case identification and psychiatric care on arrival [9], ongoing care during the period of incarceration and pre-release arrangements for ongoing care in the community following release from custody. The goals of the correctional facilities and the psychiatric system are different but they may not always be antagonistic. Improved recognition and care of persons with mental illness in prison settings may improve outcomes for affected individuals and for public security [30].

Abbreviations
CEEI: Comité d'Evaluation Ethique de L'INSERM; CNIL: Commission Nationale Informatique et Libertés; GDP: Gross Domestic Product; HIV: Human immunodeficiency virus; INSERM: Institut National de la Santé et de la Recherche Médicale; UCSA: Unité Carcérale de Soins Ambulatoires

Authors' contributions
RA, CB, MN designed the protocol; RA, GA, VA, AP collected data; MN analyzed the data and wrote first draft of the manuscript; VA, RA, GA, CB, BF, LJ, FH, AP critically reviewed the manuscript. All authors read and approved the final manuscript.

Consent for publication
All persons included gave informed consent for publication of aggregated results.

Competing interests
The authors declare that they have no competing interests.

Author details
[1]Centre d'Investigation Clinique CIC INSERM 1424, Centre Hospitalier de Cayenne, 97300 Cayenne, French Guiana. [2]Service de Psychiatrie, Centre Hospitalier de Cayenne, 97300 Cayenne, French Guiana. [3]Hôpital de Jour Adultes, Centre Hospitalier de Cayenne, 97300 Cayenne, French Guiana. [4]Unité de Consultations Ambulatoires Carcérales, 97300 Cayenne, French Guiana. [5]CESP- INSERM U1178 Equipe IPSOM, Centre Hospitalier Universitaire de Martinique, BP632, 97261 Cedex fort de France, France. [6]CESP/INSERM U1018 (Centre de Recherche en Epidémiologie et Santé des Populations), 75679 Paris cedex 14, France.

References

1. Douine M, Musset L, Corlin F, Pelleau S, Pasquier J, Mutricy L, Adenis A, Djossou F, Brousse P, Perotti F. Prevalence of Plasmodium spp. in illegal gold miners in French Guiana in 2015: a hidden but critical malaria reservoir. Malar J. 2016;15(1):1.
2. Parriault M-C, Van-Melle A, Basurko C, Valmy L, Hoen B, Cabié A, Goerger-Sow M-T, Nacher M. Sexual risk behaviors and predictors of inconsistent condom use among crack cocaine users in the French overseas territories in the Americas. Int J STD AIDS. 2017;28(13):1266–74.
3. Liste des pays et territoires par taux de croissance démographique [https://fr.wikipedia.org/wiki/Liste_des_pays_et_territoires_par_taux_de_croissance_d%C3%A9mographique]. Accessed 25 May 2018.
4. Prison population rate region taxonomy [http://www.prisonstudies.org/highest-to-lowest/prison-population-total?area=all&category=wb_poprate]. Accessed 25 May 2018.
5. Dordonne B. La prison explose. Cayenne: France Guyane; 2016.
6. Scandale pénitentiaire en Guyane [https://oip.org/communique/scandale-penitentiaire-en-guyane/]. Accessed 25 May 2018.
7. Diamond PM, Wang EW, Holzer CE, Thomas C, Cruser dA. The prevalence of mental illness in prison. Adm Policy Ment Health Ment Health Serv Res. 2001;29(1):21–40.
8. Fazel S, Seewald K. Severe mental illness in 33 588 prisoners worldwide: systematic review and meta-regression analysis. Br J Psychiatry. 2012; 200(5):364–73.
9. Ayhan G, Arnal R, Basurko C, Pastre A, Pinganaud E, Sins D, Jehel L, Falissard B, Nacher M. Suicide risk among prisoners in French Guiana: prevalence and predictive factors. BMC Psychiatry. 2017;17(1):156.
10. Lecrubier Y, Sheehan DV, Weiller E, Amorim P, Bonora I, Sheehan KH, Janavs J, Dunbar GC. The MINI international neuropsychiatric interview (MINI). A short diagnostic structured interview: reliability and validity according to the CIDI. Eur Psychiatry. 1997;12(5):224–31.
11. Sheehan D, Lecrubier Y, Sheehan KH, Janavs J, Weiller E, Keskiner A, Schinka J, Knapp E, Sheehan M, Dunbar G. The validity of the MINI international neuropsychiatric interview (MINI) according to the SCID-P and its reliability. Eur Psychiatry. 1997;12(5):232–41.
12. Aboraya A. Use of structured interviews by psychiatrists in real clinical settings: results of an open-question survey. Psychiatry (Edgmont). 2009;6(6):24.
13. Fazel S, Danesh J. Serious mental disorder in 23 000 prisoners: a systematic review of 62 surveys. Lancet. 2002;359(9306):545–50.
14. Andreoli SB, dos Santos MM, Quintana MI, Ribeiro WS, Blay SL, JGV T, de Jesus Mari J. Prevalence of mental disorders among prisoners in the state of Sao Paulo, Brazil. PLoS One. 2014;9(2):e88836.
15. Pondé MP, Freire AC, Mendonça MS. The prevalence of mental disorders in prisoners in the city of Salvador, Bahia, Brazil. J Forensic Sci. 2011;56(3):679–82.
16. Baillargeon J, Binswanger IA, Penn JV, Williams BA, Murray OJ. Psychiatric disorders and repeat incarcerations: the revolving prison door. Am J Psychiatr. 2009;166(1):103–9.
17. Yu R, Geddes JR, Fazel S. Personality disorders, violence, and antisocial behavior: a systematic review and meta-regression analysis. J Personal Disord. 2012;26(5):775–92.
18. Steadman HJ, Mulvey EP, Monahan J, Robbins PC, Appelbaum PS, Grisso T, Roth LH, Silver E. Violence by people discharged from acute psychiatric inpatient facilities and by others in the same neighborhoods. Arch Gen Psychiatry. 1998;55(5):393–401.
19. Fazel S, Bains P, Doll H. Substance abuse and dependence in prisoners: a systematic review. Addiction. 2006;101(2):181–91.
20. Huber F, Merceron A, Madec Y, Gadio G, Pastre A, Coupez I, Adenis A, Adriouch L, Nacher M. High mortality among male HIV-infected patients after prison release: ART is not enough after incarceration with HIV. PLoS One. 2017;12(4):e0175740.
21. Banks SM, Stone JL, Pandiani JA, Cox JF, Morschauser PC. Utilization of local jails and general hospitals by state psychiatric center patients. J Behav Heal Serv Res. 2000;27(4):454–9.
22. Guy G. Community-based care: deinstitutionalization or Transinstitutionalization? Except Child. 1985;32(3):137–47.
23. Primeau A, Bowers TG, Harrison MA, XuXu. Deinstitutionalization of the mentally ill: evidence for transinstitutionalization from psychiatric hospitals to penal institutions. Compr Psychol. 2013;2:16.02. 13. CP. 12.12.
24. Prins SJ. Does transinstitutionalization explain the overrepresentation of people with serious mental illnesses in the criminal justice system? Community Ment Health J. 2011;47(6):716–22.
25. Stavis PF. Why prisons are brim-full of the mentally ill: is their incarceration a solution or a sign of failure. Geo Mason UCRLJ. 2000;11:157.
26. Breton-Lerouvillois L. Atlas de la démographie médicale en France. In: Conseil National de l'ordre des médecins; 2014.
27. DREES. Les établissements de santé dans les départements et régions d'outre-mer : activité et capacités. In: DREES; 2016.
28. A. B. Strikes shut down French Guiana, with effects resonating in Paris. In: New York times; 2017.
29. Mundt AP, Chow WS, Arduino M, Barrionuevo H, Fritsch R, Girala N, Minoletti A, Mitkiewicz F, Rivera G, Tavares M. Psychiatric hospital beds and prison populations in South America since 1990: does the Penrose hypothesis apply? JAMA Psychiatry. 2015;72(2):112–8.
30. Skeem JL, Manchak S, Peterson JK. Correctional policy for offenders with mental illness: creating a new paradigm for recidivism reduction. Law Hum Behav. 2011;35(2):110.

Assessment of grief-related rumination: validation of the German version of the Utrecht Grief Rumination Scale (UGRS)

Bettina K. Doering[1*], Antonia Barke[1], Thilo Friehs[1] and Maarten C. Eisma[2]

Abstract

Background: Bereavement can result in severe mental health problems, including persistent, severe and disabling grief symptoms, termed complicated grief. Grief rumination (i.e., repetitive thought about the causes and consequences of the loss) is a malleable cognitive risk-factor in adjustment to bereavement. The Utrecht Grief Rumination Scale (UGRS) was recently developed to assess grief rumination. The present study aimed to develop and validate a German version of the UGRS.

Methods: An online survey including measures of demographic and loss-related variables, grief rumination (UGRS), depressive rumination (brooding and reflection), and symptoms of depression, anxiety, and complicated grief, was administered online among 159 persons (87% women) who had lost a first-degree relative in the past three years. UGRS item analyses, a confirmatory factor analysis and associations of grief rumination with brooding, reflection and symptom levels were performed.

Results: The internal consistency of the UGRS was good. The confirmatory factor analysis obtained a good fit for a model with five correlated grief rumination subscales. The UGRS contributed uniquely to the prediction of complicated grief symptoms even when controlling for symptoms of anxiety and depression, brooding, reflection, and demographic and loss-related variables. Discriminant validity of the UGRS was demonstrated by the fact that higher UGRS scores were found in participants with a higher likelihood of receiving a diagnosis of complicated grief ($d > 1.60$).

Conclusion: The translated UGRS showed very good psychometric properties and the correlations with maladaptive ruminative styles and complicated grief symptoms demonstrated the clinical relevance of grief rumination. Limitations concerning generalisability of the results are discussed.

Keywords: Rumination, Repetitive thinking, Bereavement, Complicated grief, Assessment, Validation

Background

Bereavement is a universal human experience. While most people react to a loss with intense pain and may even develop an increased risk of mental or physical health problems [1], a majority adjust successfully to this stressful life-event without professional help. A minority of bereaved people, however, suffer from persistent grief symptoms of clinical relevance that are accompanied by functional impairment. Both new diagnostic classification systems of mental health conditions acknowledge the syndrome. The Diagnostic and Statistical Manual for Mental Disorders in its 5th edition (DSM 5) classifies it as 'Persistent Complex Bereavement Disorder' (PCBD) and considers it a condition for further study [2]. The International Classification of Diseases in its 11th edition (ICD-11) will probably include 'Prolonged Grief Disorder' (PGD) as a stress-related disorder [3, 4]. Concerning symptom duration, ICD 11 may allow a diagnosis as early as six months after the loss occurred, whereas DSM 5 requires symptoms to last twelve months. A recent meta-analysis estimates the pooled prevalence of PGD after bereavement to

* Correspondence: doeringi@staff.uni-marburg.de
[1]Clinical Psychology & Psychotherapy, Department of Psychology, Philipps-University Marburg, Marburg, Germany
Full list of author information is available at the end of the article

be 9.8% [5]. The present article will use the well-established term 'complicated grief' to refer to clinically relevant grief symptomatology, since the present assessment of grief symptoms follows the Inventory of Complicated Grief [6]. This also allows for drawing on existing research of grief rumination and bereavement outcome.

Given the severe distress that may be experienced after bereavement, a thorough understanding of the malleable factors that may contribute to the development and persistence of mental health problems is important. Thought processes are both malleable (for a review: [7]) and are assumed to play an important role in the potential transition from 'normal' to complicated grief and its maintenance [8]. Special attention has been paid to trans-diagnostic thought processes such as repetitive thinking, i.e. the 'process of thinking attentively, repetitively or frequently about one's self and one's world' ([9], p. 909). Repetitive thinking about the deceased, the loss and its circumstances and consequences seems inherent to the acute grieving process [10]. Some forms of repetitive thinking, however, such as rumination, have been associated with poor bereavement outcome, both concurrently and prospectively (cf. [11–13]).

Two types of rumination have been studied in some detail in adjustment to loss. The first investigations in this area were conducted in the mid-nineties. They focused on clarifying the role of depressive rumination after bereavement. Depressive rumination was defined as repetitively and passively focusing on depressive symptoms and on their possible causes and consequences [11]. A frequently used theory to understand the effects of depressive rumination on psychopathological symptoms is the Response Styles Theory (RST). The RST proposes that depressive rumination fuels depression by increasing the accessibility of negative thought content, impairing instrumental behaviour and problem solving, and driving away social support [11, 14]. In an attempt to differentiate adaptive from maladaptive forms of depressive rumination (cf. [15]) and to minimise the content overlap of the assessment of rumination with that of symptoms of depression, two sub-facets of depressive rumination were introduced, namely brooding and reflection [16]. 'Brooding' implies a passive comparison of the aversive current situation with some unachieved standard, and 'reflection' indicates actively focusing inward to engage in cognitive problem solving in order to overcome depressive symptoms. Longitudinally, brooding has been associated with more depressive symptoms, whereas reflection seems to be associated with less depressive symptoms [16]. Concerning adaptation to bereavement, RST conceptualises rumination as a confrontation strategy as it entails thinking repeatedly about post-loss emotions. Previous research indicates that all three constructs (i.e. depressive rumination, brooding, and reflection) are associated with psychopathological symptoms after bereavement [17–23]. However, it also suggests that another type of rumination, namely grief rumination, is potentially more predictive of mental health problems in adjustment to bereavement, consistently explaining more variance in post-loss symptoms of depression, posttraumatic stress and complicated grief concurrently and longitudinally ([20, 24, 25]; for a review: [13]).

In contrast to depressive rumination, grief rumination is not limited to analysing feelings of depression, as negative post-loss emotions are not restricted to sadness or helplessness but may also entail many other emotions including yearning, anger or irritability [1]. Thus, rumination after loss likely focuses on a wider array of loss-related feelings [19]. Additionally, typical topics of rumination will differ in grief and depression. Similarly to rumination after traumatic events [26, 27], grief rumination may focus strongly on reconciling the event with previously held beliefs about the meaningfulness or fairness of the world (i.e., thinking about why the event happened and the injustice of the loss), and counterfactual thinking (i.e., thinking about possible courses of action that might have prevented the event's occurrence).

A model that is currently often used to understand the negative consequences of grief rumination is the Rumination as Avoidance Hypothesis (RAH [10]). The RAH conceptualises rumination as an avoidance strategy because when ruminating about, for example, alternative outcomes of the situation (counterfactual thinking), one may avoid confronting the reality and permanence of the loss. Rumination would thus impede acceptance of the loss and hinder its contextualisation within existing autobiographical knowledge [8]. Previous research suggests that experiential avoidance and thought suppression longitudinally mediate the relationship between grief rumination and symptoms of complicated grief [25]. Experimental approaches have also corroborated the link between grief rumination and avoidance [28, 29]. Additionally, grief rumination has been investigated in another longitudinal study of recently bereaved participants [20]. In this sample, while simultaneously controlling for baseline symptom levels and other loss-related variables, grief rumination was a stronger predictor of later symptom levels of grief than was depressive rumination. This analysis also provided the first evidence of a distinction between adaptive and possibly maladaptive facets of grief rumination. Rumination about emotional reactions to the loss was regarded as potentially adaptive, since it was longitudinally associated with lower symptom levels. Rumination about the injustice of the loss was considered potentially maladaptive, since it was longitudinally associated with higher symptom levels.

Given grief rumination's potential theoretical and clinical relevance, the Utrecht Grief Rumination Scale (UGRS) was recently developed to specifically assess grief rumination [19]. The UGRS is based on theories of depressive rumination [16, 30], trauma-related rumination [26], and grief-relevant rumination [8]. It captures five typical themes of post-loss rumination: (1) personal emotional reactions to the loss, (2) injustice of the death, (3) counterfactual thoughts about the circumstances of the death, (4) meaning and consequences of the loss, and (5) the reactions of others to the loss. It was originally published in Dutch [24]; an English version has been developed and its cross-cultural equivalence confirmed [19]. In confirmatory factor analyses of the data of the Dutch and British samples, a single-level factor structure with five correlated factors provided the best model fit, even though a hierarchical model with a second-order factor performed almost equally as well [19]. In English and Dutch samples, the UGRS has demonstrated very good psychometric properties. It showed excellent internal consistency ($\alpha = .90$) and, as a first indication of its validity, the UGRS contributed to the prediction of depression, posttraumatic stress and complicated grief over and above demographic and loss-related variables and other measures of rumination [19, 24].

Clearly, more international research is needed to distinguish potentially adaptive and maladaptive facets of rumination at different time points in the grieving process. We also need to elucidate the pathways via which rumination contributes to the development and maintenance of mental health problems and, specifically, complicated grief. As prerequisite to this long-term goal, the present study aimed to develop a German version of the UGRS, to investigate its psychometric properties (e.g. reliability, item-correlations, factor structure), and to test its concurrent and discriminant validity by examining associations between the UGRS, reflection and brooding, and symptoms of anxiety, depression and complicated grief.

Methods

Participants and procedures

Ethical approval was obtained from the Ethics Committee of the Department of Psychology of the Philipps University Marburg (Germany) and invitations to participate were posted on grief-related websites (e.g., peer support websites). Recruitment lasted from August to October 2016. People accepting the invitation followed a link to an online survey platform that offered information about the aims of the study, confidentiality and study eligibility criteria; after providing written informed consent, they could participate in the study. As an incentive, participants had the chance of winning one out of two 50 €-vouchers for an online store. Inclusion criteria were age over 17 years and having lost a first-degree relative or partner within the last three years. Exclusion criteria were feeling too distressed by grief to answer loss-related questions or having experienced suicidal ideation in the last month. For the analysis in the present paper, participants who indicated that German was not their first language were excluded. A total of 195 participants gave informed consent; of these, 36 were excluded (German not first language, $n = 5$; premature termination of the survey, $n = 28$; systematic data pattern, $n = 3$). The final sample therefore consisted of 159 bereaved participants, who were mostly female (87%) and aged between 18 and 77 years ($M = 47$ years, $SD = 12$). Concerning time since loss, 23% indicated that the death had taken place less than six months ago, 21% that it had happened six to twelve months ago and most (55%) reported their loss dating back to between one and three years. Most participants (54%) had lost a partner/spouse, 37% had lost a child, 6% a parent and 3% a sibling. The mean Inventory of Complicated Grief (ICG) score in the present sample was 34.33 (±13.56); most participants (75%) demonstrated ICG scores higher than the established cut-off (> 25).

Measures

Demographic and loss-related variables

In addition to the following questionnaires, participants were asked to provide demographic data (age in years; gender) and loss-related information. Loss-related variables comprised time since loss (less than 6 months; 6–12 months; 12 months to 3 years), relationship to the deceased (i.e., partner/spouse, parent, child, sibling), and cause of death (i.e., medical condition, natural death, accident, suicide, perinatal complication, unresolved cause, other).

Grief rumination

The English Utrecht Grief Rumination Scale (UGRS) [19] was translated into German following the guidelines by Beaton et al. [31]. The German version of the UGRS (UGRS-D) is provided as Additional file 1.

The UGRS consists of 15 items detailing various types of thought about the causes and consequences of the loss; participants indicate how frequently they have experienced each of these in the past month. Answers are rated on a five-point scale ranging from 1 (never) to 5 (very often). Item scores are summed to generate an overall grief rumination score. Furthermore, five subscales can be computed, consisting of three items each. 'Reactions' (items 6, 7, 13) measures how frequently participants analyse their emotional reactions to the loss (example item: 'How often in the past month did you try to analyse your feelings about this loss precisely?') The subscale 'Injustice' (items 5, 11, 12) captures thoughts about the injustice of the loss (example item: 'How often in the past month did you wonder why this had to happen to you and not to someone else?'). 'Counterfactuals' (items 4, 8, 10) assesses counterfactual thinking about the events leading to the loss (example item: 'How often in the past month did you analyse if you could have prevented the death?'). The subscale 'Meaning' (items 1, 2, 15) measures thoughts about the meaning and the consequences of the death (example item: 'How often in the past month did you analyse what the personal meaning of the loss is for you?'). The subscale 'Relationships' (items 3, 9, 14) assesses thoughts related to reactions from the social environment (example item: 'How often in the past month did you think about how you would like others to react to your loss?'). Eisma et al. [19] showed that the internal consistency was excellent for the UGRS (Cronbach's $\alpha = .90$), and reliability measures of the subscales were good to excellent (Reactions, Cronbach's $\alpha = .84$; Injustice, Cronbach's $\alpha = .88$; Counterfactuals, Cronbach's $\alpha = .89$; Meaning, Cronbach's $\alpha = .84$; Relationships, Cronbach's $\alpha = .74$).

Depressive rumination

The Response Style Questionnaire 10D (RSQ-10D) [32, 33] is the German version of the Response Style Questionnaire short form established by Treynor et al. [16]. It captures ruminative styles, i.e. the subfacets 'brooding' and 'reflection' with proposed minimal content overlap with depressive symptoms. Both facets are each assessed by five items. Participants are asked to indicate how frequently they experience certain aspects of ruminative thinking on a four-point scale ranging from 1 (never) to 4 (almost always). An example item for brooding is: 'Why do I always react this way?'. An example item for reflection is: 'I write down what I am thinking and analyse it.' The brooding and reflection scales have demonstrated adequate internal consistencies (Cronbach's α in different samples: brooding: $.60 \leq \alpha \leq .75$; reflection: $.56 \leq \alpha \leq .75$) [32]. In this sample, Cronbach's α for the subscales was .74 for brooding and .66 for reflection.

Symptoms of anxiety and depression

To measure symptoms of anxiety and depression, the Hospital Anxiety and Depression Scale (HADS) [34] was used in its validated German version (HADS-D) [35]. On subscales of seven items each, participants were asked how frequently, or to what extent, they experienced symptoms of anxiety or depression in the last week on a four-point scale with different verbal expressions for every item. An example item addressing 'anxiety' is: 'I feel tense or wound up'. An (inverted) example item addressing 'depression' is: 'I feel cheerful'. The subscales have good internal consistencies (anxiety: Cronbach's $\alpha = .80$; depression: Cronbach's $\alpha = .81$) and the scale has been validated in representative samples of the general population [35]. In this sample, Cronbach's α for the subscales was .79 for anxiety and .88 for depression.

Complicated grief

The Inventory of Complicated Grief (ICG) [6] was used in its German version (ICG-D) [36]. It contains 19 items, which describe emotional, cognitive and behavioural states relevant to persistent disabling grief. Items are rated with regard to their current occurrence on a five-point Likert scale ranging from 0 (never) to 4 (always) and added to form a total score. The ICG-D has demonstrated excellent internal consistency (Cronbach's $\alpha = .94$) and good validity [36]. In this sample, Cronbach's α was .90. A cut-off of 25 and above has been established as identifying more disabling states of grief [6] and can be used to identify potential 'cases' of complicated grief (e.g. [37, 38]). This cut-off (together with a time criterion, cf. Statistical analyses) was also used in the present study to identify 'candidates' for a diagnosis of complicated grief, bearing in mind that a self-report measure alone is not sufficient for establishing a diagnosis.

Statistical analyses

In the UGRS, no missing data were observed; single missing items in other questionnaires were replaced according to the respective questionnaire's instructions (i.e. replacement of single missing items by mean of the scale/subscale). Very few participants failed to provide answers to single items, namely: ICG $n = 5$; HADS $n = 6$; RSQ-D $n = 6$.

For the UGRS, standard item analyses were calculated to determine mean item scores and standard deviations, item difficulties, item-total correlations (with the item itself excluded from the total score) and estimations of internal consistency when the item was omitted. Mean inter-item correlations, mean item difficulties and internal consistency (standardised Cronbach's α) of the UGRS and its subscales were computed. Confirmatory factor analyses with maximum likelihood estimation were calculated to test two models previously reported for the factorial structure of the English and Dutch versions [19]: The first model (model A) assumed five correlated factors (subscales) and the second model (model B) stipulated a single higher-order factor explaining the five subscales. Goodness of fit was assessed with the chi-square test, the root mean square error of approximation (RMSEA), the standardised root mean squared residual (SRMR), the comparative fit index (CFI) and the parsimony-adjusted comparative fit index (PCFI). The following are viewed as cut-off values indicating a good fit: χ/df ratio of ≥2, RMSEA< .05, SRMR< .06 and CFI ≥

.95 [39]. The Akaike Information Criterion (AIC) was computed as an index to compare the two models; while its absolute value is not informative, smaller AIC scores indicate a better model fit when comparing several models. Correlations of the UGRS with symptoms of complicated grief (ICG), anxiety and depression (HADS) and brooding and reflection as facets of rumination (RSQ-10D) were calculated; Bonferroni-corrected significance levels are reported to account for possible alpha error cumulation due to multiple comparisons. Reported correlation coefficients are Pearson coefficients; correlation coefficients were compared with Fisher's z-test.

Various facets of validity were investigated. Convergent validity was assessed by inspecting zero-order correlations of UGRS and brooding. Divergent validity was assessed by calculating zero-order correlation of UGRS and reflection; z-tests compared the correlations of UGRS with brooding and reflection, respectively, since grief rumination should be less closely related to reflection. This prediction relies on the distinction between adaptive and maladaptive forms of repetitive thinking [15, 16, 40]. Multiple facets of the UGRS (i.e. grief rumination about injustice and social relationships) [20] have been identified as maladaptive forms of repetitive thinking; yet only one facet of the UGRS has been identified as potentially adaptive (i.e. rumination about reactions). Therefore UGRS total scores should generally demonstrate a closer association with maladaptive (i.e. brooding) than with adaptive forms of repetitive thinking (i.e. reflection). Concurrent validity was investigated by calculating zero-order correlations of UGRS and ICG and testing this correlation against other measures of psychopathology (anxiety and depression), using z-tests. To further examine concurrent validity, a hierarchical regression analysis examined the associations of the UGRS score with symptoms of complicated grief (criterion). Only participants whose loss had occurred more than six months ago were included, in order to exclude those acutely bereaved from this analysis. Using forced blockwise entry, demographic and loss-related variables were entered first. The second step additionally included symptoms of depression and anxiety (HADS), the third step entered brooding and reflection as more general rumination constructs. Lastly, grief-specific rumination (UGRS) was entered into the model. No outliers or influential cases were identified based on the leverage value criterion described by Stevens [41] or Cook's distance values [42]. VIF and tolerance statistics indicated that no multicollinearity was present.

To investigate the discriminant validity of the UGRS, we compared potential candidates for a complicated grief diagnosis with non-candidates for such a diagnosis. A potential candidate for a complicated grief diagnosis was defined as a participant with an ICG score above the cut-off of 25 [6] who also fulfilled a criterion of how much time had passed since the loss. The time restriction was necessary to avoid misclassifications of acute grievers as candidates for a diagnosis of complicated grief. Currently, two possible time criteria are considered: more than six months (ICD-11) and more than twelve months (DSM 5). In order to account for both options, we used one independent t-test to compare participants above and below the ICG cut-off whose loss had occurred more than six months ago (ICD-11 time criterion) and a second t-test to compare participants above and below the ICG cut-off whose loss dated back more than twelve months (DSM 5 time criterion). If Levene's test indicated that variances were unequal, the Welch test is reported (and the degrees of freedom were adjusted accordingly). Where appropriate, Cohen's d is reported as a measure of effect size. The data analysis was carried out with IBM SPSS statistics 24; for the confirmatory factor analysis, the SPSS AMOS version 21.0.0 was used (IBM, Meadville, USA). Unless otherwise stated, the α level was set to $p = .05$.

Results

Item analysis

Item difficulties ranged between $p_i = .37$ (item 10) and $p_i = .80$ (item 2) with a mean difficulty of $p_i = .54$. The item-whole correlations of the individual items with the total score ranged from $r_{itc} = .45$ (item 10) to $r_{itc} = .64$ (item 9); the mean item-total correlation was $r_{itc} = .57$ and the mean inter-item correlation was $r = .36$ (see Table 1). The internal consistency of the whole scale was $\alpha = .89$ and the consistency would not have benefitted

Table 1 Item analyses of the German UGRS

Item	Mean	SD	Item Difficulty p_i	Corrected item-whole correlation r_{itc}	Cronbach's alpha if item is deleted
1	4.13	1.09	.78	.52	.89
2	4.21	1.10	.80	.56	.88
3	2.57	1.39	.39	.56	.88
4	2.80	1.53	.45	.58	.88
5	2.94	1.61	.49	.63	.88
6	3.55	1.25	.64	.51	.89
7	2.65	1.49	.41	.51	.89
8	3.21	1.49	.55	.62	.88
9	2.56	1.29	.39	.64	.88
10	2.50	1.56	.37	.45	.89
11	2.73	1.64	.43	.63	.88
12	3.30	1.53	.57	.62	.88
13	3.53	1.32	.63	.51	.89
14	2.97	1.28	.49	.51	.89
15	4.14	1.03	.78	.63	.88

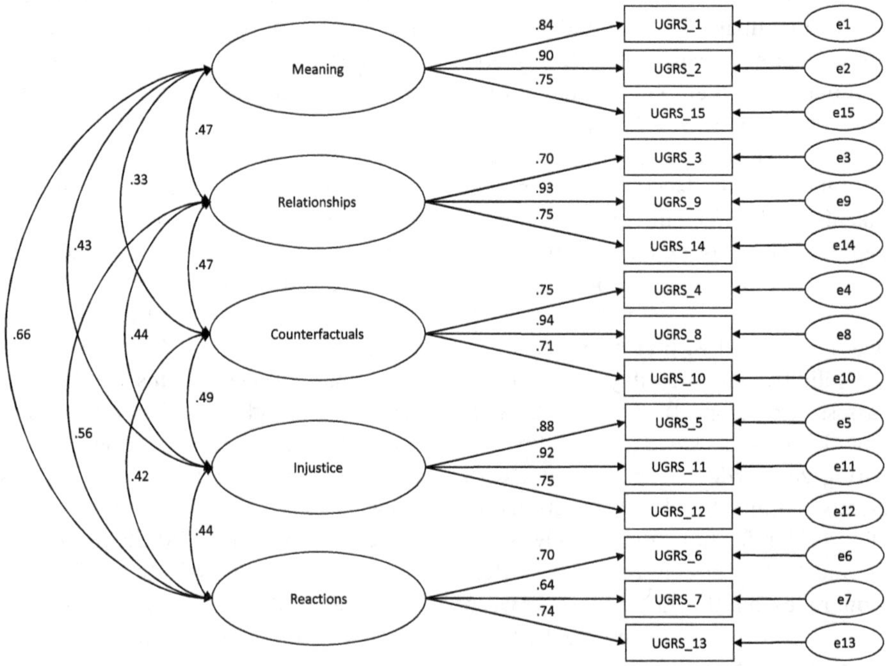

Fig. 1 Confirmatory factor analysis of the UGRS (Model A). Path diagram for confirmatory factor analysis of the UGRS with five intercorrelated, first-order factors showing standardised path coefficients (Model A). Error terms are denoted with a small 'e'. All path coefficients are significant at $p < .001$

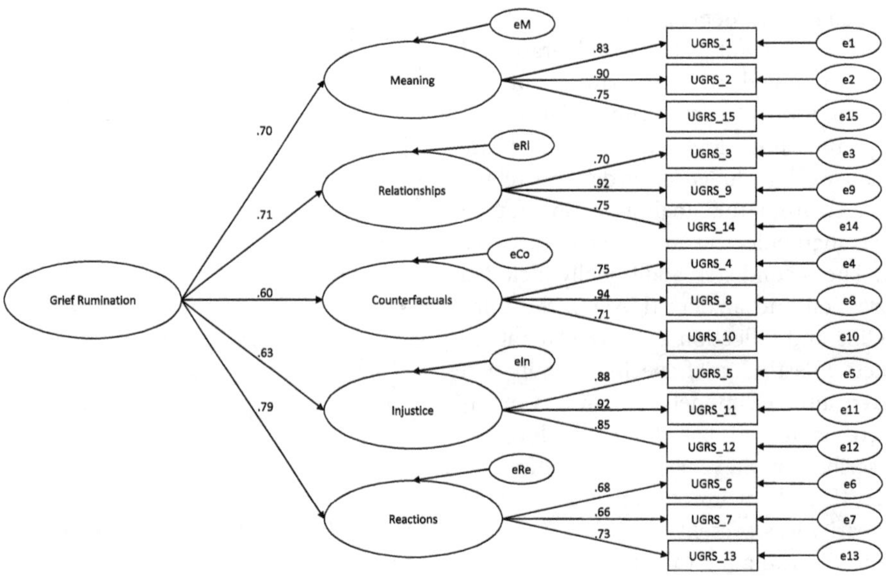

Fig. 2 Confirmatory factor analysis of the UGRS (Model B). Path diagram for confirmatory factor analysis of the UGRS with the five first-order factors and the latent construct Grief Rumination as a higher-order factor showing standardised path coefficients (Model B). Error terms are denoted with a small 'e'. All path coefficients are significant at at $p < .001$. *M* Meaning subscale, *Rl* Relationships subscale, *Co* Counterfactuals subscale, *In* Injustice subscale, *Re* Reactions subscale

Table 2 Fit indices for the models for the UGRS tested in the confirmatory factor analysis

Model	χ^2	df	p	χ^2/df	RMSEA [90% CI]	SRMR	CFI	PCFI	AIC
A	119.72	80	.003	1.50	.056 [.034; .076]	.054	.969	.738	229.72
B	132.31	85	<.001	1.59	.059 [.039; .078]	.064	.963	.780	232.31

Legend: Model A: five intercorrelated factors; Model B: five factors with one higher-order factor. *RMSEA* Root mean square error of approximation, *SRMR* Standardised root mean residual, *CFI* Comparative fit index, *PCFI* Parsimony-adjusted CFI, *AIC* Akaike information criterion

from removing any item. Internal consistencies of the UGRS subscales were: UGRS $_{\text{Meaning}}$ $\alpha = .86$; UGRS $_{\text{Relationships}}$ $\alpha = .82$; UGRS $_{\text{Counterfactuals}}$ $\alpha = .83$; UGRS $_{\text{Injustice}}$ $\alpha = .91$; and UGRS $_{\text{Reactions}}$ $\alpha = .72$.

Confirmatory factor analysis

In order to test the previously established five-factor structure [19], a confirmatory factor analysis was carried out for the UGRS. First, we examined model A, containing just five correlated factors with the respective subscale items as indicators (Fig.1 for the path diagram). Secondly, we tested a more parsimonious model B, in which the five subscales are themselves the indicators for one higher-order factor, i.e. Grief Rumination (Fig. 2 for the path diagram). Inspection of the fit indices (see Table 2) indicated that model A showed a marginally better fit than model B; this is also borne out by the comparative fit indices with the exception of the parsimony-adjusted fit index (PCFI), which favours the second model. For both models, all regression weights were significant ($p < .001$).

Validity

The UGRS sum score demonstrated significant correlations with both brooding and reflection. However, the correlation of the UGRS with brooding ($r_{\text{UGRS x Brooding}} = .56$, $p < .001$) was significantly higher than with reflection ($r_{\text{UGRS x reflection}} = .30$, $p < .001$) as indicated by the Fisher z-test [z(157) = 2.82, $p < .005$]. Interestingly though, the subscales showed varying associations with the rumination sub-facets brooding and reflection. 'Injustice' and 'Counterfactuals' were associated with brooding but not reflection, while all other subscales demonstrated significant correlations with both rumination sub-facets (see Table 3).

The UGRS sum score showed high correlations with symptoms of complicated grief symptoms as measured by the ICG. Correlations between the UGRS and indicators of anxiety and depression (HADS) were also significant. Using Fisher z-tests to compare the size of the coefficient $r_{\text{UGRS x ICG}}$ with that of the coefficient $r_{\text{UGRS x HADS-anxiety}}$ [z(157) = 3.80, $p < .001$] and $r_{\text{UGRS x HADS-depression}}$ [z(157) = 4.13, $p < .001$], demonstrated that the latter two were significantly smaller. Considering the UGRS subscales, their correlation pattern with complicated grief, anxiety and depression generally followed the sum score's pattern.

The hierarchical multiple regression on symptoms of complicated grief investigated the concurrent validity of the UGRS (see Table 4 for detailed results). It demonstrated in the first step that neither age, gender nor time since loss were significant predictors for ICG scores in this sample [$F(3,114) = 1.452$; $p = .232$, $adj.R^2 = .011$]. When entered in the next step, both symptoms of anxiety and depression contributed significantly to the prediction of ICG scores [$F(5,112) = 29.683$; $p < .001$; $adj.R^2 = .551$]. In the third model, brooding but not reflection explained a significant additional amount of variance [$F(7,110) = 24.817$; $p < .001$; $adj.R^2 = .588$]. UGRS scores were included in the model in the final step and improved the prediction of ICG scores significantly [$F(8,109) = 38.690$; $p < .001$; $adj.R^2 = .720$]. In this last model, regression coefficients for anxious and depressive symptoms remained significant predictors, while brooding lost its previous significance. This model explained 72% of variance in ICG scores.

In order to investigate the discriminant validity of the UGRS, two groups of candidates for possible diagnosis of complicated grief were established based on the ICG cut-off score and different timing criteria

Table 3 Correlations of the UGRS and its subscales with measures of grief, depression, anxiety and rumination

	ICG	HADS-Anxiety	HADS-Depression	Brooding	Reflection
UGRS Sum Score	.76***	.51***	.48***	.56***	.30***
Meaning	.54***	.38***	.39***	.24**	.19*
Relationships	.61***	.47***	.42***	.38***	.28***
Counterfactuals	.52***	.38***	.32***	.42***	.12
Injustice	.59***	.30***	.30***	.57***	.12
Reactions	.51***	.35***	.36***	.32***	.43***

Legend: * $p < .05$; ** $p < .01$; *** $p < .001$; Bonferroni-corrected threshold: $p < .0013$ (all p with *** are significant after Bonferroni correction). *HADS* Hosptial Anxiety and Depression Scale, *ICG* Inventory of Complicated Grief

Table 4 Results of the multiple hierarchical regression analysis

	B	SE B	β	ΔR^2
Step 1 (df = 3, 114)				.037
Constant	25.078	9.470	–	
Age	−0.024	0.117	−.020	
Gender	5.283	3.429	.145	
Time since loss	3.304	2.800	.109	
Step 2 (df = 2, 112)				.533***
Constant	−11.229	7.096	–	
Age	−0.051	0.080	−.041	
Gender	2.497	2.377	.068	
Time since loss	−0.977	1.923	−.032	
HADS-depression	1.487	0.219	.504***	
HADS-anxiety	1.119	0.244	.348***	
Step 3 (df = 2, 110)				.042**
Constant	−15.458	7.067	–	
Age	0.011	0.078	.009	
Gender	1.586	2.315	.043	
Time since loss	−1.639	1.866	−.054	
HADS-depression	1.446	0.216	.490***	
HADS-anxiety	0.898	0.243	.279***	
Brooding	1.012	0.298	.253**	
Reflection	−0.242	0.325	−.052	
Step 3 (df = 1, 109)				.127***
Constant	−17.326	5.824	–	
Age	−0.014	0.065	−.011	
Gender	1.496	1.906	.041	
Time since loss	−2.436	1.540	−.081	
HADS-depression	1.013	0.187	.344***	
HADS-anxiety	0.561	0.205	.174**	
Brooding	0.169	0.271	−.042	
Reflection	−0.175	0.267	−.038	
UGRS	0.511	0.070	.503***	

Legend: Results of the multiple hierarchical regression with forced blockwise entry. Criterion: complicated grief symptoms (ICG Score). Demographic characteristics and time since loss entered in the first block, depressive and anxiety symptoms in the second, brooding and reflection in the third, and grief-related rumination (UGRS Score) in the last block. ** $p < .01$, *** $p < .001$. Only participants were included whose loss occurred more than six months ago. Gender was dummy-coded; Time since loss was dummy-coded with 0 indicating a loss 12 to 36 months ago and 1 indicating a loss 6 to 12 months ago

(> 6 months for ICD-11; > 12 months for DSM 5). The UGRS sum score and its subscales differed significantly between the respective candidate groups for a diagnosis of complicated grief and groups of participants with the same time since loss but whose grief symptoms remained below the cut-off, with higher UGRS scores in the candidate groups (see Tables 5 and 6).

Discussion

This is the first study to present and validate a German version of the UGRS. In a sample of recently bereaved participants, the German UGRS was shown to have an identical factor structure to the original UGRS and the UGRS and its subscales demonstrated very good item properties, internal consistency and convergent, divergent, concurrent and discriminant validity.

The reliability of the UGRS in this study is high and comparable to those found for the English and Dutch versions. The internal consistencies of the subscales are – considering their extreme brevity – also very good. All item difficulties are in the medium range, which is recommended for maximum discriminatory power. Overall, the item-whole correlations with the total scale were high, with the exception of item 10, which was in the medium range.

Concerning the factorial structure, our analyses mirror the result of the original analyses in English and Dutch samples. They demonstrated that, even though the lower-order model with five correlated factors provided the best fit, a higher-order model with Grief Rumination as a second-order latent construct was only marginally outperformed [19]. Importantly, the fit indices of both competing models differed even less in our sample compared to the original analyses. Both absolute and comparative fit indices award a very small advantage to the lower-order model, albeit only marginally. Parsimony is an important aspect in evaluating model fit. Of note, the parsimony-adjusted fit index PCFI favours the hierarchical model. This argument for conceptualising the UGRS as containing one higher-order factor dovetails with the theoretical viewpoint, because grief rumination was intended as a unidimensional construct in which the subscales each represent a recurrent theme of repetitive thinking. Naturally, the themes will vary among bereaved people and not all themes will occur equally often in bereaved persons. However, the latent process of grief-specific rumination is thought to represent the unifying construct underlying these themes. Given the only marginal superiority of a lower-order model in the confirmatory factor analysis results of the English and Dutch UGRS [19] and our own data, it seems preferable to conceptualise the UGRS sum score as an indicator of grief-specific rumination.

The validity of the UGRS was supported further in our sample. Importantly, supporting the convergent and divergent validity of the UGRS, grief rumination was more closely associated with maladaptive types of ruminative thought (i.e. brooding) than more adaptive types (i.e. reflection). This replicates previous findings [19] even to the point that the UGRS subscales Injustice and Counterfactuals demonstrated no significant association with reflection. Both the UGRS sum score and all subscales showed high correlations with complicated grief. This concurs

Table 5 Candidates and Non-Candidates for complicated grief (time since loss > 12 months)

	CG candidates (n = 61)		Non-CG candidates (n = 27)		t	df	Cohen's d
	Mean	SD	Mean	SD			
UGRS Sum Score	50.50	12.39	33.52	7.41	7.96***	78.239	1.66
Meaning	12.87	2.75	10.04	3.04	4.31***	86	0.98
Relationships	8.72	3.58	5.33	2.09	5.55***	79.266	1.16
Counterfactuals	9.03	4.00	5.78	3.15	4.10***	62.471	0.90
Injustice	9.48	4.42	4.85	2.20	6.54***	84.773	1.32
Reactions	10.40	3.30	7.52	2.89	3.92***	86	0.93

Legend: *CG* complicated grief. Independent t-tests comparing candidates for complicated grief (ICG > 25) compared to persons below the cut-off (ICG ≤ 25), both with time since loss more than 12 months. If Levene's test indicated that variances were unequal, the Welch test is reported (and the degrees of freedom adjusted accordingly). *** $p < .001$

with theoretical accounts that view rumination as a mechanism which perpetuates complicated grief [8]. Associations between the UGRS and symptoms of anxiety and depression, which are often present concurrently in persons who suffer from complicated grief [43], were significant, yet the level of the associations also differed significantly: grief rumination was more closely associated with disabling grief than with symptoms of depression or anxiety, providing a first indication of the UGRS's discriminant validity. The regression analysis additionally demonstrated that the association between UGRS scores and symptoms of complicated grief holds even when simultaneously considering demographic and loss-related variables, depressive or anxiety symptoms, and other facets of rumination. The proportion of variance explained was high. Of note, UGRS scores explained incremental variance in ICG scores, over and above the aforementioned constructs. This speaks for the importance of grief-specific rumination as an independent construct.

Lastly, we investigated whether UGRS scores differed between participants with and without an increased likelihood of receiving a diagnosis of complicated grief. To this end, we classified participants according to the established symptom level cut-off in the ICG as candidates or non-candidates for complicated grief, applying different time criteria. The loss had to have happened at least six months ago (time criterion ICD-11) or twelve months ago (time criterion DSM 5). Irrespective of the time criterion, the UGRS scores were elevated strongly (Cohen's $d = 1.66$ and $d = 1.60$) in both candidate groups when compared with the group with less likelihood of receiving a diagnosis of complicated grief. This speaks for the discriminant validity of the UGRS.

Several limitations must be borne in mind when interpreting the results. All data are based on online self-reporting and are cross-sectional in nature. The sample consisted predominantly of conjugally bereaved females, which mirrors the over-representation of this subgroup in most grief research [44], but is not representative of the general bereaved population. While we have no reasons to assume that the associations under investigation are different for lower-educated people and men, future studies on rumination following loss should aim to recruit more representative samples. The findings refer to a convenience sample of bereaved persons, which allows comparison with previous UGRS psychometric research, but they require replication in a clinical sample of patients who suffer from complicated grief in order to ascertain that the associations remain stable across the complete range of disabling grief symptoms. Complicated grief is a diagnosis that is undergoing (re-) conceptualisations with the revisions of the classification

Table 6 Candidates and Non-Candidates for complicated grief (time since loss > 6 months)

	CG candidates (n = 89)		Non-CG candidates (n = 32)		t	df	Cohen's d
	Mean	SD	Mean	SD			
UGRS Sum Score	51.34	11.82	34.88	8.45	8.44***	76.566	1.60
Meaning	13.18	2.47	10.25	2.92	5.50***	120	1.09
Relationships	8.93	3.31	5.56	2.49	5.98***	72.635	1.15
Counterfactuals	9.01	3.88	5.84	3.34	4.41***	62.837	0.87
Injustice	9.72	4.39	5.66	3.17	5.60***	75.562	1.06
Reactions	10.51	3.13	7.56	2.77	4.70***	119	1.00

Legend: *CG* Complicated grief. Independent t-test comparing candidates for complicated grief (ICG > 25) to persons below the cut-off (ICG ≤ 25), both with time since loss more than 6 months. If Levene's test indicated that variances were unequal, the Welch test is reported (and the degrees of freedom adjusted accordingly). *** $p < .001$

systems. Even though the ICG is one of the best established and most-used instruments for assessing disabling grief symptoms, it is unclear to what extent the ICG and its established cut-offs concur with the diagnostic criteria of Persistent Complex Bereavement Disorder (DSM 5) or Prolonged Grief Disorder (ICD-11), which limits the generalisability of our results. Additionally, information on grief symptom levels in our sample was based on self-report: no clinical diagnosis can be made based solely on this information. Therefore, we have referred to our diagnostic categories based on the ICG cautiously as 'candidates for complicated grief' in order to account for this diagnostic uncertainty.

Conclusion

Further knowledge about the role of grief rumination may benefit the optimal treatment of patients who suffer from complicated grief: if grief rumination is an avoidance strategy (RAH [10]), psychotherapy should be tailored to address it, for instance by using exposure therapy. First evaluations of grief treatments that include interventions specifically targeting grief-related rumination have shown promising results concerning complicated grief [45, 46]. If, however, rumination is a confrontation strategy (RST [11]), distraction may be more beneficial. Value-oriented behavioural activation could represent one therapeutic strategy to achieve this goal; its clinical usefulness for grief treatment has already been demonstrated [46–48]. Based on these seemingly contradictory accounts, a recent review concludes that the two frameworks may be complementary and that there may be more than one way to effectively address grief rumination [13]. Thus, future research is needed to establish (1) whether grief rumination is an aetiological or a maintaining factor in complicated grief; (2) which theoretical framework best explains its role in adjustment to bereavement; and (3) whether reductions in grief rumination levels mediate the effectiveness of interventions for severely distressed bereaved persons. Establishing validated instruments to assess malleable cognitive constructs relevant to complicated grief, such as grief rumination will likely contribute to this goal.

Abbreviations

CG: Complicated grief; DSM 5: Diagnostic and Statistical Manual for Mental Disorders, 5th edition; HADS: Hospital Anxiety and Depression Scale; ICD-11: International Classification of Diseases, 11th edition; ICG: Inventory of Complicated Grief; PCBD: Persistent Complex Bereavement Disorder; PGD: Prolonged Grief Disorder; RAH: Rumination as Avoidance Hypothesis; RSQ 10D: Response Styles Questionnaire 10D; RST: Response Styles Theory; UGRS: Utrecht Grief Rumination Scale

Acknowledgements

Not applicable.

Funding

No funding source.

Authors' contributions

BKD and MCE conceptualised the project. TF carried out recruiting and data acquisition and helped prepare the manuscript. BKD and AB performed the statistical analysis. All authors contributed to the manuscript preparation and read and approved the final manuscript.

Consent for publication

Not applicable.

Competing interests

The authors declare that they have no competing interests.

Author details

[1]Clinical Psychology & Psychotherapy, Department of Psychology, Philipps-University Marburg, Marburg, Germany. [2]Department of Clinical Psychology and Experimental Psychopathology, University of Groningen, Groningen, The Netherlands.

References

1. Stroebe M, Schut H, Stroebe W. Health outcomes of bereavement. Lancet. 2007;370(9603):1960–73.
2. American Psychiatric Association: The Diagnostic and Statistical Manual of Mental Disorders: DSM 5. bookpointUS; 2013.
3. Keeley JW, Reed GM, Roberts MC, Evans SC, Robles R, Matsumoto C, et al. Disorders specifically associated with stress: a case-controlled field study for ICD-11 mental and behavioural disorders. Int J Clin Health Psychol. 2015;2: 109–27.
4. Maercker A, Brewin CR, Bryant RA, Cloitre M, Reed GM, van Ommeren M, et al. Proposals for mental disorders specifically associated with stress in the international classification of Diseases-11. Lancet. 2013;381(9878):1683–5.
5. Lundorff M, Holmgren H, Zachariae R, Farver-Vestergaard I, O'Connor M. Prevalence of prolonged grief disorder in adult bereavement: a systematic review and meta-analysis. J Affect Disord. 2017;212:138–49.
6. Prigerson HG, Maciejewski PK, Reynolds CF, Bierhals AJ, Newsom JT, Fasiczka A, et al. Inventory of complicated grief: a scale to measure maladaptive symptoms of loss. Psychiatry Res. 1995;59(1):65–79.
7. Querstret D, Cropley M. Assessing treatments used to reduce rumination and/or worry: a systematic review. Clin Psychol Rev. 2013;33(8):996–1009.
8. Boelen PA, Van Den Hout MA, Van Den Bout J. A cognitive-behavioral conceptualization of complicated grief. Clin Psychol Sci Pract. 2006;13(2): 109–28.
9. Segerstrom SC, Stanton AL, Alden LE, Shortridge BE. A multidimensional structure for repetitive thought: what's on your mind, and how, and how much? J Pers Soc Psychol. 2003;85(5):909.
10. Stroebe M, Boelen PA, Van Den Hout M, Stroebe W, Salemink E, Van Den Bout J. Ruminative coping as avoidance. Eur Arch Psychiatry Clin Neurosci. 2007;257(8):462–72.
11. Nolen-Hoeksema S. Ruminative coping and adjustment to bereavement. In: Stroebe MS, Hansson RO, Stroebe W, Schut H, editors. Handbook of bereavement research: consequences, coping and care. Washington DC: American Psychological Association; 2001. p. 545–62.
12. Watkins ER, Moulds ML. Rumination in complicated grief. In: Stroebe MA, Schut HA, van den Bout J, editors. Complicated grief: scientific foundations for health care professionals. New York: Routledge; 2013. p. 162–75.
13. Eisma MC, Stroebe MS. Rumination following bereavement: an overview. Bereave Care. 2017;36(2):58–64.
14. Nolen-Hoeksema S, Wisco BE, Lyubomirsky S. Rethinking rumination. Perspect Psychol Sci. 2003;5:400–24.
15. Watkins ER. Constructive and Unconstructive repetitive thought. Psychol Bull. 2008;134(2):163.
16. Treynor W, Gonzalez R, Nolen-Hoeksema S. Rumination reconsidered: a psychometric analysis. Cognit Ther Res. 2003;27(3):247–59.
17. van der Houwen K, Schut H, van den Bout J, Stroebe M, Stroebe W. The efficacy of a brief internet-based self-help intervention for the bereaved.

Behav Res Ther. 2010;48(5):359–67.
18. Morina N. Rumination and avoidance as predictors of prolonged grief, depression, and posttraumatic stress in female widowed survivors of war. J Nerv Ment Dis. 2011;199(12):921–7.
19. Eisma MC, Stroebe MS, Schut HA, Van Den Bout J, Boelen PA, Stroebe W. Development and psychometric evaluation of the Utrecht grief rumination scale. J Psychopathol Behav Assess. 2014;36(1):165–76.
20. Eisma MC, Schut HAW, Stroebe MS, Boelen PA, van den Bout J, Stroebe W. Adaptive and maladaptive rumination after loss: a three-wave longitudinal study. Br J Clin Psychol. 2015;54(2):163–80.
21. Ito T, Tomita T, Hasui C, Otsuka A, Katayama Y, Kawamura Y, et al. The link between response styles and major depression and anxiety disorders after child-loss. Compr Psychiatry. 2003;44(5):396–403.
22. Nolen-Hoeksema S, Parker LE, Larson J. Ruminative coping with depressed mood following loss. J Pers Soc Psychol. 1994;67(1):92–104.
23. Nolen-Hoeksema S, McBride A, Larson J. Rumination and psychological distress among bereaved partners. J Pers Soc Psychol. 1997;72(4):855–62.
24. Eisma M, Stroebe M, Schut H, Boelen P, van den Bout J, Stroebe W. 'Waarom is dit mij overkomen?'Ontwikkeling en validatie van de Utrechtse RouwRuminatieSchaal. Gedragstherapie. 2012;43:369–88.
25. Eisma MC, Stroebe MS, Schut HAW, Stroebe W, Boelen PA, van den Bout J. Avoidance processes mediate the relationship between rumination and symptoms of complicated grief and depression following loss. J Abnorm Psychol. 2013;122(4):961.
26. Michael T, Halligan SL, Clark DM, Ehlers A. Rumination in posttraumatic stress disorder. Depress Anxiety. 2007;24(5):307–17.
27. Schwartzberg SS, Janoff-Bulman R. Grief and the search for meaning: exploring the assumptive worlds of bereaved college students. J Soc Clin Psychol. 1991;10(3):270–88.
28. Eisma MC, Schut HAW, Stroebe MS, van den Bout J, Stroebe W, Boelen PA. Is rumination after bereavement linked with loss avoidance? Evidence from eye-tracking. PLoS One. 2014;9(8):e104980.
29. Eisma MC, Rinck M, Stroebe MS, Schut HAW, Boelen PA, Stroebe W, et al. Rumination and implicit avoidance following bereavement: an approach avoidance task investigation. J Behav Ther Exp Psychiatry. 2015;47:84–91.
30. Nolen-Hoeksema S, Morrow J. A prospective study of depression and posttraumatic stress symptoms after a natural disaster: the 1989 Loma Prieta earthquake. J Pers Soc Psychol. 1991;61(1):115–21.
31. Beaton DE, Bombardier C, Guillemin F, Ferraz MB. Guidelines for the process of cross-cultural adaptation of self-report measures. Spine. 2000;25(24):3186–91.
32. Huffziger S, Kühner C. Die Ruminationsfacetten brooding und reflection. Z Klin Psychol Psychother. 2012;41(1):38–46.
33. Kühner C, Huffziger S, Nolen-Hoeksema S. Response styles questionnaire: RSQ-D. Göttingen: Hogrefe; 2007.
34. Zigmond AS, Snaith RP. The hospital anxiety and depression scale. Acta Psychiatr Scand. 1983;67(6):361–70.
35. Herrmann-Lingen C, Buss U, Snaith P. Hospital Anxiety and Depression Scale-Deutsche Version (HADS-D). 3rd ed. Bern: Huber; 2011.
36. Lumbeck G, Brandstätter M, Geissner E. Erstvalidierung der Deutschen Version des "Inventory of Complicated Grief" (ICG-D). Z Klin Psychol Psychother. 2013;41(4):243–8.
37. Newson RS, Boelen PA, Hek K, Hofman A, Tiemeier H. The prevalence and characteristics of complicated grief in older adults. J Affect Disord. 2011; 132(1):231–8.
38. Kristensen P, Weisaeth L, Heir T. Predictors of complicated grief after a natural disaster: a population study two years after the 2004 south-east Asian tsunami. Death Stud. 2010;34(2):137–50.
39. Schreiber JB, Nora A, Stage FK, Barlow EA, King J. Reporting structural equation modeling and confirmatory factor analysis results: a review. J Educ Res. 2006;99(6):323–38.
40. Olatunji BO, Naragon-Gainey K, Wolitzky-Taylor KB. Specificity of rumination in anxiety and depression: a multimodal meta-analysis. Clin Psychol Sci Pract. 2013;20:225–57.
41. James S. Applied multivariate statistics for the social sciences. Mahwah, NJ: Lawrence Erlbaum Associates, Inc; 2002.
42. Cook RD, Weisberg S. Residuals and influence in regression. New York: Chapman & Hall; 1982.
43. Simon NM, Shear KM, Thompson EH, Zalta AK, Perlman C, Reynolds CF, et al. The prevalence and correlates of psychiatric comorbidity in individuals with complicated grief. Compr Psychiatry. 2007;48(5):395–9.
44. Doering BK, Eisma MC. Treatment for complicated grief: state of the science and ways forward. Curr Opin Psychiatry. 2016;29(5):286–91.
45. Bryant RA, Kenny L, Joscelyne A, Rawson N, Maccallum F, Cahill C, et al. Treating prolonged grief disorder: a randomized clinical trial. JAMA Psychiatry. 2014;71(12):1332–9.
46. Eisma MC, Boelen PA, van den Bout J, Stroebe W, Schut HA, Lancee J, et al. Internet-based exposure and behavioral activation for complicated grief and rumination: a randomized controlled trial. Behav Ther. 2015;46(6):729–48.
47. Papa A, Sewell MT, Garrison-Diehn C, Rummel C. A randomized open trial assessing the feasibility of behavioral activation for pathological grief responding. Behav Ther. 2013;44(4):639–50.
48. Papa A, Rummel C, Garrison-Diehn C, Sewell MT. Behavioral activation for pathological grief. Death Stud. 2013;37(10):913–36.

9

Psychometric properties of the Arabic version of the confusion assessment method for the intensive care unit (CAM-ICU)

Maha H. Aljuaid[1], Ahmad M. Deeb[2*], Maamoun Dbsawy[3], Daniah Alsayegh[4], Moteb Alotaibi[4] and Yaseen M. Arabi[5,6]

Abstract

Background: It is recommended that critically ill patients undergo routine delirium monitoring with a valid and reliable tool such as the Confusion Assessment Method for the Intensive Care Unit (CAM-ICU). However, the validity and reliability of the Arabic version of the CAM-ICU has not been investigated. Here, we test the validity and reliability of the Arabic CAM-ICU.

Methods: We conducted a psychometric study at ICUs in a tertiary-care hospital in Saudi Arabia. We recruited consecutive adult Arabic-speaking patients, who had stayed in the ICU for at least 24 hours, and had a Richmond Agitation-Sedation Scale (RASS) score ≥ − 2 at examination. Two well-trained examiners (ICU nurse and intensivist) independently assessed delirium in eligible patients with the Arabic CAM-ICU. Evaluations by the two examiners were compared with psychiatrist blind clinical assessment of delirium according to the Diagnostic and Statistical Manual of Mental Disorders, Fifth Edition (DSM-5). Subgroup analyses were conducted for age, invasive mechanical ventilation, and gender.

Results: We included 108 patients (mean age: 62.6 ± 17.6; male: 51.9%), of whom 37% were on invasive mechanical ventilation. Delirium was diagnosed in 63% of enrolled patients as per the psychiatrist clinical assessment. The Arabic CAM-ICU sensitivity was 74% (95% confidence interval [CI] = 0.63–0.84) and 56% (95%CI = 0.44–0.68) for the ICU nurse and intensivist, respectively. Specificity was 98% (95%CI = 0.93–1.0) and 92% (95%CI = 0.84–1.0), respectively. Sensitivity was greater for mechanically-ventilated patients, women, and those aged ≥65 years. Specificity was greater for those aged < 65 years, non-mechanically-ventilated patients and men. The median duration to complete the Arabic CAM-ICU was 2 min (interquartile range, 2–3) and 4.5 min (IQR, 3–5) for the ICU nurse and intensivist, respectively. Inter-rater reliability (kappa) was 0.66.

Conclusions: The Arabic CAM-ICU demonstrated acceptable reliability and validity to assess delirium in Arabic-speaking ICU patients.

Keywords: Delirium, CAM-ICU, Arabic, Critical care, Mechanical ventilation, Geriatric, Cognition, Inattention

* Correspondence: rn_a_deeb@hotmail.com
[2]King Abdullah International Medical Research Center, Research Office, King Abdulaziz Medical City, Ministry of National Guard Health Affairs, King Saud bin Abdulaziz University for Health Sciences, Riyadh, Saudi Arabia
Full list of author information is available at the end of the article

Background

Delirium is defined as a disturbance in attention and awareness that fluctuates over a short period of time and accompanied by changes in cognition or perceptual disturbances [1]. Delirium is extremely common in critically ill patients, resulting from the acute illness, comorbidities, and use of sedation and analgesia. Furthermore, delirium is influenced by environmental and physical factors in intensive care unit (ICU) settings, such as isolation, limited visiting hours, the use of restraint, and connection to multiple tubes, lines, and catheters [2–5].

Previous studies report that delirium occurs in between 21% and 84% of critically ill patients [6–11]. Moreover, delirium is linked to poor ICU and hospital outcomes, such as increased morbidity, increased length of stay at the ICU and hospital, self-extubation, removal of lines and catheters, and increased treatment cost [5, 10–14]. In addition, delirium is associated with increased morbidity and mortality, [11, 15, 16] and increased cognitive and functional deficits after hospital discharge [17, 18].

Routine monitoring of delirium is considered as a quality indicator for optimum care in older patients [19], and was recommended in 2013 by clinical practice guidelines for the management of pain, agitation, and delirium in adult patients in the ICU [20]. However, delirium is underdiagnosed and monitoring of delirium tends to be sporadic and underperformed [13, 21–23]. Therefore, the routine use of valid and reliable tools to assess for the presence of delirium is recommended at least once per ICU shift for patients with a high risk of delirium [20].

The Confusion Assessment Method for the ICU (CAM-ICU) is a rapid, reliable, and valid tool to assess delirium in the ICU [6]. The CAM-ICU is an adapted version of the bedside assessment tool for non-psychiatrists, the Confusion Assessment Method (CAM), which was based on the Diagnostic and Statistical Manual of Mental Disorders, Third Edition, Revised (DSM-III-R) [24]. The CAM-ICU demonstrates good validity and reliability when administered by ICU nurses and physicians for both ventilated and non-ventilated ICU patients [6, 25–27].

The CAM-ICU has been translated into several languages, with high reliability and validity [28–33]. Indeed, the CAM-ICU has been translated into Arabic by the ICU Delirium and Cognitive Impairment Study Group at Vanderbilt University Medical Center for Health Services Research [34]. However, the tool has not yet been tested for validity and reliability. The use of a valid and reliable Arabic delirium assessment tool is crucial to diagnose, prevent, and manage delirium among Arabic-speaking ICU patients.

In this study, we assess the psychometric properties of the current Arabic version of the CAM-ICU and its applicability to Arabic-speaking critical care patients' at a tertiary care hospital in Saudi Arabia.

Methods

Setting

We conducted this psychometric validation study at the Intensive Care Department (ICD) in King Abdulaziz Medical City (KAMC), Riyadh, Saudi Arabia. KAMC is a 1000-bed teaching tertiary care centre accredited by the Joint Commission International (JCI). The ICD encompasses a 21-bed medical ICU, 9-bed surgical ICU, 8-bed trauma ICU, 8-bed neuro-critical care unit, and 14-bed intermediate care unit. These units are staffed by onsite board-certified intensivists for 24 hours a day, 7 days a week. The average nurse: patient ratio is 1:1. Clinical rounds are multidisciplinary and include physicians, critical care nurses, clinical pharmacists, dieticians, physiotherapists and respiratory therapists. This study was approved by the institutional review board of KAMC and funded by the King Abdullah International Medical Research Center.

All study participants or substitute decision-makers (for patients lacking decision-making capacity) signed informed consent before participation. A consecutive sample technique was used to obtain the targeted sample size. Screening was conducted twice weekly during the day shift in the ICD between April 2016 and March 2017.

Study participants

In this study, we included Arabic-speaking critically ill patients at the ICD, aged ≥18 years and with a Richmond Agitation-Sedation Scale (RASS) ≥ -2, who had stayed for at least 24 hours in the ICU. We excluded patients with the following: pre-existing severe dementia or psychosis; neurologic diseases including traumatic brain injury, acute brain lesion, or spinal cord injury; burns; patients admitted because of drug overdose; patients with blindness or deafness; those with Glasgow Coma Scale < 9 at the time of screening; patients unable to complete assessments as they are medically unstable; and patients/substitute decision-makers who refused to sign informed consent form and participate in the study.

Sample size

Previous studies have reported that delirium occurs in between 21% and 84% of critically ill patients [6–11]. Based on previous non-English CAM-ICU validation studies, sensitivity ranges from 73% to 92% and specificity ranges from 72% to 100% [29–31, 33, 35]. Accordingly, we expected values for sensitivity and specificity of 85%. Therefore, with an estimated mid-percentage of delirium prevalence of 50%, and an acceptable width of 95% confidence interval (CI) for sensitivity and specificity to no greater than 10% (75–95%), we calculated a minimum required sample size of 98 [36]. To account for potential dropouts and to compensate for assessments that could not be done within 4 hours by all assessors or missing assessment by any assessor, we anticipated a sample size of 125 patients.

Procedures

The CAM-ICU has already been translated into Arabic by the ICU Delirium and Cognitive Impairment Study Group at Vanderbilt University Medical Center for Health Services Research. The tool (both visual and auditory sections) was translated to suit the cultural and educational background of Arabic-speaking populations. The translations were conducted independently by two members before they discussed it together. The final Arabic version was then back translated to the original language (English) by a professional independent translator [34].

The Arabic CAM-ICU comprises the same four features that are used in the English CAM-ICU to screen patients for delirium. These features include: 1) acute onset of mental status changes or a fluctuating course; 2) inattention; and 3) altered level of consciousness; or 4) disorganized thinking. For inattention, the Arabic CAM-ICU uses mainly number sequences (e.g. 6 3 1 1 4 1 5 7 1 8) instead of letter sequences (e.g. S A V E A H A A R T). However, using alternate sequences of Arabic letters is possible. In addition, some words were changed in items assessing disorganized thinking to suit the Arabic speaking culture (e.g. pounds changed to kilos) [34]. As with the CAM-ICU, a patient is considered delirious if he/she test positive for features 1 and 2, in addition to being positive for either feature 3 or 4 [34]. The Arabic CAM-ICU and the training manual are available from the ICU Delirium and Cognitive Impairment Study Group website [34].

In our validation study, two well-trained examiners (an ICU Clinical Nurse Specialist and Intensivist) independently assessed delirium in eligible ICU patients with the Arabic CAM-ICU. They performed the CAM-ICU in the same group of patients but without any specific order, with an allowed duration of up to 4 hours between two exams for each patient. All assessments were performed during the day shift.

In addition, an experienced psychiatrist specialising in geriatric psychiatry independently assessed the same ICU patients for delirium according to the Diagnostic and Statistical Manual of Mental Disorders, Fifth Edition (DSM-5) criteria [1] within the same 4 hours window of evaluation as the ICU examiners. All assessors were blinded to the results of the others until the end of the study. The results of the psychiatric screening were compared with those of the ICU examiners screening. All assessors are authors in this study.

Data collection

The following data was recorded: date and time of assessments; assessment location; gender; age; use of mechanical ventilation; RASS score [37]; and delirium assessment results (Arabic CAM-ICU and psychiatrist clinical assessment).

Statistical analysis

The psychometric properties of the Arabic CAM-ICU were calculated for the ICU nurse and intensivist separately compared with the psychiatrist clinical assessment of delirium. We calculated the sensitivity, specificity, positive likelihood ratio (LR+), negative likelihood ratio (LR-), positive predictive values, negative predictive values, pretest probability, pretest odds, posttest odds, posttest probability, accuracies, and prevalence. Subgroup analyses were conducted for age, invasive mechanical ventilation status, and gender.

Agreement (inter-rater reliability) was assessed by calculating Cohen's kappa. Continuous data are represented by mean ± standard deviation (SD) or median (quartile Q1, Q2). Calculations were performed with the Statistical Package for the Social Sciences version 24 (SPSS Inc., Chicago, IL, USA).

Results

Patient characteristics

From 129 patients, a total of 125 patients agreed to participate and were enrolled in the study. Of these, 17 patients were excluded from the study analysis for the following reasons: duration of assessments between examiners exceeded the allowed 4 hours ($n = 13$); diagnosis of chronic schizophrenia ($n = 1$); diagnosis with drug addiction ($n = 1$); psychiatrist clinical assessment of delirium not completed ($n = 1$); and psychiatrist clinical assessment of delirium missing ($n = 1$).

We included 108 patients in the final analysis, among which the CAM-ICU was conducted by a nurse and the clinical assessment of delirium by psychiatrist in 108 patients, and the CAM-ICU was conducted by an intensivist for 106 patients. Approximately half of the patients were male (51.9%), and the mean age of participants was 62.6 ± 17.6 years with a median of 66 years (interquartile range: 63.8–75 years). The majority of participants were not on invasive mechanical ventilation ($n = 68$, 63%).

With the psychiatrist clinical assessment, delirium was diagnosed in 68 patients (63%).

Psychometric properties of the Arabic CAM-ICU conducted by an ICU nurse

The Arabic CAM-ICU conducted by an ICU nurse identified 51 delirious patients (47.2%). We calculated a sensitivity of 74% (95%CI = 63–84%) and a specificity of 98% (95%CI = 93–100%). The LR+ was 29.4

(95%CI = 29.4–29.5) and the LR- was 0.27 (95%CI = 0.15–0.39). Table 1 presents the other psychometric properties of the Arabic CAM-ICU conducted by an ICU nurse. The median duration to complete the Arabic CAM-ICU by the nurse was 2 min (interquartile range: 2–3 min).

We conducted subgroup analyses for age group, mechanical ventilation status, and gender. In patients older than or equal 65 years, the sensitivity was 79% (95%CI = 67–91%) and the specificity was 95% (95%CI = 85–100%). In patients younger than 65 years, the sensitivity was 64% (95%CI = 45–83%) and the specificity was 100% (95%CI = 100–100%). Table 2 presents other psychometric properties of the Arabic CAM-ICU according to age.

In patients with invasive mechanical ventilation, the sensitivity was 75% (95%CI = 58–92%) and the specificity was 94% (95%CI = 82–100%). In patients without invasive mechanical ventilation, the sensitivity was 73% (95%CI = 60–86%) and the specificity was 100% (95%100–100%). Table 3 presents other psychometric properties of the Arabic CAM-ICU according to invasive mechanical ventilation status.

In male patients, the sensitivity was 71% (95%CI = 55–86%) and the specificity was 100% (95%CI = 100–100%). In female patients, the sensitivity was 77% (95%CI = 62–91%) and the specificity was 94% (95%CI = 84–100%). Table 4 presents other psychometric properties of the Arabic CAM-ICU according to gender.

Psychometric properties of the Arabic CAM-ICU conducted by an intensivist

The Arabic CAM-ICU conducted by an intensivist identified 41 delirious patients (38.7%), with a sensitivity of 56% (95%CI = 44–68%), and a specificity of 92% (95%CI = 84–100%). The LR+ was 7.1 (95%CI = 7–7.2) and the LR- was 0.48 (95%CI = 0.36–0.60). Table 1 presents other psychometric properties of the Arabic CAM-ICU conducted by an intensivist. The median duration to complete the Arabic CAM-ICU by an intensivist was 4. 5 min (interquartile range: 3–5 min).

We conducted subgroup analyses for age group, mechanical ventilation status, and gender. In patients older than or equal 65 years, the sensitivity was 65% (95%CI = 51–79%) and the specificity was 90% (95%CI = 76–100%). In patients younger than 65 years, the sensitivity was 40% (95%CI = 21–59%) and the specificity was 95% (95%CI = 85–100%). Table 2 presents other psychometric properties of the Arabic CAM-ICU according to age.

In patients with invasive mechanical ventilation, the sensitivity was 70% (95%CI = 51–88%) and the specificity was 88% (95%CI = 71–100%). In patients without invasive mechanical ventilation, the sensitivity was 50% (95%CI = 34–64%) and the specificity was 96% (95%CI = 87–100%). Table 3 presents other psychometric properties of the Arabic CAM-ICU according to invasive mechanical ventilation status.

In male patients, the sensitivity was 47% (95%CI = 30–64%) and the specificity was 95% (95%CI = 85–100%). In female patients, the sensitivity was 65% (95%CI = 49–81%) and the specificity was 89% (95%CI = 74–100%). Table 4 presents other psychometric properties of the Arabic CAM-ICU according to gender.

Reliability of the Arabic CAM-ICU

We assessed the level of agreement between assessments with the Arabic CAM-ICU conducted by the ICU nurse and intensivist by calculating inter-rater reliability (kappa). Assessments were matched in 88 patients (83%) with a kappa of 0.66 (standard error: 0.07; $p < 0.0001$).

Table 1 Psychometric properties of the Arabic CAM-ICU

Property	CAM-ICU by nurse (n = 108)	CAM-ICU by intensivist (n = 106)
Sensitivity (95%CI)	0.74 (0.63–0.84)	0.56 (0.44–0.68)
Specificity (95%CI)	0.98 (0.93–1.0)	0.92 (0.84–1.0)
Likelihood ratio, LR+ (95%CI)	29.4 (29.4–29.5)	7.1 (7–7.2)
Likelihood ratio, LR- (95%CI)	0.27 (0.15–0.39)	0.48 (0.36–0.60)
Positive predicted value (95%CI)	0.98 (0.94–1.0)	0.93 (0.85–1.0)
Negative predicted value (95%CI)	0.68 (0.56–0.81)	0.54 (0.42–0.66)
Pre-test probability	0.63	0.64
Pre-test odds	1.7	1.79
Post-test odds	50	12.7
Post-test probability	0.98	0.93
Delirium prevalence, CAM-ICU vs. psychiatrist clinical assessment	47.2% vs. 63%	38.7% vs. 64.2%
Accuracy	82.4%	68.9%

CAM-ICU Confusion Assessment Method for the Intensive Care Unit, *CI* Confidence interval

Table 2 Psychometric properties of the Arabic CAM-ICU according to age

Property	CAM-ICU by nurse (n = 62)	CAM-ICU by intensivist (n = 62)
Age ≥ 65 years		
Sensitivity (95%CI)	0.79 (0.67–0.91)	0.65 (0.51–0.79)
Specificity (95%CI)	0.95 (0.85–1.0)	0.90 (0.76–1.0)
Likelihood Ratio LR+ (95%CI)	15.0 (15.0–15.1)	6.2 (6.1–6.3)
Likelihood Ratio LR- (95%CI)	0.22 (0.04–0.40)	0.39 (0.22–0.56)
Positive predicted value (95%CI)	0.97 (0.92–1.0)	0.93 (0.84–1.0)
Negative predicted value (95%CI)	0.67 (0.49–0.84)	0.53 (0.36–0.70)
Pre-test probability	0.69	0.69
Pre-test odds	2.26	2.26
Post-test odds	34.00	14
Post-test probability	0.97	0.93
Delirium prevalence, CAM-ICU vs. psychiatrist clinical assessment	56.5% vs. 69.4%	48.4% vs. 69.4%
Accuracy	83.9%	72.6%
Age < 65 years		
Sensitivity (95%CI)	0.64 (0.45–0.83)	0.40 (0.21–0.59)
Specificity (95%CI)	1.0 (1.0–1.0)	0.95 (0.85–1.0)
Likelihood Ratio LR+ (95%CI)	Undefined*	7.6 (7.4–7.8)
Likelihood Ratio LR- (95%CI)	0.36 (0.20–0.52)	0.63 (0.46–0.80)
Positive predicted value (95%CI)	1.0 (1.0–1.0)	0.91 (0.74–1.1)
Negative predicted value (95%CI)	0.70 (0.54–0.86)	0.55 (0.38–0.72)
Pre-test probability	0.54	0.57
Pre-test odds	1.19	1.32
Post-test odds	Undefined**	10
Post-test probability	Undefined***	0.91
Delirium prevalence, CAM-ICU vs. psychiatrist clinical assessment	34.8% vs. 54.4%	25% vs. 56.8%
Accuracy	80.4%	63.6%

CAM-ICU Confusion Assessment Method for the Intensive Care Unit, *CI* confidence interval *Specificity value is 1; **Likelihood Ratio is undefined; ***Post-test odd is undefined

Discussion

In this study, we demonstrated the psychometric properties of the Arabic CAM-ICU. In this study, patients were assessed for delirium by an intensivist and ICU nurse with the Arabic CAM-ICU, and these assessments were compared with the psychiatrist clinical assessment according to DSM-5. In addition, subgroup analyses were conducted for age, mechanical ventilation status, and gender to determine the validity of the Arabic CAM-ICU in specific groups.

Previous studies have reported that delirium occurs in between 21% and 84% of critically ill patients [6–11]. In this study, the psychiatrist clinical assessment identified delirium in 63% of critically ill patients. This data suggests that delirium is similarly common among critically ill patients in the Arabic-speaking population. This high rate of delirium highlights the importance of a reliable and valid measure to assess delirium for critically ill patients in the ICU. In addition, it suggests the need for urgent action to establish delirium treatment and prevention measures.

Assessment of the Arabic CAM-ICU by the ICU nurse had a sensitivity of 74%. The sensitivity increased to 75% for mechanically ventilated patients, 77% for female patients, and 79% for patients aged ≥65 years. Although sensitivity in our study is less than that reported in the initial validation study for the English CAM-ICU by Ely et al. (93–100%) [6, 27], it was within the ranges reported by other validation studies for non-English versions of the CAM-ICU (73–92%) [29–33, 35]. Therefore, we believe that the sensitivity for the Arabic CAM-ICU is acceptable.

Assessment of the Arabic CAM-ICU by the ICU nurse had a specificity of 98%. The specificity increased to 100% for patients aged < 65 years, non-mechanically ventilated patients, and male patients. The specificity of

Table 3 Psychometric properties of the Arabic CAM-ICU according to mechanical ventilation status

Property	CAM-ICU by nurse (n = 40)	CAM-ICU by intensivist (n = 39)
Mechanical ventilation		
Sensitivity (95%CI)	0.75 (0.58–0.92)	0.70 (0.51–0.88)
Specificity (95%CI)	0.94 (0.82–1.0)	0.88 (0.71–1.0)
Likelihood Ratio LR+ (95%CI)	12 (11.9–12.1)	5.57 (5.4–5.7)
Likelihood Ratio LR- (95%CI)	0.27 (0.07–0.46)	0.35 (0.15–0.55)
Positive predicted value (95%CI)	0.95 (0.85–1.0)	0.89 (0.74–1.0)
Negative predicted value (95%CI)	0.71 (0.52–0.91)	0.67 (0.47–0.87)
Pre-test probability	0.60	0.59
Pre-test odds	1.5	1.44
Post-test odds	18.0	8.0
Post-test probability	0.95	0.89
Delirium prevalence, CAM-ICU vs. psychiatrist clinical assessment	47.5% vs. 60%	46.2% vs. 59%
Accuracy	82.5%	76.9%
No mechanical ventilation		
Sensitivity (95%CI)	0.73 (0.60–0.86)	0.50 (0.34–0.64)
Specificity (95%CI)	1.0 (1.0–1.0)	0.96 (0.87–1.0)
Likelihood Ratio LR+ (95%CI)	Undefined*	10.8 (10.7–10.8)
Likelihood Ratio LR- (95%CI)	0.27 (0.12–0.43)	0.54 (0.39–0.68)
Positive predicted value (95%CI)	1.0 (1.0–1.0)	0.96 (0.87–1.0)
Negative predicted value (95%CI)	0.67 (0.51–0.82)	0.48 (0.33–0.63)
Pre-test probability	0.65	0.67
Pre-test odds	1.83	2.05
Post-test odds	Undefined**	22.0
Post-test probability	Undefined***	0.96
Delirium prevalence, CAM-ICU vs. psychiatrist clinical assessment	47.1% vs. 64.7%	34.3% vs. 67.2%
Accuracy	82.4%	64.2%

CAM-ICU Confusion Assessment Method for the Intensive Care Unit, *CI* confidence interval * Specificity value is 1; ** Likelihood Ratio is undefined; *** Post-test odd is undefined

the Arabic CAM-ICU is consistent with that reported by Ely et al. (89–100%) [6, 27], which suggests that the specificity of the Arabic CAM-ICU is acceptable. Taking our results together, the Arabic CAM-ICU appears to be a valid tool for the assessment of delirium among Arabic-speaking critically ill patients.

Nonetheless, our results did show some discrepancies between raters. Although comparable values for specificity were achieved between raters (98% vs. 92%), there was greater discrepancy in sensitivity values (74% vs. 56%). These discrepancies have not been reported in other studies that have used nurses and intensivists as CAM-ICU raters [27, 32]. In the study by Ely et al., sensitivity values of the CAM-ICU for two nurses and an intensivist were 95%, 96%, and 100%, respectively, and specificity values were 93%, 93%, and 89%, respectively [27]. Moreover, in a Spanish study, sensitivity values of the CAM-ICU for an ICU nurse and an intensivist were 83% and 80%, respectively, and specificity was 96% for both raters [32]. Nonetheless, in our study, the raters' assessments were matched in 83% patients with a kappa of 0.66, which is considered moderate and acceptable inter-rater reliability [38]. We believe that the accuracy of the CAM-ICU assessment could be further improved by providing proper education about delirium and training for the CAM-ICU [33, 39, 40].

This is the first study to assess the reliability and validity of the Arabic CAM-ICU as a delirium assessment tool for critically ill patients. Our study has several strengths including a relatively large and powered sample size. In addition, it measured inclusive psychometric features of the Arabic CAM-ICU. Furthermore, we conducted subgroup analyses to measure the psychometric features of the Arabic CAM-ICU in specific groups. This is the first study to highlight delirium rate for Arabic-speaking critically ill patients. The main limitation of the

Table 4 Psychometric properties of the Arabic CAM-ICU according to gender

Property	CAM-ICU by nurse (n = 56)	CAM-ICU by intensivist (n = 54)
Male		
Sensitivity (95%CI)	0.71 (0.55–0.86)	0.47 (0.30–0.64)
Specificity (95%CI)	1.0 (1.0–1.0)	0.95 (0.85–1.0)
Likelihood Ratio LR+ (95%CI)	Undefined*	9.4 (9.3–9.5)
Likelihood Ratio LR- (95%CI)	0.29 (0.13–0.46)	0.56 (0.40–0.72)
Positive predicted value (95%CI)	1.0 (1.0–1.0)	0.94 (0.83–1.0)
Negative predicted value (95%CI)	0.69 (0.53–0.85)	0.51 (0.35–0.67)
Pre-test probability	0.61	0.63
Pre-test odds	1.55	1.70
Post-test odds	Undefined**	16
Post-test probability	Undefined***	0.94
Delirium prevalence, CAM-ICU vs. psychiatrist clinical assessment	42.9% vs. 60.7%	31.5% vs. 63%
Accuracy	82.1%	64.8%
Female		
Sensitivity (95%CI)	0.77 (0.62–0.91)	0.65 (0.49–0.81)
Specificity (95%CI)	0.94 (0.84–1.0)	0.89 (0.74–1.0)
Likelihood Ratio LR+ (95%CI)	13.8 (13.7–13.8)	5.82 (5.71–5.93)
Likelihood Ratio LR- (95%CI)	0.25 (0.07–0.43)	0.40 (0.21–0.58)
Positive predicted value (95%CI)	0.96 (0.89–1.0)	0.92 (0.81–1.0)
Negative predicted value (95%CI)	0.68 (0.50–0.86)	0.57 (0.39–0.76)
Pre-test probability	0.65	0.65
Pre-test odds	1.89	1.89
Post-test odds	26.0	11
Post-test probability	0.96	0.92
Delirium prevalence, CAM-ICU vs. psychiatrist clinical assessment	51.9% vs. 65.4%	46.2% vs. 65.4%
Accuracy	82.7%	73.1%

CAM-ICU Confusion Assessment Method for the Intensive Care Unit, *CI* confidence interval * Specificity value is 1; ** Likelihood Ratio is undefined; *** Post-test odd is undefined

study is that it assessed inattention components of the Arabic CAM-ICU with the auditory attention screening exam only. We recommend that for future studies to investigate the reliability and validity of the visual attention screening exam of the Arabic CAM-ICU. In addition, we excluded patients with neurological diseases including traumatic brain injury; such neurological diseases may dispose patients to different neuropsychiatric consequences [41]. The CAM-ICU may not be the optimal tool to assess delirium in such patients [42]. Developing specific tools to assess and differentiate delirium from other neuropsychiatric dysfunctions is recommended for future research [42].

Conclusions

The Arabic CAM-ICU demonstrated acceptable reliability and validity to assess delirium in Arabic-speaking ICU patients. We recommend researchers and clinicians to use the Arabic CAM-ICU as delirium assessment tool for Arabic-speaking ICU patients, taking into consideration the knowledge and training needed of delirium assessment. Further studies including the Arabic CAM-ICU would identify its further strengths and limitations in research and clinical fields.

Abbreviations

CAM: Confusion Assessment Method; CAM-ICU: Confusion assessment method for the intensive care unit; CI: Confidence interval; DSM-5: Diagnostic and Statistical Manual of Mental Disorders, Fifth Edition; ICU: Intensive care unit; IQR: Interquartile range; JCI: Joint Commission International; KAMC: King Abdulaziz Medical City; LR +: Positive likelihood ratio; LR-: Negative likelihood ratio; RASS: Richmond Agitation-Sedation Scale; SD: Standard deviations

Acknowledgements

We would like to thank Professor E. Wesley Ely and the ICU-Delirium and Cognitive Impairment Study Group for the support and recommendations given to our study team.

Funding
This study was supported by research grant RC15/091/R awarded to MA1 by King Abdullah International Medical Research Center (Ministry of National Guard Health Affairs, Mail Code: 1515 PO Box 3660 Riyadh 11481, Kingdom of Saudi Arabia). The study sponsor did not have any role in the study design, collection, management, analysis, or interpretation of the data, or in writing the report.

Authors' contributions
MA1, AD, MD, DA, MA2, and YA contributed to the study conception and design, data acquisition, analytical plan, and critical revision of the manuscript. MA1 and AD drafted the manuscript and contributed to interpretation of the data. AD conducted data analysis. MA1 conducted the nurse CAM-ICU assessment, MD conducted the physician CAM-ICU assessment and DA conducted the psychiatrist clinical assessment of delirium according to DSM-5. All authors have read and approved the final version of the manuscript.

Consent for publication
Not applicable.

Competing interests
The authors declare that they have no competing interests.

Author details
[1]King Abdullah International Medical Research Center, Nursing Department, King Abdulaziz Medical City, Ministry of National Guard Health Affairs, King Saud bin Abdulaziz University for Health Sciences, Riyadh, Saudi Arabia. [2]King Abdullah International Medical Research Center, Research Office, King Abdulaziz Medical City, Ministry of National Guard Health Affairs, King Saud bin Abdulaziz University for Health Sciences, Riyadh, Saudi Arabia. [3]King Abdullah International Medical Research Center, Intensive Care Department, King Abdulaziz Medical City, Ministry of National Guard Health Affairs, King Saud bin Abdulaziz University for Health Sciences, Riyadh, Saudi Arabia. [4]King Abdullah International Medical Research Center, Mental Health Department, King Abdulaziz Medical City, Ministry of National Guard Health Affairs, King Saud bin Abdulaziz University for Health Sciences, Riyadh, Saudi Arabia. [5]King Abdullah International Medical Research Center, College of Medicine, King Saud Bin Abdulaziz University for Health Sciences, Riyadh, Saudi Arabia. [6]Intensive Care Department, King Abdulaziz Medical City, National Guard Health Affairs, Riyadh, Saudi Arabia.

References

1. American Psychiatric Association. Diagnostic and statistical manual of mental disorders. 5th ed. Arlington, VA: American Psychiatric Publishing; 2013. p. 596–602.
2. Ouimet S, Kavanagh BP, Gottfried SB, Skrobik Y. Incidence, risk factors and consequences of ICU delirium. Intensive Care Med. 2007;33(1):66–73.
3. Van Rompaey B, Elseviers MM, Schuurmans MJ, Shortridge-Baggett LM, Truijen S, Bossaert L. Risk factors for delirium in intensive care patients: a prospective cohort study. Crit Care. 2009;13(3):R77.
4. McCusker J, Cole M, Abrahamowicz M, Han L, Podoba JE, Ramman-Haddad L. Environmental risk factors for delirium in hospitalized older people. J Am Geriatr Soc. 2001;49(10):1327–34.
5. Dubois MJ, Bergeron N, Dumont M, Dial S, Skrobik Y. Delirium in an intensive care unit: a study of risk factors. Intensive Care Med. 2001;27(8):1297–304.
6. Ely EW, Inouye SK, Bernard GR, Gordon S, Francis J, May L, Truman B, Speroff T, Gautam S, Margolin R, et al. Delirium in mechanically ventilated patients: validity and reliability of the confusion assessment method for the intensive care unit (CAM-ICU). JAMA. 2001;286(21):2703–10.
7. Chanques G, Payen JF, Mercier G, de Lattre S, Viel E, Jung B, Cissé M, Lefrant JY, Jaber S. Assessing pain in non-intubated critically ill patients unable to self report: an adaptation of the behavioral pain scale. Intensive Care Med. 2009;35(12):2060–7.
8. Sharma A, Malhotra S, Grover S, Jindal SK. Incidence, prevalence, risk factor and outcome of delirium in intensive care unit: a study from India. Gen Hosp Psychiatry. 2012;34(6):639–46.
9. Shehabi Y, Botha JA, Boyle MS, Ernest D, Freebairn RC, Jenkins IR, Roberts BL, Seppelt IM. Sedation and delirium in the intensive care unit: an Australian and New Zealand perspective. Anaesth Intensive Care. 2008;36(4):570–8.
10. Thomason JW, Shintani A, Peterson JF, Pun BT, Jackson JC, Ely EW. Intensive care unit delirium is an independent predictor of longer hospital stay: a prospective analysis of 261 non-ventilated patients. Crit Care. 2005;9(4):R375–81.
11. Ouimet S, Riker R, Bergeron N, Cossette M, Kavanagh B, Skrobik Y. Subsyndromal delirium in the ICU: evidence for a disease spectrum. Intensive Care Med. 2007;33(6):1007–13.
12. Lin SM, Liu CY, Wang CH, Lin HC, Huang CD, Huang PY, Fang YF, Shieh MH, Kuo HP. The impact of delirium on the survival of mechanically ventilated patients. Crit Care Med. 2004;32(11):2254–9.
13. Ely EW, Stephens RK, Jackson JC, Thomason JW, Truman B, Gordon S, Dittus RS, Bernard GR. Current opinions regarding the importance, diagnosis, and management of delirium in the intensive care unit: a survey of 912 healthcare professionals. Crit Care Med. 2004;32(1):106–12.
14. Milbrandt EB, Deppen S, Harrison PL, Shintani AK, Speroff T, Stiles RA, Truman B, Bernard GR, Dittus RS, Ely EW. Costs associated with delirium in mechanically ventilated patients. Crit Care Med. 2004;32(4):955–62.
15. Witlox J, Eurelings LS, de Jonghe JF, Kalisvaart KJ, Eikelenboom P, van Gool WA. Delirium in elderly patients and the risk of postdischarge mortality, institutionalization, and dementia: a meta-analysis. JAMA. 2010;304(4):443–51.
16. McCusker J, Cole M, Abrahamowicz M, Primeau F, Belzile E. Delirium predicts 12-month mortality. Arch Intern Med. 2002;162(4):457–63.
17. Jackson JC, Gordon SM, Hart RP, Hopkins RO, Ely EW. The association between delirium and cognitive decline: a review of the empirical literature. Neuropsychol Rev. 2004;14(2):87–98.
18. Girard TD, Jackson JC, Pandharipande PP, Pun BT, Thompson JL, Shintani AK, Gordon SM, Canonico AE, Dittus RS, Bernard GR, et al. Delirium as a predictor of long-term cognitive impairment in survivors of critical illness. Crit Care Med. 2010;38(7):1513–20.
19. Sloss EM, Solomon DH, Shekelle PG, Young RT, Saliba D, MacLean CH, Rubenstain LZ, Schnelle JF, Kamberg CJ, Wenger NS. Selecting target conditions for quality of care improvement in vulnerable older adults. J Am Geriatr Soc. 2000;48(4):363–9.
20. Barr J, Fraser GL, Puntillo K, Ely EW, Gélinas C, Dasta JF, Davidson JE, Devlin JW, Kress JP, Joffe AM, et al. Clinical practice guidelines for the management of pain, agitation, and delirium in adult patients in the intensive care unit. Crit Care Med. 2013;41(1):263–306.
21. Spronk PE, Riekerk B, Hofhuis J, Rommes JH. Occurrence of delirium is severely underestimated in the ICU during daily care. Intensive Care Med. 2009;35(7):1276–80.
22. Mac Sweeney R, Barber V, Page V, Ely EW, Perkins GD, Young JD, McAuley DF. A national survey of the management of delirium in UK intensive care units. QJM. 2010;103(4):243–51.
23. Mehta S, Burry L, Fischer S, Martinez-Motta JC, Hallett D, Bowman D, Wong C, Meade MO, Steward TE, Cook DJ. Canadian survey of the use of sedatives, analgesics, and neuromuscular blocking agents in critically ill patients. Crit Care Med. 2006;34(2):374–80.
24. Inouye SK, van Dyck CH, Alessi CA, Balkin S, Siegal AP, Horwitz RI. Clarifying confusion: the confusion assessment method. A new method for detection of delirium. Ann Intern Med. 1990;113(12):941–8.
25. Devlin JW, Fong JJ, Fraser GL, Riker RR. Delirium assessment in the critically ill. Intensive Care Med. 2007;33(6):929–40.
26. Pun BT, Gordon SM, Peterson JF, Shintani AK, Jackson JC, Foss J, Harding SD, Bernard GR, Dittus RS, Ely EW. Large-scale implementation of sedation and delirium monitoring in the intensive care unit: a report from two medical centers. Crit Care Med. 2005;33(6):1199–205.
27. Ely EW, Margolin R, Francis J, May L, Truman B, Dittus R, Speroff T, Gautam S, Bernard GR, Inouye SK. Evaluation of delirium in critically ill patients: validation of the confusion assessment method for the intensive care unit (CAM-ICU). Crit Care Med. 2001;29(7):1370–9.
28. Gaspardo P, Peressoni L, Comisso I, Mistraletti G, Ely EW, Morandi A. Delirium among critically ill adults: evaluation of the psychometric properties of the Italian 'Confusion assessment method for the intensive care Unit'. Intensive Crit Care Nurs. 2014;30(5):283–91.
29. Gusmao-Flores D, Salluh JIF, Dal-Pizzol F, Ritter C, Tomasi CD, de Lima MAS D, Santana LR, Lins RMP, Lemos PP, Serpa CV, et al. The validity and reliability of the Portuguese versions of three tools used to diagnose delirium in critically ill patients. Clinics. 2011;66(11):1917–22.

30. Pipanmekaporn T, Wongpakaran N, Mueankwan S, Dendumrongkul P, Chittawatanarat K, Khongpheng N, Duangsoy N. Validity and reliability of the Thai version of the confusion assessment method for the intensive care unit (CAM-ICU). Clin Interv Aging. 2014;9:879–85.
31. Heo EY, Lee BJ, Hahm BJ, Song EH, Lee HA, Yoo CG, Kim YW, Han SK, Shim YS, Lee SM. Translation and validation of the Korean confusion assessment method for the intensive care unit. BMC Psychiatry. 2011;11:94.
32. Tobar E, Romero C, Galleguillos T, Fuentes P, Cornejo R, Lira MT, de la Barrera L, Sánchez JE, Bozán F, Bugedo G, et al. Confusion Assessment Method for diagnosing delirium in ICU patients (CAM-ICU): cultural adaptation and validation of the Spanish version. Med Intensiva. 2010;34(1):4–13. [Article in Spanish]
33. Adamis D, Dimitriou C, Anifantaki S, Zachariadis A, Astrinaki I, Alegakis A, Mari H, Tsiatsiotis N. Validation of the Greek version of confusion assessment method for the intensive care unit (CAM-ICU). Intensive Crit Care Nurs. 2012;28(6):337–43.
34. Delirium and Cognitive Impairment Study Group: CAM-ICU Resources in Additional Language Translations. http://www.icudelirium.org/delirium/languages.html Accessed 5 Feb 2018.
35. Guenther U, Popp J, Koecher L, Muders T, Wrigge H, Ely EW, Putensen C. Validity and reliability of the CAM-ICU flowsheet to diagnose delirium in surgical ICU patients. J Crit Care. 2010;25(1):144–51.
36. Buderer NM. Statistical methodology: I. Incorporating the prevalence of disease into the sample size calculation for sensitivity and specificity. Acad Emerg Med. 1996;3(9):895–900.
37. Sessler CN, Gosnell MS, Grap MJ, Brophy GM, O'Neal PV, Keane KA, Tesoro EP, Elswick RK. The Richmond agitation-sedation scale: validity and reliability in adult intensive care unit patients. Am J Respir Crit Care Med. 2002; 166(10):1338–44.
38. McHugh ML. Interrater reliability: the kappa statistic. Biochem Med. 2012; 22(3):276–82.
39. Brummel NE, Vasilevskis EE, Han JH, Boehm L, Pun BT, Ely EW. Implementing delirium screening in the intensive care unit: secrets to success. Crit Care Med. 2013;41(9):2196–208.
40. DiLibero J, O'Donoghue SC, DeSanto-Madeya S, Felix J, Ninobla A, Woods A. An innovative approach to improving the accuracy of delirium assessments using the confusion assessment method for the intensive care unit. Dimens Crit Care Nurs. 2016;35(2):74–80.
41. Arciniegas DB, Topkoff J, Silver JM. Neuropsychiatric aspects of traumatic brain injury. Curr Treat Options Neurol. 2000;2(2):169–86.
42. Frenette AJ, Bebawi ER, Deslauriers LC, Tessier AA, Perreault MM, Delisle MS, Bertrand JC, Desjardins M, Rico P, Khwaja K, et al. Validation and comparison of CAM-ICU and ICDSC in mild and moderate traumatic brain injury patients. Intensive Care Med. 2016;42(1):122–3.

10

Psychosocial factors affecting resilience in Nepalese individuals with earthquake-related spinal cord injury

Muna Bhattarai[1*], Khomapak Maneewat[2] and Wipa Sae-Sia[2]

Abstract

Background: One of many types of injuries following an earthquake is spinal cord injury (SCI) which is a life-long medically complex injury and high-cost health problem. Despite several negative consequences, some persons with SCI are resilient enough to achieve positive adjustment, greater acceptance, and better quality of life. Since resilience is influenced by several factors and can vary by context, it is beneficial to explore factors that affect the resilience of people who sustained spinal cord injury from the 2015 earthquake in Nepal.

Methods: A descriptive cross-sectional study included 82 participants from the Spinal Injury Rehabilitation Center and communities in Nepal. Participants completed the Demographic and Injury-related Questionnaire, Connor-Davidson Resilience Scale, Multidimensional Scale of Perceived Social Support, Moorong Self-efficacy Scale, Intrinsic Spirituality Scale, and Patient Health Questionnaire-9. Pearson's correlation and point biserial correlation analyses were performed to examine associations between resilience and independent variables. A hierarchical regression analysis was used to identify the influence of certain factors.

Results: Findings indicated significant associations between resilience and social support ($r = 0.42$, $p < 0.001$), self-efficacy ($r = 0.53$, $p < 0.001$), depressive mood ($r = -0.50$, $p < 0.001$) and demographic variables which included sex ($r = 0.47$, $p < 0.001$), employment ($r = 0.27$, $p = 0.016$), and current living location ($r = 0.24$, $p = 0.029$). There was a non-significant association between resilience and spirituality ($r = -0.12$, $p > 0.05$). In hierarchical regression analysis, an overall regression model explained 46% of the variance in resilience. Self-efficacy ($\beta = 0.28$, $p = 0.007$) and depressive mood ($\beta = -0.24$, $p = 0.016$) significantly determined resilience after controlling the effect of demographic variables. Among the demographic factors, being male significantly explained the variance in resilience ($\beta = 0.31$, $p = 0.001$).

Conclusions: Multiple psychosocial and demographic factors were associated with resilience in people who sustained an earthquake-related SCI. Mental health professionals should demonstrate concern and consider such factors in allocating care in this group. Development of intervention research concerning resilience is recommended to strengthen resilience in order to improve rehabilitation outcomes and enhance reintegration of individuals with SCI into their communities.

Keywords: Resilience, Social support, Self-efficacy, Spirituality, Depressive mood, Earthquake, Spinal cord injury, Nepal

* Correspondence: bhattarai.moona@gmail.com
[1]Hope International College, Kathmandu 44600, Nepal
Full list of author information is available at the end of the article

Background

Earthquakes are devastating natural disasters that cause catastrophic impacts and extensive damage to property, residences, economics, physical and psychological health, and even human life [1]. Among the neurological injuries following an earthquake, spinal cord injury (SCI) is a life-long medically complex injury and high-cost health problem that affects physical, psychological and social health, and the well-being of an individual [2]. In Nepal, an earthquake of 7.8 magnitude and a subsequent aftershock of 7.3 magnitude in April and May 2015 left more than 173 Nepalese people suffering from SCI [3].

SCI causes complete or incomplete loss of motor and sensory functions including muscle paralysis, impairment of bladder and bowel control, and sexual function [4]. Along with physical complications, the psychosocial consequences that follow SCI are anxiety, depression, social withdrawal, low self-confidence, post-traumatic stress disorder, and suicidal thoughts and attempts. As a result, these conditions further affect and worsen rehabilitation and overall health [5–7]. Individuals who sustained disabilities, including SCI from an earthquake, reported higher psychological distress than the normal survivors of an earthquake [8]. Thus, both the earthquake and SCI are stressful traumatic events that have numerous negative consequences on survivors.

Resilience or the ability of an individual to thrive in the face of adversity [9] plays a vital role among people with SCI to overcome the catastrophic changes and negative impacts from the consequences of SCI [10, 11]. Resilience can be defined as the ability of a person with SCI to bounce back from a stressful experience and adapt to the changes resulting from a SCI [12]. Research showed that 66% of individuals who sustained a SCI were resilient [13]. As a result, they achieved positive adjustment, greater acceptance, and a better quality of life [10, 13]. However, about 34% had significant problems with resilience such as depressed mood or low self-efficacy [13]. It was recognized that resilience is influenced by numerous factors. Factors contributing to resilience can vary and have different impacts on individuals in different cultures, societies, and geographical regions or contexts [14, 15].

Several factors have been explored and evidenced to either enhance or impede resilience in persons with SCI and victims of earthquakes [6, 16–18]. Previous studies revealed that self-efficacy, social support [13, 19], and spirituality [11, 20, 21] enhanced resilience in persons with SCI, whereas depression/depressive mood [6, 11, 16, 19], stress, anxiety, and internal locus of control [6] impeded resilience of those individuals. Previous findings regarding the influence of demographic and injury-related factors on resilience are still inconclusive [6, 13, 16, 22]. Most of the aforementioned factors were also found to affect resilience in individuals surviving earthquakes or other disasters [17, 18, 23]. Nonetheless, there is still a dearth of studies exploring factors affecting resilience of persons who sustained SCI from disasters including earthquakes.

In addition, previous studies were conducted regarding resilience factors among people with SCI and survivors of earthquake but mostly in developed countries [6, 13, 17]. This leads to the question of generalizability of those results in the context of Nepal. Nepal is a developing country which has a different culture, geographical distribution, and healthcare system. Nepal is a collectivist society and many Nepalese live in rural areas that lack the availability of healthcare services [24]. Thus, factors affecting resilience among Nepalese with earthquake-related SCI could be different from people in other geographical and cultural contexts. This study hypothesized that psychosocial factors, i.e., social support, self-efficacy, spirituality, and depressive mood, determine resilience among Nepalese with the 2015 earthquake-related SCI.

Methods

Design and setting

This descriptive cross-sectional study was carried out in Nepal between December 2016 and February 2017. The participants were recruited from the Spinal Injury Rehabilitation Center (SIRC) in Kavre district, which is the major rehabilitation center for people with SCI in Nepal, and in community settings. The communities included eight districts of Nepal which were affected by the 2015 earthquake: Kathmandu, Lalitpur, Bhaktapur, Kavre, Sindupalchowk, Gorkha, Dhading, and Nuwakot.

Participants

Inclusion criteria for the participants were: (1) individuals who sustained SCI from the 2015 Nepal earthquake; (2) aged 18 years or older; (3) had been admitted to the SIRC for rehabilitation; (4) living in the community of eight districts after discharge from the SIRC; (4) understand and speak the Nepali language; and (5) conscious and absence of severe cognitive impairment (based on information obtained from the medical records and history taking). Of 117 patients with earthquake-related SCI admitted to the SIRC, the list and contact details of 101 individuals were obtained. The sample size of equal to or greater than 50 + (8 times the number of factors) was calculated based on the sample size calculation technique of multiple regression [25]. Therefore, 82 participants were recruited in this study using convenience sampling. Six participants who were readmitted for management of complications were included from the SIRC. Another 76 eligible participants were contacted via cell phone. Since all of them agreed to participate, they were approached in their communities. Written informed consent was obtained from each participant. Data collection was done via interview or self-administration of questionnaires depending on the ability of the participants to read and write.

Measurements

The demographic and injury-related questionnaire was developed by the researchers. The demographic variables included sex, ethnicity, current living location, marital status, education, employment, income, and types of caregiver. The injury-related variables comprised of injury level, completeness of injury, chronic disease, and complications related to SCI. Data related to injury level, completeness of injury, chronic disease, and complications were retrieved from the medical records, interview, observation, and physical examination.

Five standardized research instruments were used for data collection. These tools were translated into the Nepali language using the back translation process [26]. The Connor-Davidson Resilience Scale (CD-RISC) was used to measure resilience. The CD-RISC examines resilience as the ability to cope in the face of adversity and is comprised of five factors: (1) personal competence, high standards, and tenacity; (2) trust in one's instincts, tolerance of negative affect, and strengthening effects of stress; (3) positive acceptance of change and secure relationships; (4) control; and (5) spiritual influences. The CD-RISC consists of 25 items scored on a 5-point Likert scale which ranges from 0 (not true at all) to 4 (true nearly at all of the time). The range of total possible scores is from 0 to 100, where higher scores indicate greater resilience [9]. The tool has demonstrated adequate validity and reliability among persons with SCI [11] and victims of an earthquake [18]. The present study reported a Cronbach's alpha of 0.82 for the Nepali version of the CD-RISC.

The Multidimensional Scale of Perceived Social Support (MSPSS) was used to measure social support. The MSPSS measures perceived social support from three sources: family, friends, and significant other [27]. The tool consists of 12 items scored on a 7-point Likert scale ranging from 1 (very strongly disagree) to 7 (very strongly agree). Total scores range from 12 to 84, where higher scores represent greater perceived social support. Evidence of validity and reliability has been provided with adequate Cronbach's alpha among people with SCI [28]. The present study demonstrated a Cronbach's alpha of 0.89.

The Moorong Self-efficacy Scale (MSES) was used to measure self-efficacy in performing functional, social, leisure and vocational activities post-SCI [29, 30]. The MSES is comprised of 16 items with a 7-point semantic differential scale ranging from 1 (very uncertain) to 7 (very certain). The total scores range from 16 to 112, where higher scores indicate greater perceived self-efficacy. The MSES has demonstrated good validity and reliability in outpatient and inpatient individuals with SCI in a previous study [29] with a Cronbach's alpha of 0.79 in the present study.

The Intrinsic Spirituality Scale (ISS) was used to measure the spirituality. The ISS is comprised of six items and each item consists of phrase completion. The participants are asked to complete a phrase by selecting an option from a list of 11 responses ranging from 0 to 10. The score is calculated by summing the scores of the six items and dividing the total score by six. The ISS is considered an appropriate measure to assess intrinsic spirituality [11]. Cronbach's alpha was 0.76 in this study.

Depressive mood was assessed using the Patient Health Questionnaire-9 (PHQ-9) [31]. This tool consists of nine items based on diagnostic criteria of Diagnostic and Statistical Manual of Mental Health Disorder-IV for depressive disorder. The response is rated in a 4-point Likert scale ranging from 0 (not at all) to 3 (nearly every day). The total score can range from 0 to 27, where higher scores represent a higher depressive mood. The PHQ-9 has been standardized with sound psychometric properties [16, 22] and Cronbach's alpha was 0.87 in this study.

Statistical analyses

The analyses were performed using the Statistical Package for the Social Sciences Software (SPSS; version 16.0). All study variables met the assumptions of correlation and multiple regression analysis. Missing data were estimated by expectation maximization at the individual item level since data were found to be missing completely in a random pattern (Little's MCAR chi-square = 15.70, $p = 0.20$). Descriptive statistics were used to examine demographic and injury-related data. Correlations between resilience and independent variables were tested by a point-biserial correlation or Pearson's correlation depending on the level of measurement of each variable. A hierarchical regression analysis was performed to identify a unique contribution of each variable in determining resilience. Demographic and injury-related variables that were significantly correlated with resilience were entered into the first block to control for the confounding effects. Then, self-efficacy, depressive mood, and social support were entered into the second, third, and fourth blocks, subsequently based on the theoretical predictions. A statistical level of significance was set at a p value of < 0.05.

Results

Participants included 34 females with a mean age of 37.15 years (SD 12.63) and 48 males with a mean age of 33.15 (SD 10.22). Sixteen participants (19.5%) had chronic disease which included hypertension ($n = 7$), asthma, gout, and gastrointestinal problems. The reported SCI-related complications were pain ($n = 66$), spasticity ($n = 21$), pressure injury ($n = 10$), and urinary tract infection ($n = 8$) [32]. Table 1 shows the demographics and injury-related characteristics of the participants.

The average resilience score of the participants was 64.76 (SD 14.02). Descriptive statistics for social support, self-efficacy, spirituality, and depressive mood are presented in Table 2. A point-biserial correlation analysis revealed a significant correlation between sex and resilience ($r = 0.47$, $p < 0.001$). Likewise, a significant positive association was found between employment and resilience ($r = 0.27$, $p = 0.016$). In addition, current living location of the participants was positively associated with resilience ($r = 0.24$, $p = 0.029$). There were no significant associations between resilience and other demographic and injury-related variables (Table 3).

Table 1 Demographic and injury-related characteristics of participants ($N = 82$)

Variables		Number	Percent
Age (years) M = 34.80, SD = 11.38, Min-Max = 18–64			
Sex	Female	34	41.5
	Male	48	58.5
Ethnicity	Aryan	30	36.6
	Mongol	52	63.4
Current living location	Rural	51	62.2
	Urban	31	37.8
Marital status	Unmarried	32	39.0
	Married/Divorced	50	61.0
Education	Primary or lower	42	51.2
	Secondary or higher	40	48.8
Employment	Unemployed	61	74.4
	Employed	21	25.6
Income[a]	No or > Rs. 10,000	67	81.7
	≤ Rs. 10,000	15	18.3
Injury level	Tetraplegia	4	4.9
	Paraplegia	78	95.1
Completeness of injury	Complete	29	35.4
	Incomplete	53	64.6
Chronic disease	No	66	80.5
	Yes	16	19.5
Complication related to SCI	No	9	11.0
	Yes	73	89.0
Caregiver	Family members	69	84.1
	Organizational caregiver	13	15.9

Note. [a]1USD = Nepali Rupee (Rs.) 106.78

Table 2 Resilience, social support, self-efficacy, spirituality, and depressive mood of participants

Measures	Mean	SD	Possible score	Actual score
Resilience (CD-RISC)	64.76	14.02	25–100	33–95
Social support (MSPSS)	62.74	10.74	12–84	36–84
Self-efficacy (MSES)	81.63	16.88	16–112	41–111
Spirituality (ISS)	6.17	2.91	0–10	0–10
Depressive mood (PHQ-9)	8.76	5.30	0–27	0–25

Pearson's correlation matrix of resilience and psychosocial factors, i.e., social support, self-efficacy, spirituality, and depressive mood, are shown in Table 4. A significant positive correlation was found between resilience and social support ($r = 0.42$, $p < 0.001$) and self-efficacy ($r = 0.53$, $p < 0.001$). A significant negative correlation was identified between resilience and depressive mood which indicates that the participants with higher depressive mood had lower resilience ($r = -0.50$, $p < 0.001$). However, a non-significant weak negative association was found between resilience and spirituality ($r = -0.12$, $p > 0.05$).

Finally, multiple hierarchical regression analysis was performed when demographic variables, i.e., sex, employment, and current living location, were entered into the first block. Self-efficacy, depressive mood, and social support were entered into the subsequent blocks (Table 5). Since a non-significant association was found between spirituality and resilience, spirituality was excluded in the regression analysis. The full regression model was able to explain 46% of the variance in resilience (adjusted $R^2 = 0.46$, F (6, 75) = 12.53, $p < 0.001$). In

Table 3 Correlations between resilience and demographic and injury-related variables

Demographic and injury-related variables	Correlation with resilience	
	r	*P*
Age of the participants	−0.15	0.18
Sex	0.47	< 0.001**
Ethnicity	−0.07	0.52
Current living location	0.24	0.029*
Marital status	0.006	0.96
Education	0.20	0.07
Employment	0.27	0.016*
Income	0.18	0.11
Injury level	0.19	0.09
Completeness of injury	−0.09	0.43
Chronic disease	−0.10	0.34
Complication related to SCI	−0.22	0.05
Caregiver	0.06	0.59

*p value < 0.05; **p value < 0.001

Table 4 Correlation matrix between resilience and psychosocial factors

Variables	1	2	3	4	5
1. Resilience	1				
2. Social support	0.42**	1			
3. Self-efficacy	0.53**	0.37*	1		
4. Spirituality	−0.12	−0.01	−0.02	1	
5. Depressive mood	−0.50**	− 0.31*	− 0.49**	−0.04	1

*p < 0.01; **p < 0.001

the first block, sex, employment, and current living location accounted for 23% of the variance in resilience (adjusted $R^2 = 0.23$, $F\ (3,\ 78) = 8.99$, $p < 0.001$). The addition of self-efficacy into the second block greatly increased the variance explained in resilience to 40%, which was a change of 17% (adjusted R^2 change = 0.17, $p < 0.001$). Depressive mood was entered into the third block which explained the 5% additional variance in resilience (adjusted R^2 change = 0.05, $p < 0.001$). The addition of social support into the fourth block explained the additional 1% of variance; nevertheless, the increment was not significant (adjusted R^2 change = 0.01, $p > 0.05$). Overall, sex, self-efficacy, and depressive mood were statistically significant factors of resilience. Among those, sex showed a higher beta value (β = 0.31, $p = 0.001$) indicating that sex was the strongest factor of resilience in this study. Furthermore, self-efficacy was found as a significantly strong psychosocial factor of resilience (β = 0.28, $p = 0.007$), followed by depressive mood (β = − 0.24, $p = 0.016$).

Discussion

This study examined the role of psychosocial and demographic factors in determining resilience among Nepalese with earthquake-related SCI. Among psychosocial variables, self-efficacy and depressive mood significantly influenced resilience among the participants. In addition, sex, current living location, and employment of participants were also significantly related to resilience. Social support was significantly correlated; nevertheless, it could not account for the significant variance in resilience in the regression analysis. Interestingly, there was no significant association between resilience and spirituality of the study participants.

As mentioned, the study results found that self-efficacy and depressive mood had a significant association with resilience in the participants. Evidence from previous studies also revealed self-efficacy as one of the significant determinants of resilience among people with SCI [6, 13, 16]. Self-efficacy is a vital factor which motivates and reinforces individuals to adopt health-promoting behaviors [33]. Individuals who are highly self-confident of their own capabilities can better manage a stressful situation or adversity without experiencing any negative psychological consequences. A feeling of high self-confidence to have control over things that one desires can result in resilience [34].

Consistent with previous studies, depressive mood was related to low resilience among the participants in this study [6, 13, 16]. A depressive mood among people with SCI can develop as a result of long-term negative consequences such as restriction in mobility, difficulty in adjustment or re-integration into the community, financial loss, loss of independence in daily activities, chronic pain, and a perceived bias due to the disability [35, 36]. Individuals with SCI who experience depressive mood tend to diminish self-care activities, avoid eating and performing exercises, have increased risk of developing medical complications, visit the hospital more frequently, and develop suicidal ideas and thoughts which can, in turn, contribute to low resilience [37].

Similar with a previous study conducted among people with SCI in Australia, social support had no significant predictive role in resilience [13]. However, social support was found as one of the significant determinants of resilience among disaster survivors [18, 38]. According to Bandura (1998), social support is not a self-forming entity which can directly buffer against stressors.

Table 5 Hierarchical regression analyses determining resilience

Independent Variables	Block 1		Block 2		Block 3		Block 4		95% CI
	β	p	β	p	B	P	β	P	
Sex (female/male)	0.41	< 0.001	0.38	< 0.001	0.35	< 0.001	0.31	0.001*	(3.66, 13.89)
Employment (unemployed/employed)	0.10	0.30	0.001	0.99	0.02	0.87	0.02	0.87	(−5.23, 6.16)
Current living location (rural/urban)	0.14	0.16	0.03	0.70	0.007	0.94	0.04	0.65	(−3.94, 6.28)
Self-efficacy			0.45	< 0.001	0.33	0.001	0.28	0.007*	(0.07, 0.40)
Depressive mood					−0.27	0.008	−0.24	0.016*	(−1.14, − 0.12)
Social support							0.16	0.09	(−0.03, 0.45)
Adjusted R^2	0.23		0.40		0.45		0.46		
Adjusted R^2 change			0.17**		0.05**		0.01		

Model: $R^2 = 0.50$; Adjusted $R^2 = 0\ .46$; $F\ (6,75) = 12.53$; $p < 0.001$
*p value < 0.05; **p < 0.001

However, it indirectly fosters a coping ability or resilience by enhancing perceived efficacy. An individual requires a strong sense of efficacy in order to seek or obtain social support [34]. In addition, internal factors related to confidence in regulating thoughts or emotions result in resilience regardless of social support [22].

In this study, there was no significant association between spirituality and resilience. This finding is contrary to previous studies conducted among people with SCI, which reported a significant positive relationship between these two variables [11, 20]. It could be attributed to several reasons. In comparison, the differences in research settings, durations after sustaining injury, and causes of SCI could result in disparate findings since spirituality is considered dynamic and varies according to circumstances [39]. According to the compensating reciprocal causation model, it is complex to understand the role of spirituality from a cross-sectional study since spirituality is dynamic in nature [40]. Since the Nepalese participants experienced the traumatic events that occurred in 2015, it is difficult to identify whether the events developed spirituality or spirituality was affected by the events. Consequently, a cross-sectional design could have yielded non-significant results in the present study. In addition, the narrow scale range of the ISS that was used to measure spirituality in this study possibly caused difficulty for the participants to accurately identify the subtle changes in the scores and possibly led to a lack of sensitivity to measure spirituality [11].

Among the demographic variables, sex significantly explained resilience in this study which was congruent with a study conducted among survivors of an earthquake in China [18]. However, previous studies conducted among people with SCI did not support this finding [6, 22]. The inconsistencies on the role of sex on resilience possibly resulted from the differences in the contexts and cultures of the studies. Cultural context influences a gender role and priorities, their sense of self-worth, and availability of social resources [41]. Nepal is a patriarchal society, where power or authority is held by males and they are considered to be the breadwinner in the family [42]. Nepalese males have higher employment and education opportunities and incomes compared to the females [24]. Due to the important roles of males in Nepalese society, they tend to receive support from their family and society. Consequently, a sense of worth or self-esteem is greater among the Nepalese males, including the disabled. Additionally, in the Nepalese context, females are treated as secondary to males [42]. Females with a disability are less likely to get married and have a family than males with a disability since those females are considered incapable of accomplishing the reproductive activities [43]. As a result, females tend to have a low sense of self-worth [41–43]. Thus, higher self-esteem, education, and employment opportunities among males could be the reason for higher resilience among the male participants as suggested in the literature [44, 45].

The results of this study also revealed that the current living location and employment were significantly associated with resilience. In Nepal, the majority of people live in rural areas where transportation services are inaccessible due to steep mountains and hills. Healthcare and rehabilitation services are available mostly in the urban areas. It takes several hours for people (including people with SCI) living in rural Nepal to access healthcare and rehabilitation services [24]. Inaccessibility to rehabilitation and treatment for complications related to SCI further deteriorate their physical health. Physical impairments could enhance the risk of developing depression and low self-efficacy among people with SCI [44] which subsequently contribute to low resilience among people living in rural areas [6].

This study supported the results of previous studies, which found that employed individuals tended to have significantly greater resilience than unemployed individuals [17, 45, 46]. People with SCI who are employed do not have to rely financially on others for survival which enhances their sense of self-worth and satisfaction with life which further enhances resilience [36, 45].

Implications of the findings

The findings from this study offer several clinical implications for healthcare professionals, in particular, the rehabilitation nurses as well as mental health professionals. Identification of factors influencing resilience help rehabilitation nurses to plan appropriate strategies. For instance, self-efficacy strengthening interventions are beneficial to enhance resilience. Similarly, prevention or treatment of depressive mood is significant in promoting resilience of this group. Involvement of family members during the rehabilitation or nursing intervention need to be considered since social support is associated with resilience in this group. The study findings also suggest that nurses should identify or screen for low resilient groups such as females, the unemployed, rural people, and people with low self-efficacy, low social support, and unstable or depressed mood. Therefore, they can deliver interventions or care considering those vulnerable people. Community or home-based rehabilitation programs and nursing interventions would be effective since people from rural areas were found to be more vulnerable.

Limitations and future research

Despite the significance of this study in understanding the factors of resilience following earthquake-related SCI, some limitations were identified and areas for possible future study could be suggested. First, the researcher read the questions and filled the questionnaires for illiterate participants which possibly developed some biases. The participants were likely to give desirable answers rather than answering their own feelings. Next, since this cross-sectional study was conducted at two years after the earthquake, it could not identify the dynamic nature of resilience and other variables. A longitudinal study is recommended to assess the long-term changes in resilience and factors influencing resilience. Although there is evidence that supports spirituality as a determinant of resilience, it did not make a contribution to resilience in the present study. Hence, further research related to spirituality using other measures need to be conducted. Furthermore, this study did not address the pre-injury mental health status or characteristics of the participants which could influence the post-injury mental health status or resilience of those individuals. Finally, testing the psychometric properties of the resilience instrument (CD-RISC) is important to examine the feasibility and sensitivity of the tool among Nepalese.

Conclusion

Previous research findings were supported and this study reported more insight into resilience following earthquake-related SCI. The results indicated that self-efficacy, social support, and depressive mood were the significant psychosocial factors of resilience. Furthermore, demographic factors such as sex, employment, and living location were also associated with resilience. Therefore, interventions or rehabilitation should be focused on specific psychosocial factors as well as demographic factors. Future research regarding resilience interventions can aid rehabilitation nurses as well as mental health professionals to improve rehabilitation outcomes, enhance resilience, and promote successful reintegration into the community.

Abbreviations

CD-RISC: Connor-Davidson Resilience Scale; CI: Confidence interval; ISS: Intrinsic Spirituality Scale; MSES: Moorong Self-efficacy Scale; MSPSS: Multidimensional Scale of Perceived Social Support; PHQ-9: Patient Health Questionnaire-9; SCI: Spinal cord injury; SIRC: Spinal Injury Rehabilitation Center

Acknowledgements

The authors would like to acknowledge Prince of Songkla University, Dr. Charuwan Kritpracha, SIRC, and all the participants of the study.

Funding

Prince of Songkla University granted partial funding during the data collection.

Authors' contributions

MB collected data from the participants, analyzed data, and wrote the manuscript under supervision of KM and WS. WS contributed to the analysis and interpretation of the results. KM contributed to the critical revision of the manuscript. All authors read and approved the final manuscript.

Consent for publication

Not applicable

Competing interests

The authors declare that they have no competing interests.

Author details

[1]Hope International College, Kathmandu 44600, Nepal. [2]Faculty of Nursing, Prince of Songkla University, Hat Yai, Songkhla, Thailand.

References

1. World Health Organization. Earthquakes - technical hazard sheet - natural disaster profile. 2016. http://www.who.int/hac/techguidance/ems/earthquakes/en/. Accessed 15 Aug 2016.
2. World Health Organization. International perspectives on spinal cord injury. 2013. http://apps.who.int/iris/bitstream/10665/94190/1/9789241564663_eng.pdf. Accessed 17 Aug 2016.
3. Muldoon S. Nepal quakes: treating the spinally injured. BBC News. 2015; http://www.bbc.com/news/blogs-ouch-32847101. Accessed 28 Sep 2016
4. Somers MF. Spinal cord injury: functional rehabilitation. 3rd ed. Boston: Julie Levin Alexander; 2010.
5. Craig A, Tran Y, Middleton J. Psychological morbidity and spinal cord injury: a systematic review. Spinal Cord. 2009;47:108–14.
6. Kilic SA, Dorstyn DS, Guiver NG. Examining factors that contribute to the process of resilience following spinal cord injury. Spinal Cord. 2013;51(7):553.
7. Migliorini C, Sinclair A, Brown D, Tonge B, New P. Prevalence of mood disturbance in Australian adults with chronic spinal cord injury. Intern Med. 2015;45:1014–9.
8. Zhou X, Song H, Hu M, Li X, Cai Y, Huang G, Li J, Kang L, Li J. Risk factors of severity of post-traumatic stress disorder among survivors with physical disabilities one year after the Wenchuan earthquake. Psychiatry Res. 2015; 228:468–74.
9. Connor KM, Davidson JR. Development of a new resilience scale: the Connor-Davidson resilience scale (CD-RISC). Depress Anxiety. 2003;18:76–82.
10. Bonanno GA, Kennedy P, Galatzer-Levy IR, Lude P, Elfström ML. Trajectories of resilience, depression, and anxiety following spinal cord injury. Rehabil Psychol. 2012;57:236.
11. White B, Driver S, Warren AM. Resilience and indicators of adjustment during rehabilitation from a spinal cord injury. Rehabil Psychol. 2010;55:23.
12. Kornhaber R, Mclean L, Betihavas V, Cleary M. Resilience and the rehabilitation of adult spinal cord injury survivors: a qualitative systematic review. J Adv Nurs. 2017;74:23–33.
13. Guest R, Craig A, Tran Y, Middleton J. Factors predicting resilience in people with spinal cord injury during transition from inpatient rehabilitation to the community. Spinal Cord. 2015;53:682–6.
14. Kumpfer KL. Factors and processes contributing to resilience: the resilience framework. In: Glantz MD, Johnson JL, editors. Resilience and development: positive life adaptations. New York: Kluwer Academic/Plenum Press Publishers; 1999. p. 179–224.
15. Gunnestad A. Resilience in a cross-cultural perspective: how resilience is generated in different cultures. J Intercult Commun. 2006;11:1–20.
16. Driver S, Warren AM, Reynolds M, Agtarap S, Hamilton R, Trost Z, Monden K. Identifying predictors of resilience at inpatient and 3-month post-spinal cord injury. J Spinal Cord. 2016;39:77–84.
17. Kukihara H, Yamawaki N, Uchiyama K, Arai S, Horikawa E. Trauma, depression, and resilience of earthquake/tsunami/nuclear disaster survivors of Hirono, Fukushima, Japan. Psychiatry Clin Neurosci. 2014;68:524–33.
18. Ni C, Chow MCM, Jiang X, Li S, Pang SMC. Factors associated with resilience of adult survivors five years after the 2008 Sichuan earthquake in China. PLoS One. 2015;10:e0121033.
19. Guest CA, Nicholson Perry K, Tran Y, Ephraums C, Hales A, Dezarnaulds A, Crino R, Middleton J. Resilience following spinal cord injury: a prospective controlled study investigating the influence of the provision of group cognitive behavior therapy during inpatient rehabilitation. Rehabil Psychol. 2015;60:311.
20. Monden KR, Trost Z, Catalano D, Garner AN, Symcox J, Driver S, Hamilton

RG, Warren AM. Resilience following spinal cord injury: a phenomenological view. Spinal Cord. 2014;52:197–201.
21. Duggan C, Wilson C, DiPonio L, Trumpower B, Meade MA. Resilience and happiness after spinal cord injury: a qualitative study. Top Spinal Cord Inj Rehabil. 2016;22:99–110.
22. Dodd Z, Driver S, Warren AM, Riggs S, Clark M. Effects of adult romantic attachment and social support on resilience and depression in individuals with spinal cord injuries. Top Spinal Cord Inj Rehabil. 2015;21:156–65.
23. Bonanno GA, Galea S, Bucciarelli A, Vlahov D. Psychological resilience after disaster New York city in the aftermath of the September 11th terrorist attack. Psychol Sci. 2006;17:181–6.
24. Central Bureau of Statistics. Nepal living standards survey 2010/11. 2011. http://cbs.gov.np/poverty/nlssurvey2010_11. Accessed 6 Mar 2017.
25. Green SB. How many subjects does it take to do a regression analysis. Multivariate Behav Res. 1991;26:499–510.
26. Polit DF, Beck CT. Nursing research: generating and assessing evidence for nursing practice. 9th ed. Philadelphia: Lippincott Williams & Wilkins; 2012.
27. Zimet GD, Dahlem NW, Zimet SG, Farley GK. The multidimensional scale of perceived social support. J Pers Assess. 1988;52:30–41.
28. Catalano D, Chan F, Wilson L, Chiu C-Y, Muller VR. The buffering effect of resilience on depression among individuals with spinal cord injury: a structural equation model. Rehabil Psychol. 2011;56:200.
29. Middleton J, Tate RL, Geraghty TJ. Self-efficacy and spinal cord injury: psychometric properties of a new scale. Rehabil Psychol. 2003;48:281.
30. Middleton JW, Tran Y, Lo C, Craig A. Reexamining the validity and dimensionality of the moorong self-efficacy scale: improving its clinical utility. Arch Phys Med Rehabil. 2016;97:2130–6.
31. Kroencke K, Spitzer R, Williams J. The phq-9: validity of a brief depression severity measure. J Gen Intern Med. 2001;16:606–13.
32. Bhattarai M, Maneewat K, Sae-Sia W. Determinants of resilience among people who sustained spinal cord injury from the 2015 earthquake in Nepal. Spinal Cord. 2018;56:78–83.
33. Middleton J, Tran Y, Craig A. Relationship between quality of life and self-efficacy in persons with spinal cord injuries. Arch Phys Med Rehabil. 2007;88:1643–8.
34. Bandura A. Health promotion from the perspective of social cognitive theory. Psychol Health. 1998;13:623–49.
35. Craig A, Perry KN, Guest R, Tran Y, Dezarnaulds A, Hales A, Ephraums C, Middleton J. Prospective study of the occurrence of psychological disorders and comorbidities after spinal cord injury. Arch Phys Med Rehabil. 2015;96:1426–34.
36. Crew NM, Krause JS. Spinal cord injury. In: Brodwin MG, Siu FW, Howard J, Brodwin ER, editors. Medical, psychosocial and vocational aspects of disability. Athens, USA: Elliott & Fitzpatrick, Inc; 2009. p. 289–303.
37. Craig A, Perry KN. Guide for health professionals on the psychosocial care of adults with spinal cord injury. 2014. https://www.aci.health.nsw.gov.au/__data/assets/pdf_file/0019/155233/Guide-Psychosocial-Care.pdf. Accessed 3 Sept 2016.
38. Bonanno GA, Galea S, Bucciarelli A, Vlahov D. What predicts psychological resilience after disaster? The role of demographics, resources, and life stress. J Consult Clin Psychol. 2007;75:671.
39. Hodge DR. The intrinsic spirituality scale: a new six-item instrument for assessing the salience of spirituality as a motivational construct. J Soc Serv Res. 2003;30:41–61.
40. Kennedy JE, Davis RC, Taylor BG. Changes in spirituality and well-being among victims of sexual assault. J Sci Study Relig. 1998;37:322–8.
41. Niaz U, Hassan S. Culture and Mental health of women in South-East Asia. World Psychiatry. 2006;5:118–20.
42. Pokharel S. Gender discriminatory practices in Tamang and Brahmin communities. Tribhuvan university Journal. 2009;26:85–98.
43. Dhungana BM, Kusakabe K. The role of self-help groups in empowering disabled women: a case study in Kathmandu Valley, Nepal. Dev Pract. 2010;20:855–65.
44. Peter C, Müller R, Cieza A, Geyh S. Psychological resources in spinal cord injury: a systematic literature review. Spinal Cord. 2012;50:188–201.
45. Min J-A, Lee C-U, Hwang S-I, Shin J-I, Lee B-S, Han S-H, Ju H-I, Lee C-Y, Lee C, Chae J-H. The moderation of resilience on the negative effect of pain on depression and post-traumatic growth in individuals with spinal cord injury. Disabil Rehabil. 2014;36:1196–202.
46. Lowe SR, Sampson L, Gruebner O, Galea S. Psychological resilience after hurricane Sandy: the influence of individual-and community-level factors on mental health after a large-scale natural disaster. PLoS One. 2015;10:e0125761.

11

The validity of proxy-based data on loneliness in suicide research: a case-control psychological autopsy study in rural China

Lu Niu[1], Cunxian Jia[2], Zhenyu Ma[3], Guojun Wang[4], Zhenjun Yu[4] and Liang Zhou[1*]

Abstract

Background: There is a lack of evidence for the role of loneliness on suicide using psychological autopsy method, and the validity of proxy informants' reports on loneliness is not well established. This study aimed to investigate the validity of proxy respondent reports on loneliness, and the reliability and validity of the University of California Los Angeles Loneliness Scale-6 (ULS-6) as used in psychological autopsy method with rural elderly people in China.

Methods: Two hundred forty-two suicide cases and 242 normal community controls were selected, and the psychological autopsy method was utilized to collect information. Data from proxy respondents of the living controls were compared with data reported by the targets (gold standards).

Results: Subject-proxy concordance for ULS-6 was fair (ICC = 0.447) in the living controls. The suicide cases were more likely to have a higher score of ULS-6 than the living controls. Additionally, our data supported that ULS-6 had adequate psychometric properties in both suicide and control groups: factor analyses yielded one-factor component solution; Cronbach's alpha (both > 0.90) demonstrated excellent internal consistency; the Spearman correlation analysis indicated that the ULS-6 score was positively correlated with depression; and negatively correlated with QOL and social support.

Conclusions: Results support proxy-based data on loneliness in research of suicide in older adults in rural China, and the ULS-6 is a psychometrically sound instrument for measuring loneliness in psychological autopsy studies.

Keywords: Loneliness, Psychometric properties, Psychological autopsy, Chinese rural elderly, Suicide

Background

In China, a sharp decline in the official national suicide rate has been observed in the past two decades, from 15.6 per 100,000 in 2002 to 6.6 in 2015 [1]. However, the decline in suicide rate was less prominent in older age-groups compared with younger age-groups [1]. It was predicted that Chinese elderly suicide rates, especially among the rural elderly population, were likely to go up again [2]. Given the rapid aging of Chinese population, elderly suicide prevention should be given greater priority for reducing suicides in China [3]. To understand the causes and identify correlates of suicide, psychological autopsy, which gather data from postmortem proxy respondents, medical records, and other sources, is a widely used method [4, 5].

Loneliness is a feeling due to the lack of meaningful social relationships [6] or deficiency between actual and desired levels of social interaction [7]. Studies have linked loneliness to various correlates of suicidal behaviors. For example, loneliness was found as a significant predictor of depression and anxiety in the elderly [8, 9]. A high correlation was reported between loneliness and substance use as well [10]. Additionally, loneliness was found to be correlated with suicide ideation and suicide attempt [11–14]. A recent

* Correspondence: Liangzhou_csu@vip.163.com
[1]The Affiliated Brain Hospital of Guangzhou Medical University (Guangzhou Huiai Hospital), 36 Mingxin Road, Liwan District, Guangzhou 510370, China
Full list of author information is available at the end of the article

meta-analytic review found that older people experiencing loneliness were twice more likely to have suicidal ideation (OR = 2.24; 95%CI: 1.73-2.90) [15]. People suffering from loneliness also has a higher risk of suicide. In a content analysis of online suicide notes, loneliness was one of the core themes [16].

In psychological autopsy research, the supreme principle is that the greater the amount of relevant data analyzed, the more accurate the investigators' conclusions are likely to be [17]. Though loneliness has been found to be associated with suicidal behaviors, there is a lack of evidence for the role of loneliness on suicide using psychological autopsy method. Besides, the validity of psychological autopsy studies depends on the validity of the information provided by proxy informants about the deceased [18]. Previous studies have suggested that proxies are good judges of past history of suicide attempts, suicidal intent, psychiatric diagnosis, depression, life events, and social support [4, 5, 19, 20]. As loneliness is a subjective and personal inner experience or feeling, is it amenable to detection by others? The validity of proxy informants' reports on loneliness is not yet well established.

With different operationalizations of the construct of loneliness, there are several established instruments, such as the Rasch-Type Loneliness Scale [21], the Social and Emotional Loneliness Scale [22], and the University of California Los Angeles Loneliness Scale (ULS) [23]. The ULS with 20 items was firstly developed by Russell et al. in 1978 [23]. A four-item (ULS-4) and an eight-item (ULS-8) short form of ULS was later developed by Russell et al. [24] and Hays et al. [25], respectively. In 2002, Zhou et al. [26] has translated the ULS-8 into Chinese and revised the scale into 6 items (ULS-6). The Chinese version ULS-6 has shown good internal reliability, test-retest reliability, construct validity, and concurrent validity in Chinese rural community-dwelling elderly [26]. Thus, the ULS-6 was adopted to measure loneliness in this study.

In this case-control psychological autopsy study, we aimed to assess the concordance of subject and proxy reports on loneliness in the Chinese rural elderly; and to evaluate the psychometric properties of ULS-6 in individuals who died by suicide and, separately, in matched community-based control subjects in rural China.

Methods

Participants and procedures

This case-control psychological autopsy study was conducted, during June 2014 to September 2015, in Shandong Province, Hunan Province, and Guangxi Province. A total of 12 counties from the three provinces were randomly selected. In each county, suicide cases aged 60 and above were collected consecutively based on the death certification system. All village doctors and local public health professionals involved in death certification were given brief training and required to report all elderly suicide death to local Centers for Disease Control and Prevention (CDCs). After all relevant and available information was collected, the manner of death was determined by trained investigators.

For each suicide case, we randomly selected community living comparison based on age (±3 years old), gender, and living location. When a suicide case was identified, investigators would list and numerate all matched older adults. One living comparison was then selected from the list randomly by a computer program. Besides, for each suicide case and living comparison, we selected two informants: generally, the first informant was one next-to-kin who lived with the individual who died by suicide or the living comparison; and the second informant was always a friend, a neighbor, or a remote relative.

The information provided by two informants was combined as the proxy data for suicide cases and living comparisons. For demographic characteristics, information provided by the first informant was relied on. For each item of ULS-6, GDS, QOL, and DSSI, answers that were hypothetically associated with elevated risk of suicide were used, because a targeting symptom or behavior might exist as long as either informant had observed it. Thus, positive answer of an item of GDS was used when one of the two informants reported positive; similarly, higher score, and lower score of QOL and DSSI were used.

This study was approved by the Human Research Ethics Committees of Shandong University, Central South University, and Guangxi Medical University. Written informed consent has been obtained from participants in the living comparison group, and all informants of both suicide cases and living comparisons.

Measurements

Demographic characteristics

Demographic data were collected such as gender, age, educational level, marital status, employment, and living arrangements. In this study, people that were married and living with spouse, or cohabiting were classified as "currently married"; while people with other marital status (including single, divorced, widowed, and married but living apart) were classified as "non-currently married". Being left-behind was defined was during the last 12 months prior to death/investigation, all adult children had lived out of the original township for at least 10 months, and had visited their parents no more than twice.

University of California Los Angeles Loneliness Scale-6 (ULS-6)

Loneliness was assessed by the Chinese version of ULS-6. In 2002, the original ULS-8 was translated by Zhou et al. [26], and validated in elderly samples in a rural community. By exploratory factor analysis, a 6-item ULS (ULS-6) with one factor was generated. The ULS-6 has shown good internal reliability, test-retest reliability, construct validity, and concurrent validity in Chinese rural community-dwelling elderly [26].Each item is rated on a 4-point scale ranging from 1 (never) to 4 (often feel this way). The total score ranges from 6 to 24, with higher scores indicating higher levels of loneliness.

Geriatric Depression Scale (GDS)

Depression was measured by GDS, a 30-item screening instrument developed by Brink et al. [27]. It is a validated and reliable scale upon 30 yes-or-no questions that was developed to assess depressive symptoms in the past week among elderly people. Higher scores indicate higher levels of depression. A cut-off score of 10 and 20 represents mild and severe levels of depression, respectively. The GDS-30 has shown adequate properties in the Chinese elderly [28].

Quality of Life (QOL)

QOL was assessed by 6 items developed by Phillips et al. [29], regarding physical health, psychological health, economic circumstances, work, family relationships, and relationships with non-family associates in the past month. Each item is rated on a 5-point scale ranging from 1 (very poor) to 5 (excellent), with higher scores indicating better QOL.

Duke Social Support Index (DSSI)

Social support was measured by the 23-item DSSI [30]. It consists of three subscales: social interaction, subjective support, and instrumental support. The total score ranges from 11 to 45, with higher scores indicating higher levels of social support. The 23-item DSSI has shown good reliability and validity in Chinese elderly samples [31].

Statistical analysis

First, in the living controls, proxy-based data were compared with subject-based data (gold standard). The Spearman correlation analysis, the pair-sample t-test, and intraclass correlation coefficients (ICC) were used. ICC values were evaluated based on the following benchmarks: poor, less than 0.40; fair, 0.40 – 0.59; good, 0.60 – 0.74; and excellent, greater than 0.75 [18, 32].

Then, the combined data were adopted to evaluate the psychometric properties of the ULS-6 for suicide cases and living controls, respectively. The exploratory factor analysis (EFA) was conducted to explore the underlying factor structure of the ULS-6. The sample adequacy was assessed by the Kaiser-Meyer-Olkin (KMO) test and Bartlet's test. Internal reliability was assessed using the criterion of Cronbach's alpha ≥0.70 and split-half reliability coefficient (Spearman-Brown coefficient) ≥ 0.70 [33, 34]. Independent-samples t-tests and one-way ANOVA were used for comparison among different demographic groups (gender, age groups, education, marital status, employment, living alone, and being left-behind). Concurrent validity was evaluated by correlations between the depression, quality of life, and social support.

All analyses were performed with SPSS version 23.0 (SPSS Inc., Chicago, IL, USA). Significance levels of this study were set at 0.05.

Results

Demographic characteristics

Altogether 242 suicide cases and 242 living comparisons were obtained. In the suicide cases, 43.8% were female, and the mean age was74.4 years (SD = 8.2). In the living controls, 43.8% were female, and the mean age was 74.1 years (SD = 8.2). As presented in Table 1, compared with the living controls, the suicide cases were more likely to be non-currently married, unemployed, living alone, and left-behind. Besides, suicides cases reported higher scores of depression, but lower scores of QOL and social support than the living controls.

Subject-proxy agreement on loneliness

In the living controls, the mean score of ULS-6 reported by the subjects themselves was 9.8 (SD = 3.9). The mean score of ULS-6 from the proxy data was 11.0 (SD = 4.0). The Spearman correlation analysis indicated a low correlation between the self-reported and proxy data ($r = 0.308$, $p = 0.000$). The paired-sample T-test showed a significant difference ($t = 4.045$, $p = 0.000$). As shown in Table 2, there was moderate agreement on self-reported and proxy data of the ULS-6 based on the ICC value of 0.447 ($p = 0.000$). The consistency was low to moderate for each item, as the ICCs ranged from 0. 295 to 0.503 (Table 3).

Construct validity

In the suicide cases, the KMO value was 0.910, and the Bartlett's test of Sphericity was statistically significant ($\chi^2 = 1245.214$, $p = 0.000$), indicating the adequacy of proceeding with factor analysis. The EFA results yielded an one-factor solution that accounted for 66.092% of the variance. Item loadings ranged from 0.844 to 0.916 (Table 3).

In the living controls, the KMO value was 0.871, and the Bartlett's test of Sphericity was statistically

Table 1 Demographic characteristics of suicide cases and living controls

Variable	Suicide cases (n = 242)	Living controls (n = 242)	χ^2/t	P
Gender			–	–
Male	135 (55.8)	135 (55.8)		
Female	107 (44.2)	107 (44.2)		
Age groups			0.913	0.633
60-69	73 (30.2)	70 (28.9)		
70-79	100 (41.3)	110 (45.5)		
≥ 80	69 (28.5)	62 (25.6)		
Education			1.920	0.383
Below primary school	111 (45.9)	96 (39.7)		
Primary school	105 (43.4)	116 (47.9)		
Above primary school	26 (10.7)	30 (12.4)		
Marital status			19.890	0.000
Currently married	122 (50.4)	170 (70.2)		
Non-currently married	120 (49.6)	72 (29.8)		
Employment			8.274	0.016
Employed	41 (16.9)	61 (25.2)		
Unemployed	194 (80.2)	167 (69.0)		
Retired	7 (2.9)	14 (5.8)		
Living alone			10.679	0.002
Yes	64 (26.4)	35 (14.5)		
No	178 (73.6)	207 (85.5)		
Being left-behind			4.491	0.046
Yes	41 (16.9)	25 (10.3)		
No	201 (83.1)	217 (89.7)		
Depression [mean (SD)]	21.40 (5.95)	9.22 (6.42)	21.654	0.000
QOL [mean (SD)]	15.40 (3.06)	19.50 (3.11)	14.629	0.000
Social support [mean (SD)]	22.88 (5.98)	27.47 (6.82)	7.868	0.000

significant ($\chi^2 = 921.187$, $p = 0.000$), indicating the adequacy of proceeding with factor analysis. The EFA results yielded an one-factor solution that accounted for 68.425% of the variance. Item loadings ranged from 0.781 to 0.880.

Reliability

In the suicide cases, the Cronbach's α for ULS-6 was 0.940. The Spearman-Brown coefficient was 0.919.

In the living controls, the Cronbach's α for ULS-6 was 0.905. The Spearman-Brown coefficient was 0.878.

Table 2 Subject-proxy agreement on loneliness among living controls (n = 242)

Items of ULS-6	Self-reported data Mean (SD)	Proxy data Mean (SD)	Paired t-test	p	ICC	p
1. I lack companionship.	1.75 (0.94)	1.98 (0.92)	3.297	0.001	0.446	0.000
2. There is no one I can turn to.	1.66 (0.84)	1.85 (0.83)	2.913	0.004	0.372	0.000
3. I feel left out.	1.61 (0.77)	1.81 (0.82)	3.099	0.002	0.315	0.002
4. I feel isolated from others.	1.55 (0.72)	1.77 (0.75)	3.724	0.000	0.345	0.001
5. I am unhappy being so withdrawn.	1.52 (0.69)	1.72 (0.71)	3.418	0.001	0.295	0.003
6. People are around me but not with me.	1.67 (0.85)	1.85 (0.83)	2.849	0.005	0.503	0.000
The total score of ULS-6	9.76 (3.90)	10.99 (4.01)	4.045	0.000	0.447	0.000

Table 3 Factor matrix for the ULS-6 in suicide cases and living controls

Item description	Suicide cases (n = 242)		Living controls (n = 242)	
	Mean (SD)	Factor 1	Mean (SD)	Factor 1
1. I lack companionship.	2.75 (0.99)	0.849	1.98 (0.92)	0.793
2. There is no one I can turn to.	2.60 (0.94)	0.856	1.85 (0.83)	0.839
3. I feel left out.	2.67 (0.94)	0.916	1.81 (0.82)	0.880
4. I feel isolated from others.	2.52 (0.94)	0.898	1.77 (0.75)	0.875
5. I am unhappy being so withdrawn.	2.47 (0.90)	0.844	1.72 (0.71)	0.789
6. People are around me but not with me.	2.54 (0.99)	0.898	1.85 (0.83)	0.781
The total score of ULS-6	15.55 (5.00)		10.99 (4.01)	
Eigenvalue		4.619		4.106
Proportion of explained variance (%)		76.991		68.425

Convergent validity

In the suicide cases, the mean score of ULS-6 was 15.55 (SD = 5.00), which was significantly higher than that of the living controls ($t = 11.054$, $p = 0.000$).

As shown in Table 4, people, who had non-currently married, were living alone, and were left-behind, were more likely to report higher ULS-6 scores in both suicides and living controls. There was no significant difference on the ULS-6 scores between different groups of gender, age groups, education, and employment ($p > 0.05$). As presented in Table 5, the Spearman correlation analysis indicated that the ULS-6 score was significantly and positively correlated with depression; and negatively correlated with QOL and social support (all $p < 0.01$).

Discussion

The aim of this study was to assess whether information derived without input from the targets themselves was valid for identifying the feeling of loneliness using a Chinese version of ULS-6 in rural China. In this case-control psychological autopsy study, we used the data of the living control group to compare the information from proxy respondents with the data reported by the targets themselves (gold standard). The agreement was fair between the living targets and proxy respondents about the degree of loneliness with an ICC value of 0.447. This finding was consistent with previous research on factors related to internal and emotional experience; the subject-proxy agreement on internal emotional experience were found to be moderate or poor, such as anxiety [4] and perceived emotional support [5, 19].

The estimates of the proxy respondents were significantly and slightly higher than subject reports with about a mean difference of 1.23 (SD = 4.72). Symptoms and behaviors that are prominent, noticeable, and recurrent are the most detectable [20]. With increasing age, social networks of older adults will become smaller (e.g., loss of spouse and friends), and social contracts will decrease as well due to worsen physical health and reduced physical activity performance. Thus, from external perception, proxy respondents may easily overestimate the subject's feeling of loneliness. Still, the significant

Table 4 Demographic factors related to loneliness in suicides cases and living controls

Variable	Suicide cases (n = 242) ULS-6 Mean (SD)	*t*	*P*	Living controls (n = 242) ULS-6 Mean (SD)	*t*	*P*
Marital status		3.539	0.000		3.925	0.000
Currently married	14.44 (5.20)			10.35 (3.78)		
Non-currently married	16.67 (4.55)			12.50 (4.15)		
Living alone		5.082	0.000		3.565	0.000
Yes	18.14 (4.47)			13.17 (4.50)		
No	14.61 (4.86)			10.62 (3.81)		
Being left-behind		2.587	0.010		3.125	0.002
Yes	17.37 (5.21)			13.32 (4.34)		
No	15.17 (4.89)			10.72 (3.89)		

There was no significant difference on the ULS-6 score between different groups of gender, age groups, education, and employment ($p > 0.05$)

Table 5 Correlations of the ULS-6 to validating scales in suicide cases and living controls

Scale	Suicide cases (n = 242)	Living controls (n = 242)
	ULS-6 (Spearman's rho)	ULS-6 (Spearman's rho)
GDS score	0.277[a]	0.516[a]
QOL score	−0.344[a]	-0.382[a]
DSSI score	-0.443[a]	-0.466[a]

[a]Correlation is significant at the 0.01 level

correlation coefficients between the proxy respondents and the living targets themselves indicate comparatively accurate estimates of the proxy respondents on the reality of the loneliness feeling of the targets.

The information bias could exist in both suicide cases and living controls. The case-control design could minimize the effect of information bias. By comparison of proxy data between suicide cases and living controls, it could better estimate the role of risk factors for suicide [35]. In the suicide cases, the mean score of ULS-6 was significantly higher than that of the living controls, which indicates that loneliness should be considered as a risk factor of suicide in Chinese rural elderly.

Moreover, this study presents the psychometric characteristics of the ULS-6 as used in psychological autopsy method. Exploratory Factor Analysis was adopted to assess the construct validity of the ULS-6, and the one-factor structure was found for both suicide and control groups. The reliability findings supported that the ULS-6 has good internal consistency with the Cronbach's α value over 0.90 in both suicide and control groups. It was similar to the previous study conducted in the elderly in rural China [26].

The association between social support and loneliness has been showed in abundant studies that a high level of social support can reduce the feeling of loneliness [36–38]. The results of the present study are consistent with the previous findings. People, who were non-currently married, living alone, and left behind by children, and had a lower score of social support, were more likely to report higher ULS-6 scores in both suicide and control groups. Emotional loneliness could be caused by the absence of a secure attachment person in one's life such as a spouse [37], and close relationships are long-term predictors of loneliness in older age [38]. Rural elderly people that live alone, are non-currently married, and left behind by children, should be evaluated as a high-risk group. Interventions targeted social support systems, especially intimate relationships are needed to alleviate loneliness feeling among the rural elderly in China.

The concurrent validity was additionally evaluated by correlations between the ULS-6 and depression and QOL. As mentioned above, many elderly people experienced loneliness either as a result of living alone, a lack of close family ties or social support. It is not surprising to find a positive correlation between loneliness and depression in both suicide and control groups. A similar correlation was reported in the previous literature [8, 9, 39]. Our study also indicated that there was a significant correlation between loneliness and QOL in both suicide and control groups. In other words, the QOL decreases along with increased feelings of loneliness, which is also supported by previous evidence [37, 40]. Thus, the construct validity of the ULS-6 was supported and demonstrates the expected link between loneliness and depression and QOL in both suicide and control groups.

There are some limitations. In this study, we used the data from the community normal living controls as the gold standard to assess the validity of their informants' responses. As suggested in previous studies [5, 19], the informants of suicide cases are most likely to be in grief, which may influence their responses to the information of the deceased. It might be asymmetrical to generalize the response from the non-grieving normal people in the living controls. Future studies may need to find ways to adjust this imbalance. Further, this study focuses on rural elderly. Future study of this type should be conducted with other age groups, and continue to evaluate its psychometric properties in psychological autopsy studies.

Conclusions

This study helps to establish the validity of proxy respondent based data on loneliness in research on suicide in older adults in rural China. Proxy respondents are generally fair judges of targets' loneliness. The ULS-6, with adequate reliability and validity, can be used in psychological autopsy research to collect data that may be ultimately inform prevention efforts, and the role of loneliness in suicide should be further studied. In addition, the ULS-6 shows potential for identifying elderly people that may be at risk for suicide. Rural elderly people that live alone, are left behind by children, non-currently married, and have higher depression and poor quality of life, are more likely to suffer from loneliness, and should be evaluated as a high-risk group.

Abbreviations

CDC: Center for Disease Control and Prevention; DSSI: Duke Social Support Index; EFA: Exploratory factor analysis; GDS: Geriatric Depression Scale; ICC: Intraclass correlation coefficient; KMO: Kaiser-Meryer-Olkin test; QOL: Quality of life; SD: Standard deviation; ULS-6: University of California Los Angeless Loneliness Scale with 6 items

Acknowledgments

We would like to thank all fieldworkers and participants for this study.

Funding
This study was funded by the American Foundation of Suicide Prevention to Dr. Liang Zhou (Grant No. SRG – 0-169-12).

Authors' contributions
LN drafted the manuscript and contributed the design and completion of the data analyses. CJ, ZM, and LZ contributed the study design and provided substantial editorial imput in the drafting of the manuscript. GW and ZY participated in the data collection, and assisted in performance of the statistical analyses. All authors read and approved the final manuscript.

Competing interests
The authors declare that they have no competing interests.

Author details
[1]The Affiliated Brain Hospital of Guangzhou Medical University (Guangzhou Huiai Hospital), 36 Mingxin Road, Liwan District, Guangzhou 510370, China. [2]School of Public Health, Shandong University, Jinan, China. [3]School of Public Health, Guangxi Medical University, Nanning, China. [4]Xiangya School of Public Health, Central South University, Changsha, China.

References

1. Liu Z, Huang Y, Ma C, Shang L, Zhang T, Chen H. Suicide rate trends in China from 2002 to 2015. Chin Ment Health J. 2017;31(10):756–67.
2. Zhong BL, Chiu HF, Conwell Y. Elderly suicide trends in the context of transforming China, 1987–2014. Sci Rep. 2016;6:37724.
3. Zhang D, Yang Y, Sun Y, Wu M, Xie H, Wang K, Zhang J, Jia J, Su Y. Characteristics of the Chinese rural elderly living in nursing homes who have suicidal ideation: a multiple regression model. Geriatr Nurs. 2017;38(5):423–30.
4. Conner KR, Duberstein PR, Conwell Y. The validity of proxy-based data in suicide research: a study of patients 50 years of age and older who attempted suicide. I. Psychiatric diagnoses. Acta Psychiatr Scand. 2001;104(3):204–9.
5. Zhang J, Conwell Y, Wieczorek WF, Jiang C, Jia S, Zhou L. Studying Chinese suicide with proxy-based data: reliability and validity of the methodology and instruments in China. J Nerv Ment Dis. 2003;191(7):450–7.
6. Fees BS, Martin P, Poon LW. A model of loneliness in older adults. J Gerontol. 1999;54(4):P231.
7. Peplau LA, Perlman D, Peplau LA, Perlman D. Blueprint for a social psychological theory of loneliness. Love Attraction. 1979:101–10.
8. Ahmed D, El Shair IH, Taher E, Zyada F. Prevalence and predictors of depression and anxiety among the elderly population living in geriatric homes in Cairo, Egypt. J Egypt Public Health Assoc. 2014;89(3):127–35.
9. Singh A, Misra N. Loneliness, depression and sociability in old age. Ind Psychiatry J. 2009;18(1):51–5.
10. Segrin C, McNelis M, Pavlich CA. Indirect effects of loneliness on substance use through stress. Health Commun. 2018:33(5)513–8.
11. Minayo MC, Cavalcante FG. Suicide attempts among the elderly: a review of the literature (2002/2013). Cien Saude Colet. 2015;20(6):1751–62.
12. Goodman ML, Serag H, Keiser PK, Gitari S, Raimer BG. Relative social standing and suicide ideation among Kenyan males: the interpersonal theory of suicide in context. Soc Psychiatry Psychiatr Epidemiol. 2017;52(10):1307–16.
13. Chang EC, Wan L, Li P, Guo Y, He J, Gu Y, Wang Y, Li X, Zhang Z, Sun Y, et al. Loneliness and suicidal risk in young adults: does believing in a changeable future help minimize suicidal risk among the lonely? J Psychol. 2017;151(5):453–63.
14. Sharma B, Lee TH, Nam EW. Loneliness, insomnia and suicidal behavior among school-going adolescents in western Pacific Island countries: role of violence and injury. Int J Environ Res Public Health 2017,14(7):791.
15. Chang Q, Chan CH, Yip PSF. A meta-analytic review on social relationships and suicidal ideation among older adults. Soc Sci Med. 2017;191:65.
16. Synnott J, Ioannou M, Coyne A, Hemingway S: A Content Analysis of Online Suicide Notes: Attempted Suicide Versus Attempt Resulting in Suicide. Suicide Life Threat Behav 2017. https://doi.org/10.1111/sltb.12398. [Epub ahead of print]
17. Knoll JL. The psychological autopsy, part I: applications and methods. J Psychiatr Pract. 2008;14(6):393–7.
18. An J, Phillips MR, Conner KR. Validity of proxy-based reports of impulsivity and aggression in Chinese research on suicidal behavior. Crisis. 2010;31(3):137.
19. Conner KR, Conwell Y, Duberstein PR. The validity of proxy-based data in suicide research: a study of patients 50 years of age and older who attempted suicide. II. Life events, social support and suicidal behavior. Acta Psychiatr Scand. 2001;104(6):452.
20. Conner KR, Beautrais AL, Brent DA, Conwell Y, Phillips MR, Schneider B. The next generation of psychological autopsy studies. Part I. Interview content. Suicide Life Threat Behav. 2011;41(6):594–613.
21. Jonggierveld JD, Kamphuls F. The development of a Rasch-type loneliness scale. Appl Psychol Measur. 1985;9(3):289–99.
22. Ditommaso E, Spinner B. The development and initial validation of the social and emotional loneliness scale for adults (SELSA). Personal Individ Differ. 1993; 14(1):127–34.
23. Russell D, Peplau LA, Ferguson ML. Developing a measure of loneliness. J Pers Assess. 1978;42(3):290.
24. Russell D, Peplau LA, Cutrona CE. The revised UCLA loneliness scale: concurrent and discriminant validity evidence. J Pers Soc Psychol. 1980;39(3):472–80.
25. Hays RD, Dimatteo MR. A short-form measure of loneliness. J Pers Assess. 1987;51(1):69–81.
26. Zhou L, Li Z, Hu M, Xiao S. Reliability and validity of ULS-8 loneliness scale in elderly samples in a rural community. J Cent South Univ (Medical Sciences). 2012;37(11):1124–8.
27. Brink TL, Yesavage JA, Lum O, Heersema PH, Adey M, Rose TL. Screening tests for geriatric depression. Clin Gerontol. 1982;1(1):37–43.
28. He X, Xiao S, Zhang D. Reliability and validity of the Chinese version of geriatric depression scale: a study in a population of Chinese rural community-dwelling elderly. Chin J Clin Psych. 2008;16(5):473–5.
29. Phillips MR, Yang G, Zhang Y, Wang L, Ji H, Zhou M. Risk factors for suicide in China: a national case-control psychological autopsy study. Lancet. 2002; 360(9347):1728–36.
30. Koenig HG, Westlund RE, George LK, Hughes DC, Blazer DG, Hybels C. Abbreviating the Duke social support index for use in chronically ill elderly individuals. Psychosomatics. 1993;34(1):61.
31. Mao H, Qiu P, Wen P, Yang Y, Hao T, Gao X, Yuan P. Reliability and validity of DSSI-23 scale in a rural elderly population. J Sichuan Univ (Medical Science Edition). 2015;46(1):90–3.
32. Cicchetti DV. Guidelines, criteria, and rules of thumb for evaluating normed and standardized assessment instruments in psychology. Psychol Assess. 1994;6(4):284–90.
33. Niu L, Qiu Y, Luo D, Chen X, Wang M, Pakenham KI, Zhang X, Huang Z, Xiao S. Cross-culture validation of the HIV/AIDS stress scale: the development of a revised Chinese version. PLoS One. 2016;11(4):e0152990.
34. Hu Y, Zhang Z, Xie J, Wang G. The outpatient experience questionnaire of comprehensive public hospital in China: development, validity and reliability. International J Qual Health Care. 2017;29(1):40–6.
35. Isometsa ET. Psychological autopsy studies–a review. Eur Psychiatry. 2001; 16(7):379–85.
36. Wang G, Zhang X, Wang K, Li Y, Shen Q, Ge X, Hang W. Loneliness among the rural older people in Anhui, China: prevalence and associated factors. Int J Geriatr Psychiatry. 2011;26(11):1162–8.
37. Arslantaş H, Adana F, Abacigil EF, Kayar D, Acar G. Loneliness in elderly people, associated factors and its correlation with quality of life: a field study from western Turkey. Iran J Public Health. 2015;44(1):43–50.
38. Dahlberg L, Andersson L, Lennartsson C. Long-term predictors of loneliness in old age: results of a 20-year national study. Aging Ment Health. 2018;22(2):190–6.
39. van den Brink RH, Schutter N, Hanssen DJ, Elzinga BM, Rabeling-Keus IM, Stek ML, Comijs HC, Penninx BW, Oude Voshaar RC. Prognostic significance of social network, social support and loneliness for course of major depressive disorder in adulthood and old age. Epidemiol Psychiatr Sci. 2017:1–12.
40. Chalise HN, Saito T, Takahashi M, Kai I. Relationship specialization amongst sources and receivers of social support and its correlations with loneliness and subjective well-being: a cross sectional study of Nepalese older adults. Arch Gerontol Geriatr. 2007;44(3):299–314.

12

Insomnia as an independent predictor of suicide attempts: a nationwide population-based retrospective cohort study

Han-Ting Lin[1], Chi-Huang Lai[1], Huey-Jen Perng[2], Chi-Hsiang Chung[2], Chung-Ching Wang[3], Wei-Liang Chen[3] and Wu-Chien Chien[1,2,4*]

Abstract

Background: Numerous studies have verified that insomnia is associated with suicidal ideation, suicide attempts, and death by suicide. Limited population-based cohort studies have been conducted to examine the association. The present study aimed to analyze whether insomnia increases the risk of suicide attempts and verify the effects of insomnia on suicide risk.

Methods: This study is a cohort study using 2000–2013 hospitalization data from the National Health Insurance Research Database (NHIRD) to track the rate of suicide attempts among insomnia patients aged 15 years or older. In addition, a 1:2 pairing based on sex, age, and date of hospitalization was conducted to identify the reference cohort (patients without insomnia). Cox proportional hazard model was used to assess the effects of insomnia on suicide risk.

Results: The total number of hospitalized patients aged 15 years or older was 479,967 between 2000 and 2013 (159,989 patients with insomnia and 319,978 patients without insomnia). After adjusting for confounders, suicide risk in insomnia patients was 3.533-fold that of patients without insomnia (adjusted hazard ratio [HR] = 3.533, 95% confidence interval [CI] = 3.059–4.080, $P < 0.001$). Suicide risk in low-income patients was 1.434-fold (adjusted HR = 1.434, 95% CI = 1.184–1.736, $P < 0.001$) that of non-low-income patients. Suicide risk in patients with drug dependence and with mental disorders was 1.592-fold (adjusted HR = 1.592, 95% CI = 1.220–2.077, $P < 0.001$) and 4.483-fold (adjusted HR = 4.483, 95% CI = 3.934–5.109, $P < 0.001$) that of patients without drug dependence and without mental disorders, respectively. In the female population, suicide risk in insomnia patients was 4.186-fold (adjusted HR = 4.186, 95% CI = 3.429–5.111, $P < 0.001$) that of patients without insomnia. Among patients aged 25–44 years, suicide risk in insomnia patients was 5.546-fold (adjusted HR = 5.546, 95% CI = 4.236–7.262, $P < 0.001$) that of patients without insomnia. Furthermore, the suicide risk of insomnia patients with mental disorders was 18.322-fold that of patients without insomnia and mental disorders ($P < 0.001$).

Conclusion: Insomnia, low income, drug dependence, and mental disorders are independent risk factors for suicide attempts. Female patients and those aged 25–44 years are at high risk of suicide due to insomnia. Insomnia, mental disorders, and low income exhibit a synergistic effect on suicide attempts. Clinicians should pay attention to mental status and income level of insomnia patients.

Keywords: Insomnia, Suicide, National Health Insurance Research Database (NHIRD)

* Correspondence: chienwu@ndmctsgh.edu.tw
[1]National Defense Medical Center, School of Public Health 4325R, No. 161, Section 6, Min-Chuan East Road, Neihu District, Taipei City 11490, Taiwan, Republic of China
[2]National Defense Medical Center, Graduate Institute of Life Sciences 7115R, No. 161, Section 6, Min-Chuan East Road, Neihu District, Taipei City 11490, Taiwan, Republic of China
Full list of author information is available at the end of the article

Background

Suicide is a serious public health problem around the world. The World Health Organization (WHO) reported that approximately 800,000 people worldwide die from suicide every year (an average of one death every 40 s). In addition, suicide is the second leading cause of death among those aged 15–29 years globally, and the fifth leading cause of death among those aged 30–49 years [1]. Compared with death by suicide, there are many more suicide attempts every year [2], and according to a meta-analysis from Japan in 2008, a prior suicide attempt is the most important predictor of suicide [3]. Suicide, moreover, causes immense socioeconomic burdens on families, communities, and nations [4]. In 2016, the number of deaths from suicide in Taiwan was 3765 (a suicide death rate of 16.0 persons per 100,000 population), making suicide the twelfth leading cause of death in Taiwan. The suicide death rate among men was approximately 2.1-times higher than that among women (17.0 men and 7.7 women per 100,000 population). The suicide death rate in all age groups increased with age [5].

Insomnia is one of the most prevalent sleeping disorders in the world [6]. According to epidemiological studies around the world, the prevalence of insomnia in general populations is 10%–25% [7–10]. A 2017 report by the Taiwan Society of Sleep Medicine indicated that a tenth of the population across Taiwan suffers from chronic insomnia (prevalence rate of 11.3%) [11]. Insomnia refers to difficulty falling asleep, remaining awake while trying to sleep, waking up often during the night, or still feeling tired after sleeping for a brief period, factors that subsequently influence daytime activities of daily living for more than four weeks. If insomnia persists for more than six months, it becomes a chronic condition influencing not only the person's psychology and physiology but also his or her health and activities of daily living (e.g., learning and working) [12].

Numerous studies have indicated that insomnia is associated with suicidal ideation [13–16], suicide attempts [17–19], and death by suicide [20–22] among adolescents and adults. These studies laid the foundation for the relationship between insomnia and suicide. However, there are some weakness in methodology and need future research to fill this gap. For example, some studies used a questionnaire asking a single question as criteria for determining insomnia or suicide [22]. Furthermore, mental disorders are a major confounding factor for insomnia and suicide, and over 90% of suicide decedents have at least one mental disorder [23]; however, some studies assessing the link between insomnia and suicide did not adjust for mental disorders [17, 20].

There are still different arguments about whether insomnia is an independent factor of suicide or if insomnia, as a symptom of mental disorders such as depression, increases the risk of suicide. Some studies have found that the relationship between insomnia and suicide is fully mediated by mental disorders [13, 14, 24]. Other studies have shown that insomnia remains an independent factor of suicidal ideation [15, 16], suicide attempt [19], and death by suicide [21, 22] after adjustments for mental disorders, substance abuse and alcohol abuse.

A meta-analysis by Pigeon et al. indicated that insomnia is still a predictor of suicide even after other factors have been adjusted for. However, the authors asserted that the samples collected are non-homogeneous, and samples for observational and clinical studies are confined to adolescents or adults only. Additionally, numerous studies are cross-sectional studies [25], which cannot be used to elucidate whether insomnia increases suicide risk. Hence, we employed the National Health Insurance Research Database (NHIRD) in Taiwan to conduct a retrospective cohort study of whether insomnia increases the risk of suicide attempts.

Methods

Data source

Introduced in Taiwan in 1995, the NHRID contains the medical records of all insured. The database encompasses the information of more than 99% of the 23 million people who live in Taiwan; thus, the health care information contained therein represents evidence-based data in the medicine and healthcare sector [26]. This study analyzed the 2000–2013 inpatient expenditure files and the registry for contracted medical facilities in the NHRID.

Design and sample

The retrospective cohort study design method was adopted in this study. Inpatients aged 15 years or older who were newly diagnosed with insomnia (International.

Classification of Diseases, 9th Revision, Clinical Modifications [ICD-9-CM]: 307.41, 307.42, 780.52) were allocated to the study cohort. To ensure that the patients were newly diagnosed, we also excluded patients who were diagnosed with insomnia between 1997 and 1999. The study period began on January 1, 2000 and ended on December 31, 2013. In total, 159,989 participants were included. The average of follow-up for the diagnosis of insomnia was 6.47 years. To facilitate comparison of the study cohort, propensity score-matching based on sex, age group, and date of hospitalization was performed for a 1:2 pairing to identify the reference cohort (n = 319,978 inpatients who were diagnosed as not having insomnia). Furthermore, there was no difference in the cause of hospitalization at baseline (Additional file 1: Table S1).

Outcome assessment

All research participants were observed until the incidence of suicide attempts (ICD-9-CM E code: 950–959), loss to follow up, or until the end of December 31, 2013.

Covariates of interested

The participants in this study were allocated into four groups by age: 15–24, 25–44, 45–64, and ≥ 65 years. Urbanization levels were categorized into high, moderate, and low levels of urbanization [27]. Low income included insured individuals in Category 5 (those to which laws and regulations governing social relief apply). Catastrophic illness was indicated in the copayment remarks of inpatient expenditure files. The Charlson comorbidity index (CCI) was used to weigh the 19 types of diseases by assigning each with a score of 1, 2, or 6, and the scores were summed according to whether each patient had any of these diseases [28, 29]. Because drug dependence, alcohol dependence, and mental disorders are risk factors for suicide attempts, drug dependence (ICD-9-CM 292, 304), alcohol dependence (ICD-9-CM 291, 303), and mental disorders (ICD-9-CM 290–319, excluding 291, 292, 303, 304) were incorporated in the regression model for adjustments.

Statistical analysis

All analyses were performed using SPSS 22 (SPSS, Inc., Chicago, IL, U.S.). The χ^2 test and Fisher exact test were used to compare the categorical variables of the two groups, and a t-test was conducted to compare the continuous variables of the two groups. With adjustments for sex, age, low income, catastrophic illness, urbanization, CCI, drug dependence, alcohol dependence, and mental disorders, Cox proportional hazards regression analyses were performed to assess the effects of insomnia on the risk of suicide attempts and presented as hazard ratio (HR) with a 95% confidence interval (CI). Furthermore, differences in the risk of suicide attempts between the study and reference cohort were estimated using the Kaplan-Meier method with the log-rank test. A 2-tailed p-value < 0.05 was considered to indicate statistical significance.

Results

Figure 1 shows the case-screening process (inclusion and exclusion) and follow-up results as well as the cumulative risk of suicide incidence between the two groups (patients with/without insomnia). Between 2000 and 2013, 16,716,547 patients were hospitalized, 178,589 of which had insomnia. After exclusion criteria were applied (18,600 excluded), there were a total of 159,989 insomnia

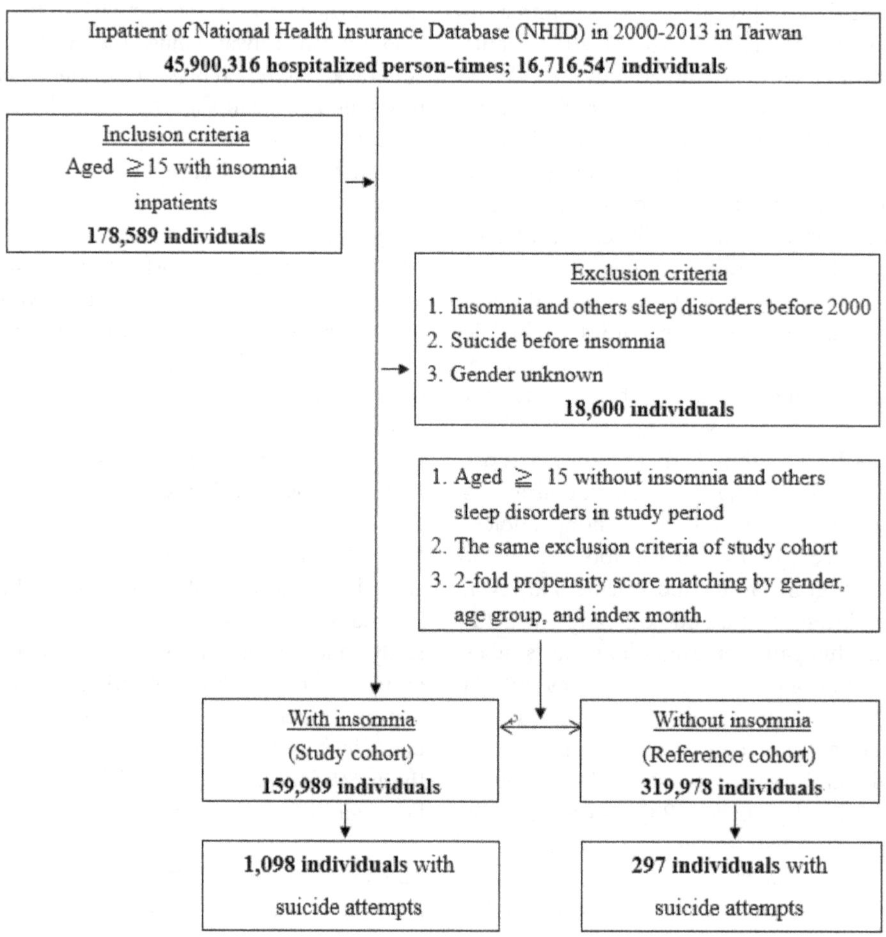

Fig. 1 Flowchart of study sample selection from the National Health Insurance Research Database in Taiwan

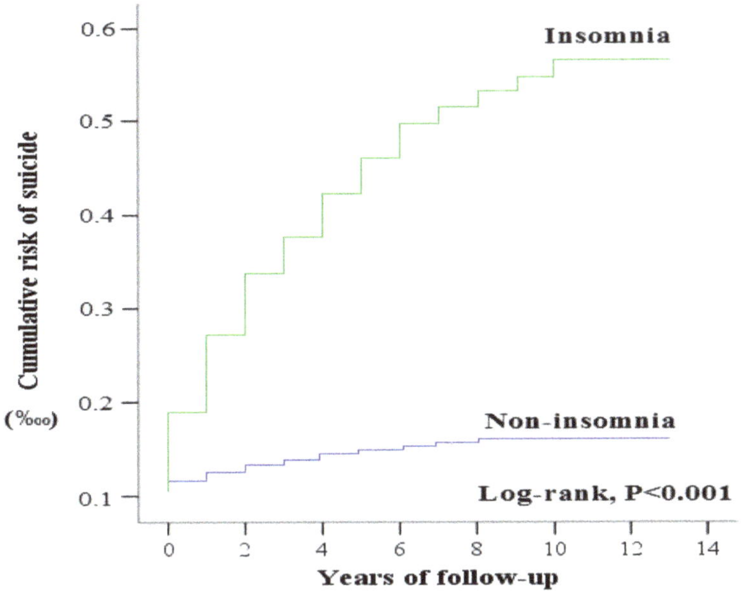

Fig. 2 Kaplan-Meier analysis of the cumulative risk of suicide attempts in 13 years of tracking stratified by insomnia with log-rank test

cases (319,978 patients were placed in the reference cohort based on 1:2 pairing) with a subsequent suicide incidence of 0.69% (1098/159,989), whereas the reference cohort exhibited a suicide incidence of 0.09% (297/319,978). The groups demonstrated significant difference (log-rank $P < 0.001$). In other words, the probability (risk) of suicide attempts in insomnia patients was considerably higher than that in patients without insomnia. In addition, both groups exhibited a statistically significant difference after one year follow up (Fig. 2, Table 1). Furthermore, an average follow-up period for the diagnosis of insomnia to suicide attempts was 2.38 years.

Table 2 presents the basic characteristics of the 479,967 patients at the endpoint of the follow-up process (study cohort = 159,989 insomnia patients; reference cohort = 319,978 non-insomnia patients). The study cohort exhibited a substantially higher incidence of suicide attempts compared with the reference cohort (0.7% vs 0.1%; $P < 0.001$). The study cohort comprised significantly higher numbers of low income patients (4.0% vs 1.5%; $P < 0.001$), patients with catastrophic illness (31.2% vs 19.8%; $P < 0.001$), and those who lived in working class urbanized townships (33.4% vs 22.3%; $P < 0.001$) than the reference cohort. The numbers of patients with drug dependence (1.0% vs 0.1%; $P < 0.001$), alcohol dependence (3.5% vs 0.7%; $p < 0.001$), and mental disorders (33.5% vs 7.1%; $p < 0.001$) and other comorbidities in the study cohort were significantly higher than those of the reference cohort.

Table 3 shows the univariate and multivariate analysis results of the factors of suicide attempts. After the research variables (sex, age, low income, catastrophic illness, urbanization, CCI, drug dependence, alcohol dependence, and mental disorders) were adjusted for, the risk of suicide attempts among insomnia patients was 3.533-fold that of non-insomnia patients ($P < 0.001$). The risk of suicide attempts among female patients was 1.522-fold ($P < 0.001$) that of male patients. The risk of suicide attempts among patients aged 15–24, 25–44, 45–64 years was 6.000-fold, 3.581-fold, and 1.595-fold ($P < 0.001$) that of patients aged 65 years or older, respectively. The risk of suicide attempts among low-income patients and patients with catastrophic

Table 1 Kaplan-Meier analysis of the cumulative risk of suicide attempts in 13 years of tracking stratified by insomnia with log-rank test

Insomnia	With ($N = 159{,}989$)	Without ($N = 319{,}979$)	*P*-value
X-year(s) of suicide attempts	Numbers of suicide attempts		
1	285	101	< 0.001
2	525	157	< 0.001
3	700	195	< 0.001
4	808	222	< 0.001
5	890	248	< 0.001
6	965	265	< 0.001
7	1020	276	< 0.001
8	1052	286	0.001
9	1070	295	< 0.001
10	1084	296	< 0.001
11	1198	297	< 0.001
12	1198	297	< 0.001
13	1198	297	< 0.001

Table 2 Characteristics of study in the endpoint

Variables	Total n	Total %	With insomnia n	With insomnia %	Without insomnia n	Without insomnia %	*P*-value
Total	479,967	100.0	159,989	33.3	319,978	66.7	
Suicide attempts							< 0.001
with	1395	0.3	1098	0.7	297	0.1	
without	478,572	99.7	158,891	99.3	319,681	99.9	
Gender							0.880
male	235,771	49.1	78,615	49.1	157,156	49.1	
female	244,196	50.9	81,374	50.9	162,822	50.9	
Age group (years)							0.958
15–24	15,901	3.3	5330	3.3	10,571	3.3	
25–44	99,058	20.6	33,030	20.6	66,028	20.6	
45–64	172,650	36.0	57,504	35.9	115,146	36.0	
≧65	192,358	40.1	64,125	40.1	128,233	40.1	
Low income							< 0.001
yes	11,251	2.3	6441	4.0	4810	1.5	
no	468,716	97.7	153,548	96.0	315,168	98.5	
Catastrophic illness							< 0.001
yes	113,150	23.6	49,914	31.2	63,236	19.8	
no	366,817	76.4	110,075	68.8	256,742	80.2	
Urbanization							< 0.001
high	150,124	31.3	41,562	26.0	108,562	33.9	
medium	205,154	42.7	65,049	40.7	140,105	43.8	
low	124,689	26.0	53,378	33.4	71,311	22.3	
CCI	2.36 ± 3.82		2.97 ± 4.10		2.06 ± 3.63		< 0.001
Drug dependence							< 0.001
yes	2051	0.4	1597	1.0	454	0.1	
no	477,916	99.6	158,392	99.0	319,524	99.9	
Alcohol dependence							< 0.001
yes	7846	1.6	5674	3.5	2172	0.7	
no	472,121	98.4	154,315	96.5	317,806	99.3	
Mental disorders							< 0.001
yes	76,322	15.9	53,537	33.5	22,785	7.1	
no	403,645	84.1	106,452	66.5	297,193	92.9	

P-value (category variable: Chi-square/Fisher exact test; continue variable: t-test)

illness was 1.434-fold and 1.286-fold that of their counterparts, respectively ($P < 0.001$). The risk of suicide attempts among patients with drug dependence and mental disorders was 1.592-fold and 4.483-fold that of their counterparts, respectively ($P < 0.001$).

Table 4 shows the hierarchical analysis of various variables to elucidate the difference in risk of suicide attempts between insomnia and non-insomnia patients. The results indicated that (after other factors were adjusted for), in the female population, suicide risk in insomnia patients was 4.186-fold (adjusted HR = 4.186, 95% CI = 3.429–5.111, $P < 0.001$) that of patients without insomnia. Among patients aged 25–44 years, suicide risk in insomnia patients was 5.546-fold (adjusted HR = 5.546, 95% CI = 4.236–7.262, $P < 0.001$) that of patients without insomnia.

Figures 3 and 4 show the interactive effects of insomnia, mental disorders, and low income after other factors were adjusted for. The risk of suicide attempts in insomnia patients without mental disorders was 4.960-fold that of patients without insomnia and mental disorders. The risk of

Table 3 Factors of suicide attempts by Cox proportional hazard model analysis

Variables	Crude HR	95% CI		*P*-value	Adjusted HR	95% CI		*P*-value
Insomnia								
no	reference				reference			
yes	7.416	6.524	8.431	< 0.001	3.533	3.059	4.080	< 0.001
Gender								
female	reference				reference			
male	1.289	1.159	1.433	< 0.001	1.522	1.361	1.702	< 0.001
Age group (years)								
≧65	reference				reference			
15–24	6.477	5.292	7.928	0.001	6.000	4.876	7.383	< 0.001
25–44	4.909	4.238	5.687	< 0.001	3.581	3.069	4.177	< 0.001
45–64	1.747	1.487	2.052	< 0.001	1.595	1.357	1.876	< 0.001
Low income								
no	reference				reference			
yes	3.940	3.267	4.751	< 0.001	1.434	1.184	1.736	< 0.001
Catastrophic illness								
No	reference				reference			
Yes	1.972	1.771	2.196	< 0.001	1.286	1.143	1.446	< 0.001
Urbanization								
high	reference				reference			
medium	1.045	0.916	1.193	0.510	1.013	0.887	1.157	0.847
low	1.569	1.372	1.795	< 0.001	1.073	0.937	1.230	0.309
CCI	0.983	0.969	0.998	0.025	0.989	0.973	1.005	0.179
Drug dependence								
no	reference				reference			
yes	9.614	7.407	12.479	< 0.001	1.592	1.220	2.077	0.001
Alcohol dependence								
no	reference				reference			
yes	5.872	4.899	7.038	< 0.001	1.164	0.955	1.420	0.133
Mental disorders								
no	reference				reference			
yes	9.742	8.723	10.879	< 0.001	4.483	3.934	5.109	< 0.001

suicide attempts in non-insomnia patients with mental disorders was 8.237-fold that of patients without insomnia and mental disorders. The risk of suicide attempts in insomnia patients with mental disorders was 18.322-fold that of patients without insomnia and mental disorders ($P < 0.001$) (Fig. 3). The risk of suicide attempts in non-low-income patients with insomnia was 3.521-fold that of non-insomnia patients who were not in the low-income group. The risk of suicide attempts in low-income patients without insomnia was 1.330-fold that of non-insomnia patients who were not in the low-income group. The risk of suicide attempts in low-income patients with insomnia was 5.084-fold that of non-insomnia patients who were not in the low-income group ($P < 0.001$) (Fig. 4).

Discussion

Our study found that insomnia remained an independent risk factor for suicide attempts after adjustments for mental disorders, alcohol dependence, and drug dependence. To the best of our knowledge, our study is the first retrospective cohort study to use population-based data and clinical diagnosis as the criteria for determining insomnia and suicide. The findings can reinforce the deficiencies of other relevant studies.

In recent years, some studies found that mental disorders, alcohol abuse, and drug abuse do not fully mediate the association between insomnia and suicide. A study conducted in 2012 regarding members of the military in the United States reported that insomnia was an independent risk

Table 4 Factors of suicide attempts stratified by variables listed in the table by Cox proportional hazard model analysis

Variables	With insomnia			Without insomnia			Ratio	Adjusted HR	95%CI		*P*-value
	Event	PYs	Rate (per 10^3 PYs)	Event	PYs	Rate (per 10^3 PYs)					
Total	1098	953,594	115.143	297	1,913,519	15.521	7.418	3.533	3.059	4.080	< 0.001
Gender											
female	633	468,954	134.981	153	941,910	16.244	8.310	4.186	3.429	5.111	< 0.001
male	465	484,640	95.948	144	971,609	14.821	6.474	2.861	2.323	3.523	< 0.001
Age group (years)											
15–24	119	42,625	279.179	33	85,435	38.626	7.228	2.778	1.747	4.417	< 0.001
25–44	546	198,523	275.031	80	400,512	19.974	13.769	5.546	4.236	7.262	< 0.001
45–64	264	317,825	83.065	105	637,466	16.471	5.043	2.637	2.053	3.389	< 0.001
≧65	169	394,621	42.826	79	790,106	9.999	4.283	2.900	2.188	3.844	< 0.001
Low income											
no	987	915,626	107.795	288	1,884,404	15.283	7.053	3.487	3.009	4.040	< 0.001
yes	111	37,968	292.351	9	29,115	30.912	9.458	4.069	2.012	8.228	< 0.001
Catastrophic illness											
no	635	645,939	98.306	220	1,504,259	14.625	6.722	3.769	3.171	4.479	< 0.001
yes	463	307,655	150.493	77	409,260	18.814	7.999	2.916	2.255	3.770	< 0.001
Urbanization											
high	291	243,831	119.345	84	661,398	12.700	9.397	3.911	2.964	5.161	< 0.001
medium	398	369,572	107.692	132	835,185	15.805	6.814	3.320	2.655	4.153	< 0.001
low	409	340,191	120.227	81	416,936	19.427	6.188	3.355	2.592	4.342	< 0.001
Drug dependence											
no	1044	942,877	110.725	292	1,910,198	15.286	7.243	3.569	3.086	4.127	< 0.001
yes	54	10,717	503.872	5	3321	150.557	3.347	2.079	0.817	5.286	0.207
Alcohol dependence											
no	978	916,596	106.699	288	1,899,319	15.163	7.037	3.513	3.032	4.072	< 0.001
yes	120	36,998	324.342	9	14,200	63.380	5.117	3.844	1.936	7.634	< 0.001
Mental disorders											
no	300	618,043	48.540	181	1,763,589	10.263	4.730	4.798	3.968	5.801	< 0.001
yes	798	335,551	237.818	116	149,930	77.369	3.074	2.223	1.823	2.711	< 0.001

factor for suicidal ideation after adjustments for depression, hopelessness, post-traumatic stress disorder, anxiety, drug abuse, and alcohol abuse. However, there were no significant associations between insomnia and suicide attempts [15]. Different from the above study [15] using a 3-item questionnaire as the criteria for insomnia, our study used the clinical diagnosis as the criteria for determining insomnia. Another study conducted in the United States in 2016 revealed that insomnia symptoms increase the risk of suicidal ideation and attempts in adolescents with adjustments for mental disorders and substance use disorders [19]. However, the above study [19] had several limitations. First, the study was cross-sectional. No temporal relationships could be established. Second, all measures were based on self-report, thus the data were subject to response and recall bias. Therefore, based on above study [19], we established insomnia as an independent predictor of suicide attempts.

Our study found that insomnia and mental disorders have a synergistic effect on the risk of suicide attempts. The risk of suicide attempts in insomnia patients with mental disorders was 18-fold that of patients without insomnia and mental disorders. However, no comparison with past studies can be made because investigations concerning the interactive effects of insomnia and mental disorders on suicide attempts are lacking. A cross-sectional study conducted in 2018 in the United States reported that poor sleep quality will increase the risk of suicide after adjusting for depression among adolescents. However, sleep problems and depression do not interact with the risk of suicide [30]. Different from above study [30] focus on the association between sleep problems and suicide, our study

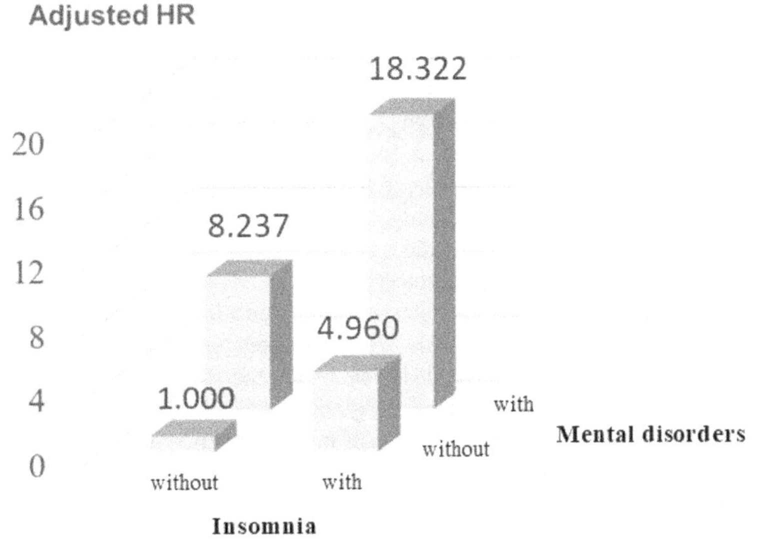

Fig. 3 Interaction for risk of suicide attempts by insomnia and mental disorders

focused on insomnia and suicide attempts. Therefore, it cannot be compared.

The mechanisms underlying the relationship between insomnia and suicide remain unclear. In 2013, a systematic literature review of adult insomnia and suicide conducted in the United States indicated that the mechanisms of insomnia and suicide involve both physiological and psychological dimensions [31]. The physiological mechanism includes a reduction in serotonin [32] and hypothalamic-pituitary-adrenal (HPA) axis dysfunction [33]. The psychological mechanism is associated with dysfunctional beliefs and attitudes about sleep (DBAS) [15] and depression [34]. Furthermore, a previous study found that fatigue resulting from sleep disorders may lead to hopelessness and decrease impulse control, both demonstrated risk factors for suicide [35]. The above possible mechanisms between insomnia and suicide require further studies for confirmation.

Our study determined that the risk of suicide attempts in patients with drug dependence was 1.592-fold that of patients without drug dependence. Several studies have indicated that the abuse of drugs such as marijuana [36], heroin [37, 38], and nicotine [39] are risk factors for suicide. A review article reported that 25% to 50% of people who

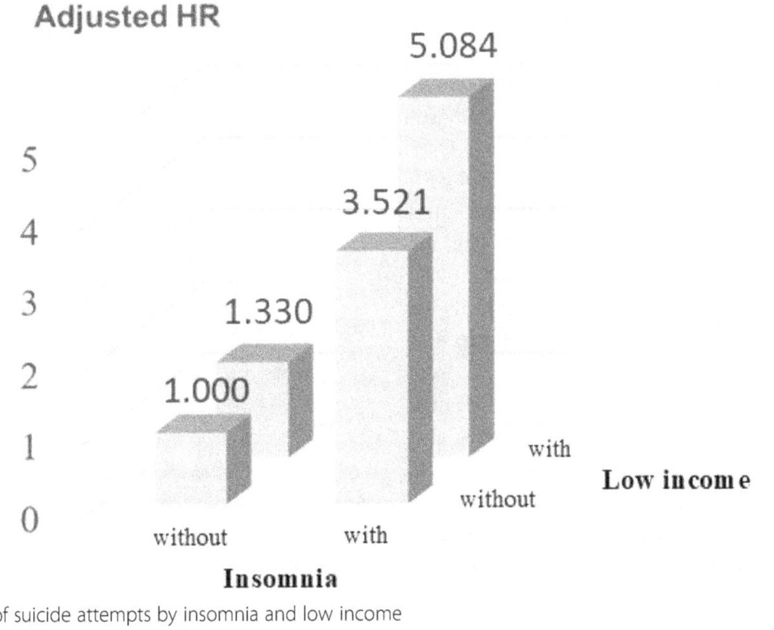

Fig. 4 Interaction for risk of suicide attempts by insomnia and low income

are suicidal are dependent on alcohol or drugs, and the risk of suicide increases if these people have mental disorders [40]. A study conducted in 1995 regarding indigenous peoples in Taiwan reported that the risk of suicide in people with substance dependence and depression was 470.2-fold that of people without substance dependence and depression [41]. In our study, we found that the risk of suicide attempts in patients with both substance dependence and depression was 22.7-fold that of their counterparts who did not fact these issues, which is lower than the finding of the aforementioned study. This difference might be attributable to social group, population, and cultural discrepancies. Another study conducted in the United States in 1993 revealed that the risk of suicide in patients with substance dependence and an emotional disorder was 17.0-fold that of their counterparts [42]. By contrast, we determined that the risk of suicide attempts in patients with both substance dependence and emotional disorder was 23.4-fold that of their counterparts. Similar to the Taiwan study [41], the focus of substance abuse in this study was alcohol and drugs; however, we reported a lower rate of substance abuse (alcohol abuse = 9.2% and drug abuse = 4.3%) compared with that of [41] (alcohol abuse = 24.3% and drug abuse = 13. 4%). This difference is possibly attributed to the more stringent standard of substance abuse (individuals exhibiting substance dependence) adopted in the present study.

Our study found that the risk of suicide attempts in patients with mental disorders was 4.483-fold that of patients without mental disorders. In western countries such as the United Kingdom, a study reported that 90% of suicides were associated with a history of mental disorders [43]. In Asian countries such as China, 40% to 70% of suicides were associated with a history of mental disorders [44, 45]. Multiple studies have indicated that different types of mental disorders predict different levels of suicide risk [46–49]. In particular, schizophrenia has the highest risk for suicide [50]. In our study, depression had the highest risk for suicide attempts, followed by schizophrenia. Another study revealed that the risk of suicide in patients with more than one mental disorders was 1.5–2.5-fold that of patients with only one type of mental disorders [43]. We incorporated depression, anxiety, bipolar disorder, and schizophrenia for further analysis and found that for every increase in the number of mental disorders, the risk of suicide attempts increased by 0.6-fold. This finding is somewhat similar to that reported in the aforementioned study.

In 2016, a United Kingdom systematic literature review indicated that low income, low socioeconomic status, and unemployment predicted higher levels of suicidal ideation, suicidal behavior, and death by suicide [51]. Our study found that risk of suicide attempts in low-income patients was 1.434-fold that of their counterparts (adjusted HR = 1. 431, 95% CI = 1.182 1.732, $P < 0.001$). Furthermore, the risk of suicide attempts in insomnia patients who earn low levels of income was 4.960-fold that of their counterparts ($P < 0.001$). This result implies that under the interactive effects of an economic stressor (low income) and insomnia, suicide became a major option for this particular population (particularly women, people aged 25–44 years, and breadwinners in the family), thereby leading to regrettable circumstances.

Our study has the following limitations. First, due to the limited types of data provided in the NHIRD, we were unable to acquire important suicide-related information (e.g., stigma, family history of suicide, occurrence of material events, and network of support). Second, our study adopted inpatient expenditure files from the NHIRD for analysis; therefore, our study findings may not be generalizable to the entire population without including outpatient cases. Third, all information was collected from medical record (NHIRD). The possibility of information bias cannot be ruled out.

Conclusions

Insomnia is a risk factor for suicide attempts and, indeed, increases the risk for suicide. In addition, low income, drug dependence, and mental disorders are risk factors for suicide attempts. Female patients and those aged 25–44 years are high-risk groups. Risk of suicide attempts is higher in low-income individuals with insomnia and mental disorders. Clinicians should pay attention to the mental status and income level of insomnia patients and implement early suicide prevention intervention. If members of the general public have friends who suffer from insomnia, they should pay attention to the mental and financial status of their friends in order to reduce the probability of suicide.

Abbreviations

CCI: The Charlson comorbidity index; CI: Confidence interval; HR: Hazard ratio; ICD-9-CM: The International Classification of Diseases, 9th Revision, Clinical Modifications; NHIRD: National Health Insurance Research Database; WHO: World Health Organization

Acknowledgments

This study was supported by grants from Tri-service Hospital Research Foundation (TSGH-C107-004), and the sponsor has no role in study design, data collection and analysis, decision to publish, or preparation of the manuscript.

Authors' contributions

CCH, LCH and CWC contributed to the study design. Data analyses and interpretation were performed by LHT, PHJ, WCC, CWL and CWC. LHT, LCH and CWC drafted and revised the manuscript. All authors read and approved the final manuscript.

Competing interests

The authors declare that they have no competing interests.

Author details

[1]National Defense Medical Center, School of Public Health 4325R, No. 161, Section 6, Min-Chuan East Road, Neihu District, Taipei City 11490, Taiwan, Republic of China. [2]National Defense Medical Center, Graduate Institute of Life Sciences 7115R, No. 161, Section 6, Min-Chuan East Road, Neihu District, Taipei City 11490, Taiwan, Republic of China. [3]Department of Family and Community Medicine, National Defense Medical Center, Tri-Service General Hospital Taipei, No. 325, Section 2, Cheng-Kung Road, Taipei City 11490, Taiwan, Republic of China. [4]Department of Medical Research 7115R, National Defense Medical Center, Tri-Service General Hospital Taipei, No. 325, Section 2, Cheng-Kung Road, Taipei City 11490, Taiwan, Republic of China.

References

1. World Health Organization. Suicide: Fact sheet. 2017 [http://www.who.int/mediacentre/factsheets/fs398/en/].
2. Nock MK, Borges G, Bromet EJ, Cha CB, Kessler RC, Lee S. Suicide and suicidal behavior. Epidemiol Rev. 2008;30:133–54.
3. Yoshimasu K, Kiyohara C, Miyashita K. Stress research Group of the Japanese Society for hygiene. Suicidal risk factors and completed suicide: meta-analyses based on psychological autopsy studies. Environ Health Prev Med. 2008;13(5):243–56.
4. World Health Organization. Preventing suicide: A global imperative. 2014 [http://www.who.int/mental_health/suicide-prevention/world_report_2014/en/].
5. Ministry of Health and Welfare, Taiwan. 2016 statistical results on causes of death in Taiwan. 2016 [https://www.mohw.gov.tw/cp-16-33598-1.html].
6. Unbehaun T, Spiegelhalder K, Hirscher V, Riemann D. Management of insomnia: update and new approaches. Nat Sci Sleep. 2010;28(2):127–38.
7. Doghramji K. The epidemiology and diagnosis of insomnia. Am J Manag Care. 2006;12(Suppl 8):S214–20.
8. Cho YW, Shin WC, Yun CH, Hong SB, Kim J, Earley CJ. Epidemiology of insomnia in korean adults: prevalence and associated factors. J Clin Neurol. 2009;5(1):20–3.
9. Chan-Chee C, Bayon V, Bloch J, Beck F, Giordanella JP, Leger D. Epidemiology of insomnia in France. Rev Epidemiol Sante Publique. 2011; 59(6):409–22.
10. Ikeda M, Kaneita Y. The newest epidemiology trend of insomnia. Nihon Rinsho. 2014;72(3):573–7.
11. Taiwan Society of Sleep Medicine. 2017 trend in prevalence of sleep problems in Taiwan: a 10-years cross sectional study. 2017 [http://www.tssm.org.tw/file/1494489550.pdf].
12. Chung WS, Li FC, Ho FM. Classification and Treatment of insomnia. Taiwan Med J. 2013;56(12):642–5.
13. Nadorff MR, Nazem S, Fiske A. Insomnia symptoms, nightmares, and suicidal ideation in a college student sample. Sleep. 2011;34(1):93–8.
14. Nadorff MR, Fiske A, Sperry JA, Petts R, Gregg JJ. Insomnia symptoms, nightmares, and suicidal ideation in older adults. J Gerontol B Psychol Sci Soc Sci. 2013;68(2):145–52.
15. Ribeiro JD, Pease JL, Gutierrez PM, Silva C, Bernert RA, Rudd MD, et al. Sleep problems outperform depression and hopelessness as cross-sectional and longitudinal predictors of suicidal ideation and behavior in young adults in the military. J Affect Disord. 2012;136(3):743–50.
16. Richardson JD, Thompson A, King L, Corbett B, Shnaider P, St Cyr K, et al. Insomnia, psychiatric disorders and suicidal ideation in a National Representative Sample of active Canadian forces members. BMC Psychiatry. 2017;17(1):211.
17. Hall RC, Platt DE, Hall RC. Suicide risk assessment: a review of risk factors for suicide in 100 patients who made severe suicide attempts. Evaluation of suicide risk in a time of managed care. Psychosomatics. 1999;40(1):18–27.
18. Kay DB, Dombrovski AY, Buysse DJ, Reynolds CF, Begley A, Szanto K. Insomnia is associated with suicide attempt in middle-aged and older adults with depression. Int Psychogeriatr. 2016;28(4):613–9.
19. Wong MM, Brower KJ, Craun EA. Insomnia symptoms and suicidality in the National Comorbidity Survey - adolescent supplement. J Psychiatr Res. 2016; 81:1–8.
20. Fujino Y, Mizoue T, Tokui N, Yoshimura T. Prospective cohort study of stress, life satisfaction, self-rated health, insomnia, and suicide death in Japan. Suicide Life Threat Behav. 2005;35(2):227–37.
21. Goldstein TR, Bridge JA, Brent DA. Sleep disturbance preceding completed suicide in adolescents. J Consult Clin Psychol. 2008;76(1):84–91.
22. Bjorngaard JH, Bjerkeset O, Romundstad P, Gunnell D. Sleeping problems and suicide in 75,000 Norwegian adults: a 20 year follow-up of the HUNT I study. Sleep. 2011;34(9):1155–9.
23. Bertolote JM, Fleischmann A, De Leo D, Wasserman D. Psychiatric diagnoses and suicide: revisiting the evidence. Crisis. 2004;25(4):147–55.
24. Bernert RA, Joiner TE, Cukrowicz KC, Schmidt NB, Krakow B. Suicidality and sleep disturbances. Sleep. 2005;28(9):1135–41.
25. Pigeon WR, Pinquart M, Conner K. Meta-analysis of sleep disturbance and suicidal thoughts and behaviors. J Clin Psychiatry. 2012;73(9):e1160–7.
26. National Health Research Institutes, Taiwan. The National Health Insurance Research Database: background. 2003 [https://nhird.nhri.org.tw/en/index.html].
27. Liu CY, Hung YT, Chuang YL, Chen YJ, Weng WS, Liu JS, et al. Incorporating development stratification of Taiwan townships into sampling Design of Large Scale Health Interview Survey. J Health Manag. 2006;4(1):1–22.
28. Charlson ME, Pompei P, Ales KL, MacKenzie CR. A new method of classifying prognostic comorbidity in longitudinal studies: development and validation. J Chronic Dis. 1987;40(5):373–83.
29. Deyo RA, Cherkin DC, Ciol MA. Adapting a clinical comorbidity index for use with ICD-9-CM administrative databases. J Clin Epidemiol. 1992;45(6):613–9.
30. Becker SP, Dvorsky MR, Holdaway AS, Luebbe AM. Sleep problems and suicidal behaviors in college students. J Psychiatr Res. 2018;99:122–8.
31. McCall WV, Black CG. The link between suicide and insomnia: theoretical mechanisms. Curr Psychiatry Rep. 2013;15(9):389.
32. Elmenhorst D, Kroll T, Matusch A, Bauer A. Sleep deprivation increases cerebral serotonin 2A receptor binding in humans. Sleep. 2012;35(12):1615–23.
33. Bonnet MH, Arand DL. 24-hour metabolic rate in insomniacs and matched normal sleepers. Sleep. 1995;18(7):581–8.
34. Kitamura S, Hida A, Watanabe M, Enomoto M, Aritake-Okada S, Moriguchi Y, et al. Evening preference is related to the incidence of depressive states independent of sleep-wake conditions. Chronobiol Int. 2010;27(9–10):1797–812.
35. Joiner TE, Brown JS, Wingate LR. The psychology and neurobiology of suicidal behavior. Annu Rev Psychol. 2005;56:287–314.
36. Borges G, Benjet C, Orozco R, Medina-Mora ME, Menendez D. Alcohol, cannabis and other drugs and subsequent suicide ideation and attempt among young Mexicans. J Psychiatr Res. 2017;91:74–82.
37. Kazour F, Soufia M, Rohayem J, Richa S. Suicide risk of heroin dependent subjects in Lebanon. Community Ment Health J. 2016;52(5):589–96.
38. Darke S, Ross J, Marel C, Mills KL, Slade T, Burns L, et al. Patterns and correlates of attempted suicide amongst heroin users: 11-year follow-up of the Australian treatment outcome study cohort. Psychiatry Res. 2015;227(2–3):166–70.
39. Bohnert KM, Ilgen MA, McCarthy JF, Ignacio RV, Blow FC, Katz IR. Tobacco use disorder and the risk of suicide mortality. Addiction. 2014;109(1):155–62.
40. Schneider B. Substance use disorders and risk for completed suicide. Arch Suicide Res. 2009;13(4):303–16.
41. Cheng AT. Mental illness and suicide. A case-control study in East Taiwan. Arch Gen Psychiatry. 1995;52(7):594–603.
42. Brent DA, Perper JA, Moritz G, Allman C, Friend A, Roth C, et al. Psychiatric risk factors for adolescent suicide: a case-control study. J Am Acad Child Adolesc Psychiatry. 1993;32(3):521–9.
43. Cavanagh JT, Carson AJ, Sharpe M, Lawrie SM. Psychological autopsy studies of suicide: a systematic review. Psychol Med. 2003;33(3):395–405.
44. Zhang J, Xiao S, Zhou L. Mental disorders and suicide among young rural Chinese: a case-control psychological autopsy study. Am J Psychiatry. 2010; 167(7):773–81.
45. Jia CX, Wang LL, Xu AQ, Dai AY, Qin P. Physical illness and suicide risk in rural residents of contemporary China: a psychological autopsy case-control study. Crisis. 2014;35(5):330–7.
46. Indu PS, Anilkumar TV, Pisharody R, Russell PSS, Raju D, Sarma PS, et al. Prevalence of depression and past suicide attempt in primary care. Asian J Psychiatr. 2017;27:48–52.
47. Thibodeau MA, Welch PG, Sareen J, Asmundson GJ. Anxiety disorders are independently associated with suicide ideation and attempts: propensity score matching in two epidemiological samples. Depress Anxiety. 2013; 30(10):947–54.

48. McGrady A, Lynch D, Rapport D. Psychosocial factors and comorbidity associated with suicide attempts: findings in patients with bipolar disorder. Psychopathology. 2017;50(2):171–4.
49. Jakhar K, Beniwal RP, Bhatia T, Deshpande SN. Self-harm and suicide attempts in schizophrenia. Asian J Psychiatr. 2017;30:102–6.
50. Limosin F, Loze JY, Philippe A, Casadebaig F, Rouillon F. Ten-year prospective follow-up study of the mortality by suicide in schizophrenic patients. Schizophr Res. 2007;94(1–3):23–8.
51. Iemmi V, Bantjes J, Coast E, Channer K, Leone T, McDaid D, et al. Suicide and poverty in low-income and middle-income countries: a systematic review. Lancet Psychiatry. 2016;3(8):774–83.

13

Assessment of subjective emotional valence and long-lasting impact of life events: development and psychometrics of the Stralsund Life Event List (SEL)

Johanna König[1*], Andrea Block[1,2], Mathias Becker[1,3], Kristin Fenske[1], Johannes Hertel[1], Sandra Van der Auwera[1,4], Kathleen Zymara[1], Henry Völzke[5], Harald Jürgen Freyberger[1,3] and Hans Jörgen Grabe[1,4]

Abstract

Background: Life events (LEs) are associated with future physical and mental health. They are crucial for understanding the pathways to mental disorders as well as the interactions with biological parameters. However, deeper insight is needed into the complex interplay between the type of LE, its subjective evaluation and accompanying factors such as social support. The "Stralsund Life Event List" (SEL) was developed to facilitate this research.

Methods: The SEL is a standardized interview that assesses the time of occurrence and frequency of 81 LEs, their subjective emotional valence, the perceived social support during the LE experience and the impact of past LEs on present life. Data from 2265 subjects from the general population-based cohort study "Study of Health in Pomerania" (SHIP) were analysed. Based on the mean emotional valence ratings of the whole sample, LEs were categorized as "positive" or "negative". For verification, the SEL was related to lifetime major depressive disorder (MDD; Munich Composite International Diagnostic Interview), childhood trauma (Childhood Trauma Questionnaire), resilience (Resilience Scale) and subjective health (SF-12 Health Survey).

Results: The report of lifetime MDD was associated with more negative emotional valence ratings of negative LEs (OR = 2.96, $p < 0.0001$). Negative LEs ($b = 0.071$, $p < 0.0001$, $\beta = 0.25$) and more negative emotional valence ratings of positive LEs ($b = 3.74$, $p < 0.0001$, $\beta = 0.11$) were positively associated with childhood trauma. In contrast, more positive emotional valence ratings of positive LEs were associated with higher resilience ($b = -7.05$, $p < 0.0001$, $\beta = 0.13$), and a lower present impact of past negative LEs was associated with better subjective health ($b = 2.79$, $p = 0.001$, $\beta = 0.05$). The internal consistency of the generated scores varied considerably, but the mean value was acceptable (averaged Cronbach's alpha > 0.75).

Conclusions: The SEL is a valid instrument that enables the analysis of the number and frequency of LEs, their emotional valence, perceived social support and current impact on life on a global score and on an individual item level. Thus, we can recommend its use in research settings that require the assessment and analysis of the relationship between the occurrence and subjective evaluation of LEs as well as the complex balance between distressing and stabilizing life experiences.

Keywords: Positive life events, Negative life events, General population, Emotional valence, Depressive disorder

* Correspondence: johanna.koenig@uni-greifswald.com
[1]Department of Psychiatry and Psychotherapy, University Medicine Greifswald, Ellernholzstraße 1-2, 17489 Greifswald, Germany
Full list of author information is available at the end of the article

Background

Negative life events (LEs) have been associated with enhanced biological stress reactions and enhanced risk of physical and mental diseases. For example, as part of gene-environment-interactions (GxE interactions), childhood and adulthood trauma have been described as an important environmental factor [1–7]. Thus, Grabe et al. [7] demonstrated that the s-allele of the 5-HTTLPR polymorphism was highly associated with higher depression scores only in subjects who reported both childhood and adulthood traumatic LEs. On the other hand, positive LEs have been associated with lower biological stress levels and increased resilience [8–12]. Hence, Haeffel and Vargas [9] reported positive LEs to buffer the negative impact of negative LEs on depressive symptoms. In addition, various studies have demonstrated that the impact of LEs on long-term health outcomes depends on the experience's characteristics, e.g., experience time as well as individual protective resources [11, 13–17]. Thus, Kleiman et al. [18] reported optimistic subjects to be less affected by negative LEs, and Asselmann et al. [19] observed that coping efficacy mediated the impact of negative LEs on mental health. Further, Brown and McGill [16, 17] found subjects with low self-esteem to benefit less from the buffering effect of positive LEs, and Staufenbiel et al. [11] reported positive LEs to moderate the association between social support and hair cortisol levels. However, it is unclear whether the experience, and thus the number of LEs, or the subjective emotional perception of the LE is more important in this regulation.

The substantial importance of LEs for long-term health has stimulated the development of scales measuring the experience of positive and negative LEs. For example, one of the first known scales is Meyer's *Life Chart,* which uses a lifeline to collect and organize the onset and duration of LEs as well as physical and mental diseases [20, 21]. Likewise, Caspi et al. [22] developed the *Life History Calendar (LHC),* which records LEs and diseases graphically linked to a calendar. However, both scales focus on the LE and life history but do not include an evaluation of the emotional valence of the LEs [20–22]. The *Social Readjustment Rating Scale (SRRS)* assesses 43 LEs associated with fixed life change units, which correspond to standardized ratings of subjective stress reactions and are summed to evaluate the risk of disease [23]. In contrast, the German language *Munich Event List (MEL)* assesses the subjective stress level and emotional valence for each LE individually [24, 25]. However, both the *SRRS* and the *MEL* focus on the assessment and evaluation of LEs but do not include explicitly an assessment of accompanying dimensions such as social support. Within the *Life Events and Difficulties Schedule (LEDS),* the interviewee is guided to a comprehensive LE story covering the surrounding situation during the LE experience [26, 27]. Later, these stories are rated regarding the "emotional arousal", "general contextual threat" and "specific aspects of the threat" by an evaluator who was uninvolved during the interview [26–28]. Within the German language *Inventar zur Erfassung lebensverändernder Ereignisse (ILE),* all LEs are rated by the individual in terms of controllability and predictability as well as personal coping skills and perceived social support [29, 30]. Another German-language scale, the *Leipziger Ereignis- und Belastungsinventar (LEBI),* focusses on the impact of LEs on major aims in life and assesses social support, subjective burden and subjective controllability [31]. However, the *SRRS, LEDS, ILE* and *LEBI* only assess the individual burden caused by the LEs but do not assess the subjective emotional valence (positive/negative/neutral) associated with the LEs.

Within the "Study of Health in Pomerania" (SHIP), a comprehensive health assessment, our working group aimed to investigate the influences of LEs and GxE interactions on mental and physical health outcomes. This research approach requires an advanced assessment tool to evaluate various aspects of LEs:

1. We aimed to assess positive, negative and neutral LEs covering the whole lifespan.
2. Similar to the *LHC,* we aimed to assess the time of occurrence, the frequency and the duration of LEs using a life history method to be able to relate the LEs to mental and physical diseases.
3. In contrast to the SRRS, we aimed to assess the subjective burden caused by the LEs individually, as it is unclear to what extent this could be represented properly by a priori standardized values [28]. In addition to what is assessed in the *LEDS, ILE* and *LEBI,* we aimed to assess the subjective emotional valence of all LEs (positive/negative/neutral).
4. In addition to what is assessed in the *MEL,* we aimed to assess the perceived social support received during the LE experience, as accompanying circumstances have been demonstrated to influence the impact of LEs on future life and health status [5, 11, 28, 32].

No single measurement was available that covered all the abovementioned requirements. Hence, we set out to develop a new interview that aimed to optimize and extend the already existing measurements: the *Stralsund Life Event List (Stralsunder Lebensereignisliste, SEL).* The *SEL* is a standardized interview assessing not only the occurrence and frequency of LEs but also the perceived social support and the impact of past LEs on current life. In contrast to existing measurements, the emotional valence of LEs was not determined a priori but was rated individually by the interviewees. These emotional valence ratings were assessed for all LEs at the time of their occurrence as well as at the time of the interview. The present article describes the development, structure, first descriptive statistics and preliminary validity and reliability data of the *SEL*.

Methods

Study populations

We analysed data from the study "Life Events and Gene-Environment-Interaction in Depression" (SHIP-LEGEND), which is a sub-sample of the "Study of Health in Pomerania" (SHIP) [33]. SHIP is a two-stage stratified population-based cohort study conducted in West Pomerania that comprises a baseline sample of 4308 Caucasian participants (SHIP-0, 20-79 years), who were drawn from local registers between 1997 and 2001. Three follow-up measurements (SHIP-1: 2002-2006, SHIP-2: 2008-2012, SHIP-3: 2015-2017) were conducted. SHIP-LEGEND was conducted in parallel to SHIP-2. All participants from the baseline sample (SHIP-0) still alive in 2006 were asked to participate in SHIP-LEGEND. A total of 2400 subjects participated in SHIP-LEGEND between 2007 and 2010. SHIP-LEGEND comprised a comprehensive psychological assessment by fully qualified psychologists or advanced psychology students based on diagnostic interviews for mental disorders and LEs (SEL) as well as questionnaires that were sent to the participant's home before the interviews. The interviews occurred in the Departments of Psychiatry and Psychotherapy in Greifswald and Stralsund or at the participant's home. The presented data are based on a rectified sample (n = 2265) that excluded participants whose response behaviours were rated as highly unreliable or inconsistent by the interviewer (n = 106) and/or participants who did not complete the interview (n = 117).

All participants had given written informed consent. The study protocol and methods of SHIP and SHIP-LEGEND were approved by the local Institutional Review Board of the University of Greifswald and conformed to the principles of the Declaration of Helsinki.

For preliminary reliability analyses, a second, clinical sample (n = 19) was drawn. All participants were patients in the day hospital of the Department of Psychiatry and Psychotherapy of the University Medicine Greifswald in 2012 and 2013. To assess the test-retest reliability, half of the participants (n = 9) were re-interviewed approximately 28 days (mean (M) = 28.7, standard deviation (SD) = 4.7) after the initial interview by the same interviewer. The remaining participants (n = 10) were re-interviewed approximately two days (M = 1.8, SD = 0.4) after the initial interview by another interviewer. All participants in the reliability sample gave written informed consent. The reliability sample was used to estimate the inter-rater and test-retest reliabilities. The corresponding analyses are presented in the Additional file 1 and Additional file 2: Table S3, Additional file 3: Table S4 and Additional file 4: Table S5.

Stralsund life event list (Stralsunder Lebensereignisliste, SEL)

The SEL comprises 81 LEs structured in 14 sections (Additional file 5: Table S1). The created LE items are partially based on existing LE measurements [22, 24, 26, 29, 31], supplemented by further positive LEs and sample-specific, major historical LE questions concerning, for example, forced displacement in the post-war era (World War II) and the German reunification in 1990. In addition to 70 standardized LEs, 11 open questions were added, giving the participant the opportunity to report additional previously unmentioned LEs.

For each LE, the participants were asked to report if they had ever experienced the given LE (*occurrence of LE*). If a LE had not been experienced, the interviewer continued with the next one. If a LE had been experienced, the frequency and respective onsets of the LE were coded. To standardize the onset coding process, onsets were categorized in 5-year periods starting with 5 to 10 years up to 81 to 85 years. If there were multiple experiences of the same LE, only the one with the highest subjective meaning for the participant was rated in detail. The exact age at the occurrence was noted (Additional file 6: Figure S1). Further, to improve the coding of the time of the occurrence (*occurrence time coding*), LEs were embedded in the context of developmental milestones (e.g., graduation, marriage, childbirth). For each experienced LE, participants rated the *emotional valence* of the LE at the time of the occurrence and at the time of the interview on a 5-point scale (1 = very positive, 2 = positive, 3 = neutral, 4 = negative, 5 = very negative). Similar to the *emotional valence* ratings, the perceived *social support* at the time of the occurrence was rated (0 = no social support desired, 1 = no social support, 2 = minimal social support, 3 = moderate social support, 4 = considerable social support). The rating scales for *emotional valence* and perceived *social support* were given to the participants during the interview. Finally, the participants were asked to decide whether the past LE still had an impact on their emotional and social life currently (*present impact*). If a LE was not applicable (e.g., items about children if the participant had never had children), the item was skipped. For a coding example, see Additional file 6: Figure S1. Note that there are LEs where some of the ratings were not appropriate.

Because this article aims to provide a first overview of the SEL and its psychometric criteria, all analyses will focus on lifespan measurements. Further, to ensure the comparability of the SEL scores, open questions (unstandardized items) were excluded from all analyses.

Further interviews and psychometric data

To associate LEs with pathogenic mechanisms of mental and physical diseases, valid diagnoses are essential. Therefore, prior to the SEL interview, the Munich Composite International Diagnostic Interview [34] was used. The M-CIDI is a structured and standardized interview evaluating the individual lifetime prevalence of mental diseases according to the internationally used classification systems ICD-10 and DSM-IV. The M-CIDI has been shown to be highly reliable and valid in assessing the onset and duration of the disorders [35]. To assess subjective health, the SF-12 Health Survey [36] was used. Additionally, depressive symptoms and childhood trauma were assessed using the Beck Depression Inventory-II [37] and Childhood Trauma Questionnaire [38], respectively. Resilience and social support were assessed by the Resilience Scale [39] and the Social Support Questionnaire [40, 41], respectively. All questionnaires have been shown to be highly reliable [36, 41–44].

Statistical analyses

For descriptive analyses, metric variables are reported in means (M) and standard deviations (SD). Categorical variables are reported in frequencies. All p-values (p) reported are two-tailed. Statistical analyses were performed in STATA/SE 14.

Classification process of LEs

To aggregate LE information but sustain inter-individual and inter-LE comparability, we a posteriori applied a classification process that resulted in three classes of LEs (valence categories) typifying positive, negative and neutral LEs. The classification process was based on the average *emotional valence* rating for each LE within the SHIP-LEGEND sample. Every LE's mean *emotional valence* at the time of its occurrence rated retrospectively was tested for the deviation from 3 (3 = neutral) using a one-sample t-test. Means that were significantly smaller were classified as positive, and means that were significantly higher, as negative. Means that did not vary significantly from 3 were classified as neutral. As the *emotional valence* at the time of the occurrence was not assessed in seven items where this information was not appropriate (items S9, B15, K28, L35, A47, F50 and D57), these LEs were typified as positive, negative and neutral using the mean *emotional valence* rating at the time of the interview. Only four LEs (H2, K22, A43, G63) were classified as neutral. Thus, the neutral valence category was neglected in further analyses.

SEL scores

Since we aimed to aggregate the rating information assessed by the SEL, we calculated scores based on the classification process described. For every participant, the *basic number of LEs* was calculated for positive and negative LEs. The *basic number of LEs* represents the number of different LEs experienced over the whole lifespan. Further, the *proportion* of positive and negative LEs in fact rated as positive or negative, respectively, was calculated to determine the individual *emotional valence* at the time of the occurrence. To develop a score that reveals not only the number of different experienced LEs (*basic number of LEs*) but also the total number of experienced LEs including repeated occurrences of the same LE, a *total frequency of LEs* was calculated per valence category for every participant by adding up the individual frequency of each experienced LE. To compare the *emotional valence* ratings at the time of the interview inter-individually, the mean individual *emotional valence* for positive and negative LEs was determined for every participant. Therefore, a quotient of the sum of the individual *emotional valence* ratings of experienced LEs and the individual *basic number of LEs* was calculated for each valence category. This procedure was repeated for the *social support* and *present impact* ratings.

Verification analyses

To verify the explanatory power of the SEL, well-studied relations between LEs, childhood trauma, health and individual resources were replicated. Using univariate multivariable linear regression analyses, the associations between the *basic number, total number, proportion, emotional valence* at the time of the interview and *present impact* of positive and negative LEs were considered with the following questionnaires: SF-12 Health Survey (SF-12) [36], Resilience Scale (RS-25) [39], and Childhood Trauma Questionnaire (CTQ) [38]. To validate the *social support* scores, the Social Support Questionnaire (F-SozU) [40] was used. Using a univariate multivariable linear logistic regression, the impact of the *basic number, total number, proportion, emotional valence* and *present impact* of LEs on the probability of reporting a lifetime diagnosis of major depressive disorder (MDD) was also assessed. As depressive symptoms repeatedly have been associated with recognition biases concerning LE reports [45–48], the BDI-II total score was used as a covariate for all analyses [37] in addition to age, sex and educational level. Hence, 12 multivariable regression analyses were calculated for each verification scale.

Internal consistency

To analyse the internal consistency of the SEL scores, Cronbach's alpha was calculated using the SHIP-LEGEND sample [49, 50]. As sufficient observations are needed for calculation, nine LEs reported by less than 5% of the sample (n = 113) were excluded from analysis.

Statistical analyses concerning the inter-rater and test-retest reliabilities are presented in the Additional file 1.

Results

Descriptive statistics

The following analyses are based on 2265 participants (47.7% male, M = 55.3 years, SD = 13.9 years, age range: 29-89 years). A sample description is provided in Table 1. The BDI-II, CTQ, RS-25, SF-12 and F-SozU scores are similar to scores reported for the general population [41–43, 51, 52]. The descriptive statistics of all SEL items including the mean *frequencies*, mean *emotional valence* ratings, mean *social support* ratings and *present impact* ratings are presented in Additional file 7: Table S2. The descriptive statistics of the SEL scores are provided in Table 2.

Verification analyses

Participants reporting lifetime MDD reported higher *basic numbers of negative LEs* (odds ratio (OR) = 1.17, 95%-CI = 1.13;1.21, $p < 0.001$) than those reported by participants without lifetime MDD. Lifetime MDD was also associated with more negatively rated life events in both valence categories, even though only the proportion of negatively rated negative LEs reached significance (OR = 4.61, 95%-CI = 2.20;9.64, $p < 0.001$); see Fig. 1a. Further, lifetime MDD was associated with a more negative current emotional valence rating of negative LEs (OR = 2.96, 95%-CI = 2.29;3.84, $p < 0.001$) and a higher present impact of negative LEs (OR = 2.80, 95%-CI = 1.67;4.63, $p < 0.001$) (Fig. 1b and c). Similarly, childhood trauma was associated with more negative LEs (b = 0.71, 95%-CI = 0.59;0.83, $p < 0.001$, $\beta = 0.25$) and reduced proportions of positively rated positive LEs (b = – 7.12, 95%-CI = – 10.97;-3.27, $p = 0.0003$, $\beta = -0.08$). However, childhood trauma was related to neither the basic number of positive LEs (b = 0.08, 95%-CI = – 0.15;0.31, $p = 0.487$, $\beta = 0.02$) nor to the proportion of negatively rated negative LEs (b = 0.74, 95%-CI = – 1.62;3.09, $p = 0.540$, $\beta = 0.01$). Further, with increasing severity of childhood traumas, positive LEs were currently rated more negatively (b = 3.74, 95%-CI = 2.28;5.19, $p < 0.001$, $\beta = 0.11$), but this was not true for negative LEs (b = 0.50, 95%-CI = – 0.37;1.38, $p = 0.259$, $\beta = 0.02$). Interestingly, childhood trauma was negatively associated with the perceived social support during the LE occurrence for positive (b = – 1.34, 95%-CI = – 1.81;-0.86, $p < 0.001$, $\beta = 0.13$) and negative LEs (b = – 2.15, 95%-CI = – 2.62;-1.68, $p < 0.001$, $\beta = 0.20$). In contrast to lifetime MDD and childhood trauma, high resilience was associated with higher proportions of positively rated positive LEs (b = 11.62, 95%-CI = 5.91;17.33, $p < 0.001$, $\beta = 0.08$) as well as increased present impact of positive life events (b = 9.93, 95%-CI = 5.61;14.25, $p < 0.001$, $\beta = 0.09$) but was not related to any score for negative LEs. Higher proportions of positively rated positive LEs (b = 2.79, 95%-CI = 1.07;4.51, $p = 0.001$, $\beta = 0.05$) and fewer reported negative LEs (b = – 0.12, 95%-CI = – 0.18;-0.07, $p < 0.001$, $\beta = 0.07$) were associated with better subjective health. Accordingly, better subjective health was associated with a lower present impact of negative LEs (b = – 2.14, 95%-CI = – 2.99;-1.29, $p < 0.001$, $\beta = -0.07$). Higher social support reported in the F-SozU questionnaire was associated with higher SEL *social support* scores for both positive (b = 0.05, 95%-CI = 0.03;0.08, $p < 0.001$, $\beta = 0.10$) and

Table 1 Descriptive statistics for 2265 analysed participants of SHIP-LEGEND

	SHIP-LEGEND		No Lifetime MDD[a]		Lifetime MDD[a]		*p*-value
	Missing (#)		Missing (#)		Missing (#)		
N	–	2265	–	1876	–	386	–
Male (%)	0	47.7	0	51.2	0	30.8	< 0.0001[h]
Age (years)	0	55.3 (13.9)	0	55.8 (14.1)	0	52.6 (12.8)	< 0.0001[g]
Education (%)	3		2		1		0.011[h]
< 10 years		26.9		28.1		21.0	
10 years		53.1		52.8		54.2	
> 10 years		20.0		19.0		24.6	
Lifetime MDD (%)[a]	3	17.0	–	–	–	–	–
Current Depressive Sympoms (BDI-II)[b]	102	6.3 (7.1)	82	5.3 (5.8)	20	11.3 (9.9)	< 0.0001[g]
Childhood Trauma (CTQ)[c]	101	43.9 (11.2)	83	43.0 (5.8)	18	48.3 (15.1)	< 0.0001[g]
Resilience (RS-25)[d]	44	145.5 (18.4)	35	147.2 (17.2)	9	137.5 (21.6)	< 0.0001[g]
Subjective Health (SF-12)[e]	161	49.3 (7.1)	130	50.1 (6.6)	31	45.6 (8.3)	< 0.0001[g]
Social Support (F-SOzU)[f]	43	4.3 (0.6)	34	4.3 (0.6)	9	4.1 (0.7)	< 0.0001[g]

[a]*MDD* Major Depressive Disorder, [b]*BDI-II* Beck Depression Inventory-II, [c]*CTQ* Childhood Trauma Questionnaire
[d]*RS-25* Resilience Scale, [e]*SF-12* SF-12 Health Survey, [f]*F-SozU* Social Support Questionnaire, [g]p-value of Welch t-test
[h]*p*-value of Fisher's exact test

Table 2 Descriptive statistics of the SEL scores for 2265 analysed participants of SHIP-LEGEND

	Positive			Negative		
	N	M	(SD)	*N*	M	(SD)
Basic number of Life Events	2265	14.75	(2.21)	2265	9.02	(3.88)
Proportion of Life Events rated as positive/negative[a]	2265	0.83	(0.12)	2262	0.77	(0.19)
Total Number of Life Events	2265	13.73	(4.41)	2265	14.10	(8.31)
Emotional Valence (Time of the Interview)[b]	2264	1.88	(0.32)	2260	3.65	(0.52)
Present Impact[c]	2264	0.79	(0.16)	2260	0.30	(0.25)
Social Support (Undesired)[d]	386	17.04%		139	6.14%	
Desired[e]	1873	2.11	(1.13)	2118	2.45	(1.02)

[a]Rating not available for all life event items, [b]Rating: 1 (very positive) – 5 (very negative), [c]Rating: 0 (no) vs. 1 (yes)
[d]Rating: 0 (no social support desired), [e]participants reporting undesired social support excluded; Rating: 1 (no social support) – 4 (much social support)

negative LEs (b = 0.12, 95%-CI = 0.09;0.14, $p < 0.001$, β = 0.20). For an overview of the regression coefficients, see Table 3.

Reliability

Internal consistency

The SHIP-LEGEND sample was used to assess Cronbach's alpha (α). The calculated α varied between 0.38 and 0.94 for positive and negative scores (Table 4). Only the *emotional valence* of positive LEs (α = 0.73), the present impact of positive LEs (α = 0.69) and both total numbers of LE frequency (α = 0.38 resp. α = 0.54) had an α lower than 0.76, which is the average α over all SEL scores for our data.

The results of the inter-rater and test-retest analyses are presented in the Additional file 1 and in Additional file 2: Tables S3, Additional file 3: Table S4 and Additional file 4: Table S5.

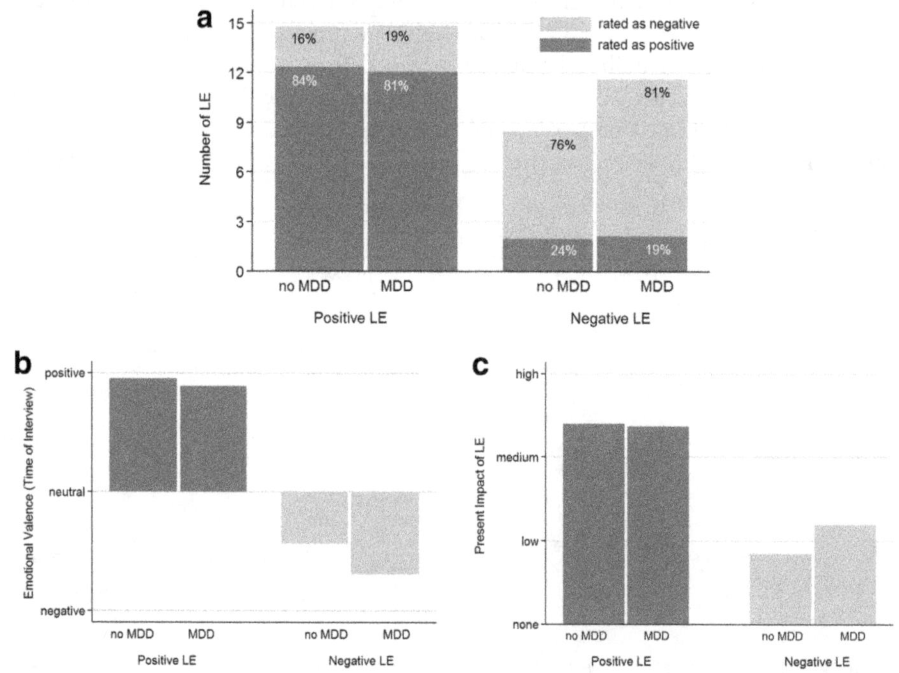

Fig. 1 Associations of lifetime major depressive disorder (MDD) and life event (LE) Ratings. All LE ratings are stratified for lifetime major depressive disorder (MDD) as well as for positive and negative LEs according to the classification process. **a** Proportions of LEs actually rated as positive and negative, respectively. *Participants with lifetime MDD have equal proportions of positively rated positive LEs (OR = 0.63, 95%-CI = 0.22;1.75, p = 0.317) but higher proportions of negatively rated negative life events (OR = 4.61, 95%-CI = 2.20;9.64, p < 0.001).* **b** Emotional valence ratings at the time of the interview. *For participants reporting lifetime MDD ratings are more negative for negative LEs (OR = 2.96, 95%-CI = 2.29;3.84, p < 0.001) but do not differ from participants without lifetime MDD for positive LEs (OR = 1.26, 95%-CI = 0.85;1.85, p = 0.252).* **c** The present impact of past LEs. *Participants with lifetime MDD are reporting more impact of past negative LEs on their current emotional and social life (OR = 2.80, 95%-CI = 1.69;4.63, p < 0.001) but do not differ from participants without lifetime MDD for positive LEs (OR = 0.68, 95%-CI = 0.31;1.50, p = 0.343)*

Table 3 Regression coefficients of the verification analyses

	MDD[a]	CTQ[b]		RS-25[c]		SF-12[d]		F-SozU[e]	
	OR(95%-CI)	b(95%-CI)	β	b(95%-CI)	β	b(95%-CI)	β	b(95%-CI)	β
Positive Life Events									
Basic number of Life Events	1.14(1.06;1.22)***	0.08(−0.15;0.31)	0.02	0.06(−0.28;0.41)	0.01	0.17(0.07;0.28)***	0.05	0.04(0.03;0.05)****	0.15
Proportion of Life Events rated positive	0.63(0.22;1.75)	−7.12(−10.97;-3.27)***	−0.08	11.62(5.91;17.33)****	0.08	2.79(1.07;4.51)**	0.05	0.70(0.50;0.90)****	0.14
Total Number of Life Events	1.07(1.04;1.10)****	0.28(0.17;0.39)****	0.11	0.13(−0.03;0.29)	0.03	−0.03(− 0.08;0.02)	−0.02	0.01(0.01;0.02)****	0.08
Emotional Valence (Time of the Interview)[f]	1.26(0.85;1.85)	3.74(2.28;5.19)****	0.11	−7.05(−9.20;-4.90)****	−0.13	−0.95(−1.61;-0.30)**	0.04	− 0.52(− 0.59;-0.45)****	−0.28
Present Impact[g]	0.68(0.31;1.50)	−3.94(−5.96;-0.11)*	−0.04	9.93(5.6;14.025)****	0.09	1.22(−0.08;2.52)	0.03	0.46(0.31;0.61)****	0.12
Social Support[h]	1.00(0.89;1.13)	−1.34(−1.81;-0.86)****	−0.13	−0.08(− 0.76;0.60)	0.00	−0.02(− 0.22;0.19)	0.00	0.05(0.03;0.08)****	0.10
Negative Life Events									
Basic number of Life Events	1.17(1.13;1.21)****	0.71(0.59;0.83)****	0.25	−0.06(−0.25;0.12)	− 0.01	−0.12(− 0.18;− 0.07)****	-0.07	−0.01(− 0.01;-0.00)*	−0.05
Proportion of Life Events rated negative	4.61(2.20;9.64)****	0.74(−1.62;3.09)	0.01	−1.44(−4.94;2.05)	−0.02	0.21(−0.84;1.26)	0.01	0.06(−0.06;0.18)	0.02
Total Number of Life Events	1.04(1.03;1.06)****	0.30(0.24;0.35)****	0.22	−0.04(− 0.13;0.04)	−0.02	− 0.06(− 0.08;-0.03)****	−0.07	0.00(− 0.01;0.0)	−0.04
Emotional Valence (Time of the Interview)[f]	2.96(2.29;3.84)****	0.50(−0.37;1.38)	0.02	−0.69(−1.99;0.60)	− 0.02	−0.46(− 0.85;-0.07)*	−0.03	0.03(− 0.02;0.07)	0.03
Present Impact[g]	2.80(1.69;4.63)****	0.89(−1.037;2.82)	0.02	2.65(−0.20;5.51)	0.04	−2.14(−2.99;-1.29)****	−0.07	0.03(− 0.07;0.13)	0.01
Social Support[h]	1.02(0.89;1.16)	−2.15(− 2.62;-1.68)****	−0.20	0.03(− 0.67;0.74)	0.00	− 0.02(− 0.23;0.19)	0.00	0.12(0.09;0.14)****	0.20

All analyses adjusted for age, sex, educational level and BDI-II. * p-value < 0.05; ** p-value < 0.01; *** p-value < 0.001; **** p < 0.0001
[a]Lifetime Major Depressive Disorder (yes vs. no), [b]Childhood Trauma Questionnaire, [c]Resilience Scale, [d]SF-12 Health Survey, [e]Social Support Questionnaire
[f]Rating: 1 (very positive) – 5 (very negative), [g]Rating: 0 (no) vs. 1 (yes)
[h]Participants reporting undesired social support excluded; Rating: 1 (no social support) – 4 (much social support)

Table 4 Cronbach's alpha[a] of the SEL scores

	Positive	Negative
Basic number of Life Events	0.78	0.91
Total Number of Life Events	0.38	0.54
Emotional Valence (Time of the Interview)	0.73	0.87
Present Impact	0.69	0.88
Social Support	0.83	0.94
Averaged	0.68	0.83

[a]SHIP-LEGEND sample (N = 2265) without Life Events reported by less than 5% of the sample (n = 113)

Discussion

The SEL is a standardized interview that assesses positive and negative LEs over the whole lifespan using a life history method [22]. Thereby, the SEL combines an assessment of the time of the LE *occurrence* and the LE *frequency* with an assessment of the subjective *emotional valence*. In contrast to existing LE scales, within the SEL, the *emotional valence* is not determined a priori by normative assumptions but rather individually rated by each participant. To aggregate LE information for practical reasons, an empirical classification process was performed a posteriori to identify positive, negative and neutral LEs based on the mean *emotional valence* ratings of our large, population-based sample (N = 2265). Further, the desired and perceived *social support* as well as the *present impact* of past LEs on current life were assessed.

Verification analyses

For verification analyses, we assessed well-established relations between LEs and mental health. As suggested by former research, lifetime MDD was associated with more negative LEs [48]. However, we demonstrated that not only the kind of LE (positive/negative) but also the subjective evaluation of the LE impacts future health outcomes. Thus, MDD was more strongly associated with the *emotional valence* ratings of LEs than with the *occurrence of LEs* per se [48, 53, 54]. In line with former research describing hyperactive emotional responses in maltreated subjects [55–57], we observed more negative *emotional valence* ratings also to be associated with more childhood trauma. In contrast, higher scores on the RS-25 and SF-12, assessing resilience and subjective health, respectively, were associated with more positive *emotional valence* ratings, which is supported by former research regarding LEs, chronic strain and resilience [58–60].

Internal consistency

Tavakol and Dennick [50] summarized that alphas between 0.70 and 0.90 are desirable. According to these authors, lower values might be based on a low number of items, low inter-item correlations or a heterogeneous construct [50]. The latter two factors are desired and inherent facts of the SEL scores, as the SEL was designed to cover a high variety of LEs, and the classification process aimed to aggregate but not unitise the SEL items. Nevertheless, for the SHIP-LEGEND sample, Cronbach's alpha was smaller than 0.70 only for the *total number of positive and negative LEs*. This might be a result of the coding process used for repeated LE occurrences. Because rare LEs are better remembered than typical ones [61], LE frequencies higher than 10 were universally coded as 11. This led to a ceiling effect and an inaccurate estimate of the *total number of LEs* that probably reduced Cronbach's alpha values. In future research, this rating might be reconstructed for future assessments, which might also enhance the reliability of these scores.

Limitations

First, the whole interview took about one to two h depending on the interviewee's life history, willingness for disclosure and cognitive speed. Especially for subjects with low concentration and endurance levels, this led to a decrease in quality with ongoing interview time. Further, recall biases had to be considered, as autobiographical memory is reconstructive and affected by cognitive mechanisms [62, 63]. We intended to improve the recall accuracy using a life history method [22]. Second, the classification procedure was based on the entire population-based sample (N = 2265) including participants reporting lifetime MDD and high current depressive symptoms. Research suggests that a cognitive vulnerability for depression leads to a more negative interpretation of LEs in depressed individuals [45–47]. However, only 17% (n = 386) of the SHIP-LEGEND sample reported lifetime MDD, and the descriptive statistics of the whole sample were more similar to participants not reporting lifetime MDD. To compensate for a cognitive response bias due to current depressed mood, we adjusted the analyses for current depressive symptoms. Nevertheless, the classification procedure is highly dependent on the study sample. Thus, one must mention that the SHIP-LEGEND sample is a subsample of the SHIP-0, which has the risk for selection bias (e.g., mortality, willingness for participation) and an elevated age range. Third, seven items (S9, B15, K28, L35, A47, F50 and D57) indicated a positive *emotional valence* through the wording of the description of the LE, as reported by 70-98% of the SHIP-LEGEND participants. This indicated both low specificity and low sensitivity, and future assessments should decide whether to reformulate or exclude these items. Fourth, in addition to several striking effect sizes (e.g., *proportion* of negatively rated negative LEs and lifetime MDD, *basic number* of negative LEs and childhood trauma, *emotional valence rating* of positive LEs at the time of the interview and resilience), we also observed small effect sizes, which are significant due to the large study sample size. Odds ratios and beta values determine the effect sizes depending on the used covariates within the regression model. All verification analyses were adjusted for the BDI-II total score, as depression has been associated with a recognition and evaluation bias [45–48]. As the scales used to verify the SEL are related to depression as well as, current depressive symptoms [7, 59, 60, 64–68], the inclusion of the BDI-II total score in the analyses may have diminished the effect sizes. Further, a putative selection bias might have impacted the results. As we analysed the second follow-up of a general population sample, healthier subjects might be relatively overrepresented. Hence, the variance within the responses on the verification scales would be decreased, which would also have an impact on the effect sizes. Fifth, the SEL must still be compared to other LE measurements. As several LE items used in the SEL are shared with other instruments [22, 24, 26, 29, 31], we generally assume a good agreement between the SEL and other life event scales. However, validation is still required. Finally, all analyses conducted are cross-sectional. Thus, causality should be discussed with caution. Further, the value of the SEL for prospective analysis remains to be elucidated. Longitudinal analyses are conceivable as soon as the data from the third follow-up measurement of the SHIP studies (SHIP-3) are available. Further, note that no adjustments for multiple tests were used in the present analyses. Due to the large sample size of the SHIP-LEGEND sample, the *p*-values of the verification analyses were very small and robust against multiple testing.

Future implications

Within a therapeutic setting, the SEL could be used to assess LEs occurring immediately before a disease onset. Although we focussed on the whole lifespan in the present manuscript, the SEL could be adapted to assess any period of life of interest. Within the SHIP-LEGEND study, the SEL interview was used to assess the 12-month and 5-year periods before the interview and the 5-year period before the onset of the first subclinical depressive episode as well as the first and the worst clinical depressive episodes. Furthermore, the 5-year period before the onset of a obsessive-compulsive disorder and the 5-year period before and after an initial panic attack were assessed. By integrating the subjective *emotional valence* and *present impact*, the most afflicting LEs could be selected as a central theme within the therapeutic process. Moreover, in LE research, the SEL could be a valuable measurement to associate subjective emotional ratings with future health status, to identify subgroups of LEs as well as their differential impacts on diseases, and to integrate personal circumstances and LE evaluations. Within our own working group, the SEL will be used for longitudinal analyses regarding physical and mental health based on future follow-up measurements of the SHIP studies. Moreover, the SEL can inform research on the interplay between life experiences and biological factors, e.g., in GxE interactions (e.g., [7, 64, 69, 70]).

Conclusion

Previous studies have demonstrated the impact of subjective emotional evaluations in addition to objective valence assessments [71], and LEs have been repeatedly demonstrated to enhance the risk of various mental and physical diseases, especially if interacting with genetic dispositions [4, 8, 10, 13, 14]. The SEL not only enables the testing of the impact of LEs on the pathology of diseases but also integrates the impact of the experience with the individual emotional valence and subjective long-lasting life impact. Thus, the SEL could help generate and test new models of the pathogenesis of various disorders and facilitate research on potential mechanisms of stress balance. Moreover, the SEL is adaptable not only in the lifetime period measured but also in the individuality of the appraisal. The described SEL scores are only one way of analysing the data. More individualized analyses can be generated and are desirable in future research. Therefore, we recommend the SEL as a valuable instrument in life event research on disorder and health outcomes.

Additional files

Additional file 1: Reliability Analyses. To estimate the inter-rater and test-retest reliability, a small second, clinical sample was used. The methods, results, discussion and limitations of these analyses are presented within this supplementary material.

Additional file 2: Table S3. Inter-rater and test-retest intraclass coefficient (ICC) reliabilities of the SEL scores. * p-value < 0.05; ** p-value < 0.01; *** p-value < 0.001. [b]Averaged Intraclass Coefficient based on the reliability samples (N = 10 resp. 9).

Additional file 3: Table S4. Occurrence agreement of the life event items. [a]Based on the inter-rater reliability sample (N = 10), [b]Based on the test-retest reliability sample (N = 9), [c]Number of subjects with identical occurrence ratings (yes/no), [d]Sum of life events with identical occurrence ratings for all subjects, [e]Sum of life events with identical occurrence ratings for 90% of the subjects (n = 9 resp. n = 8).

Additional file 4: Table S5. Reliability of the occurrence time coding of selected life events[1]. [1] Life events were selected if present at both time points of reliability measurement for at least 5 interviewees. * p-value < 0.05; ** p-value < 0.01; *** p-value < 0.001

Additional file 5: Table S1. Life event items and corresponding abbreviations of the SEL interview. [a] open questions.

Additional file 6: Figure S1. Coding Example. A fictive person moved out of its childhood home twice (18 and 28 years). The most important experience was at the age of 18. The person had one subclinical depressive episode at the age of 32 and an initial panic attack at the age of 20. Hence, life event ratings concern the age of 18 for the whole lifespan and the 5-year period before the initial panic attack. For the 5-year period before the subclinical depressive episode, life event ratings concern the age of 28. LT = Lifetime; 12 = 12 months prior to the interview; 5Y = 5 years prior to the interview; 1SuD = 5 years prior to the first subclinical depressive episode; 1DE = 5 years prior to a clinical depressive episode; WDE = 5 years prior to the worst depressive episode; OCD = 5 years prior to an obsessive-compulsive disorder; IPA- = 5 years prior to an initial panic attack; IPA+ = 5 years after an initial panic attack.

Additional file 7: Table S2. Descriptive statistics of the life event items for 2265 analysed participants of SHIP-LEGEND. Note: Due to the life event items some information is unavailable. Due to a low using frequency and in desire to improve the inter-individual comparability, open questions were not considered in the classification process. [a]without missing values, [b]open questions, [c]Rating: 1 (very positive) – 5 (very negative), [d]Rating: 0 (no social support desired), 1(no social support) – 4 (much social support).

Abbreviations

BDI-II: Beck Depression Inventory II; CI: Confidence Interval; CTQ: Childhood Trauma Questionnaire; F-SozU: Social Support Questionnaire; GxE interaction: Gene-Environment Interaction; ICC: Intraclass Coefficient; LE: Life Event; M: Mean; MDD: Major Depressive Disorder; p: *p*-value; RS-25: Resilience Scale; SD: Standard Deviation; SEL: Stralsund Life Event List; SF-12: SF-12 Health Survey; SHIP: Study of Health in Pomerania; SHIP-LEGEND: Study of Health in Pomerania - Life Events and Gene-Environment-Interaction in Depression; α: Cronbach's Alpha; κ: Cronbach's Kappa

Acknowledgments

We would like to thank Christopher Gray for the translation of the German SEL interview into English.

Funding

SHIP is part of the Community Medicine Research net of the University Greifswald, Germany, which is funded by the Federal Ministry of Education and Research (grants no. 01ZZ9603, 01ZZ0103, and 01ZZ0403), the Ministry of Cultural Affairs and the Social Ministry of the Federal State of Mecklenburg-West Pomerania. None of these funding bodies had any influence on the design of the SHIP-studies, nor on the collection, analysis and interpretation of data. SHIP provided the recruiting population for SHIP-LEGEND but further was unrelated to SHIP-LEGEND.

All assessments of SHIP-LEGEND were funded by the German Research Foundation (GR 1912/5-1). The German Research Foundation had no influence on the design of SHIP-LEGEND, nor on the collection, analysis and interpretation of data.

As JK is employed at the University Medicine Greifswald, the statistical analyses and the writing of the manuscript were funded by the University Medicine Greifswald. The interpretation of the data was not influenced by any funding.

Authors' contributions

HV and HJG had substantial contributions to the concept and design of SHIP and were main leaders in data acquisition. HJF and HJG had substantial contributions on the development of the SEL and on the concept and design of SHIP-LEGEND. AB, MB, KF and KZ have done major parts of the SEL interviews. JK has developed and written the manuscript including all analyses. AB, MB, JH and SVdA critically revised the analytic procedures. All authors gave final approval to the version to be published.

Consent for publication

Not applicable.

Competing interests

The authors declare that they have no competing interests.

Author details

[1]Department of Psychiatry and Psychotherapy, University Medicine Greifswald, Ellernholzstraße 1-2, 17489 Greifswald, Germany. [2]Department of Health Sciences, Institute of Sociology of Health and Physical Activity, University of Potsdam, Potsdam, Germany. [3]Department of Psychiatry and Psychotherapy, Helios Clinic, Stralsund, Germany. [4]German Centre of Neurodegenerative Diseases (DZNE), Site Rostock/Greifswald, Greifswald, Germany. [5]Institute for Community Medicine, University Medicine Greifswald, Greifswald, Germany.

References

1. Karg K, Burmeister M, Shedden K, Sen S. The serotonin transporter promoter variant (5-HTTLPR), stress, and depression meta-analysis revisited: evidence of genetic moderation. Arch Gen Psychiatry. 2011;68:444–54. https://doi.org/10.1001/archgenpsychiatry.2010.189.
2. Zannas AS, Binder EB. Gene-environment interactions at the FKBP5 locus: sensitive periods, mechanisms and pleiotropism. Genes Brain Behav. 2014; 13:25–37. https://doi.org/10.1111/gbb.12104.
3. Binder EB, Bradley RG, Liu W, Epstein MP, Deveau TC, Mercer KB, et al. Association of FKBP5 polymorphisms and childhood abuse with risk of posttraumatic stress disorder symptoms in adults. JAMA. 2008;299:1291–305. https://doi.org/10.1001/jama.299.11.1291.
4. Nugent NR, Tyrka AR, Carpenter LL, Price LH. Gene-environment interactions: early life stress and risk for depressive and anxiety disorders. Psychopharmacology. 2011;214:175–96. https://doi.org/10.1007/s00213-010-2151-x.
5. Kaufman J, Yang B-Z, Douglas-Palumberi H, Grasso D, Lipschitz D, Houshyar S, et al. Brain-derived neurotrophic factor-5-HTTLPR gene interactions and environmental modifiers of depression in children. Biol Psychiatry. 2006;59: 673–80. https://doi.org/10.1016/j.biopsych.2005.10.026.
6. Hosang GM, Shiles C, Tansey KE, McGuffin P, Uher R. Interaction between stress and the BDNF Val66Met polymorphism in depression: a systematic review and meta-analysis. BMC Med. 2014;12:7. https://doi.org/10.1186/1741-7015-12-7.
7. Grabe HJ, Schwahn C, Mahler J, Schulz A, Spitzer C, Fenske K, et al. Moderation of adult depression by the serotonin transporter promoter variant (5-HTTLPR), childhood abuse and adult traumatic events in a general population sample. Am J Med Genet B Neuropsychiatr Genet. 2012;159B: 298–309. https://doi.org/10.1002/ajmg.b.32027.
8. Broeren S, Newall C, Dodd HF, Locker R, Hudson JL. Longitudinal investigation of the role of temperament and stressful life events in childhood anxiety. Dev Psychopathol. 2014;26:437–49. https://doi.org/10.1017/S0954579413000989.
9. Haeffel GJ, Vargas I. Resilience to depressive symptoms: the buffering effects of enhancing cognitive style and positive life events. J Behav Ther Exp Psychiatry. 2011;42:13–8. https://doi.org/10.1016/j.jbtep.2010.09.003.
10. Lumeng JC, Wendorf K, Pesch MH, Appugliese DP, Kaciroti N, Corwyn RF, Bradley RH. Overweight adolescents and life events in childhood. Pediatrics. 2013;132:e1506–12. https://doi.org/10.1542/peds.2013-1111.
11. Staufenbiel SM, Koenders MA, Giltay EJ, Elzinga BM, Manenschijn L, Hoencamp E, et al. Recent negative life events increase hair cortisol concentrations in patients with bipolar disorder. Stress. 2014;17:451–9. https://doi.org/10.3109/10253890.2014.968549.
12. Cohen LH, McGowan J, Fookas S, Rose S. Positive life events and social support and the relationship between life stress and psychological disorder. Am J Community Psychol. 1984;12:567–87.
13. Brown GW, Harris TO. Depression and the serotonin transporter 5-HTTLPR polymorphism: a review and a hypothesis concerning gene-environment interaction. J Affect Disord 2008;111:1–12. https://doi.org/10.1016/j.jad.2008.04.009.
14. Horesh D, Solomon Z, Zerach G, Ein-Dor T. Delayed-onset PTSD among war veterans: the role of life events throughout the life cycle. Soc Psychiatry Psychiatr Epidemiol. 2011;46:863–70. https://doi.org/10.1007/s00127-010-0255-6.
15. Pe ML, Brose A, Gotlib IH, Kuppens P. Affective updating ability and stressful events interact to prospectively predict increases in depressive symptoms over time. Emotion. 2016;16:73–82. https://doi.org/10.1037/emo0000097.
16. Shimizu M, Pelham BW. The unconscious cost of good fortune: implicit and explicit self-esteem, positive life events, and health. Health Psychol. 2004;23: 101–5. https://doi.org/10.1037/0278-6133.23.1.101.
17. Brown JD, McGill KL. The cost of good fortune: when positive life events produce negative health consequences. J Pers Soc Psychol. 1989;57:1103–10. https://doi.org/10.1037/0022-3514.57.6.1103.
18. Kleiman EM, Chiara AM, Liu RT, Jager-Hyman SG, Choi JY, Alloy LB. Optimism and well-being: a prospective multi-method and multi-dimensional examination of optimism as a resilience factor following the

occurrence of stressful life events. Cogn Emot. 2017;31:269–83. https://doi.org/10.1080/02699931.2015.1108284.

19. Asselmann E, Wittchen H-U, Lieb R, Höfler M, Beesdo-Baum K. Does low coping efficacy mediate the association between negative life events and incident psychopathology? A prospective-longitudinal community study among adolescents and young adults. Epidemiol Psychiatr Sci. 2016;25:171–80. https://doi.org/10.1017/S204579601500013X.
20. Leys R. Types of one: Adolf Meyer's life chart and the representation of individuality. Representations. 1991;34:1–28. https://doi.org/10.2307/2928768.
21. Paykel ES. The evolution of life events research in psychiatry. J Affect Disord. 2001;62:141–9.
22. Caspi A, Moffitt TE, Thornton A, Freedman D, Amell JW, Harrington H, et al. The life history calendar: a research and clinical assessment method for collecting retrospective event-history data. Int J Methods Psychiatr Res. 1996;6:101–14.
23. Holmes TH, Rahe RH. The social readjustment rating scale. J Psychosom Res. 1967;11:213–8.
24. Maier-Diewald W, Wittchen H-U, Hecht H, Werner-Eilert K. Die Münchner Ereignisliste (MEL). Anwendungsmanual. München: Max-Planck-Institut; 1983.
25. ZPID Leibniz Institut. MEL - Münchner Ereignisliste. 2006. https://www.zpid.de/retrieval/PSYNDEXTests.php?id=9001799. Accessed 22 Mar 2017.
26. Brown GW. Life events and measurement. In: Brown GW, Harris TO, editors. Life events and illness. New York: Guilford Press; 1989. p. 3–48.
27. Wethington E, Brown GW, Kessler RC. Interview measurement of stressful life events. In: Cohen S, editor. Measuring stress: a guide for health and social scientists. New York: Oxford Univ. Press; 1995. p. 59–79.
28. Filipp S-H, Aymanns P. Kritische Lebensereignisse und Lebenskrisen: Vom Umgang mit den Schattenseiten des Lebens. 1st ed. Stuttgart: Verlag W. Kohlhammer; 2010.
29. Siegrist J, Geyer S. Inventar lebensverändernder Ereignisse: Zusammenstellung sozialwissenschaftlicher Items und Skalen. ZIS - GESIS Leibniz Institute for the Social Sciences 1997. https://doi.org/10.6102/zis92.
30. Richter G, Richter J. Kritische Lebensereignisse - Inventar zur Erfassung lebensverändernder Ereignisse (ILE). In: Richter G, Richter J, editors. Komplexität von Depressivität: Explorative Analyse von Verlaufsdaten, erhoben an stationär behandelten psychiatrischen Patienten. Münster: Waxmann; 1995. p. 97–8.
31. Richter V, Guthke J. Leipziger Ereignis-und Belastungsinventar (LEBI): Hogrefe, Verlag für Psychologie; 1996.
32. Staufenbiel SM, Penninx BWJH, Spijker AT, Elzinga BM, van Rossum EFC. Hair cortisol, stress exposure, and mental health in humans: a systematic review. Psychoneuroendocrinology. 2013;38:1220–35. https://doi.org/10.1016/j.psyneuen.2012.11.015.
33. Völzke H, Alte D, Schmidt CO, Radke D, Lorbeer R, Friedrich N, et al. Cohort profile: the study of health in Pomerania. Int J Epidemiol. 2011;40:294–307. https://doi.org/10.1093/ije/dyp394.
34. Wittchen H-U. DIA-X-Interviews: Manual für Screening Verfahren und Interview; Interviewheft Längsschnittuntersuchung (DIA-X-Lifetime); Ergänzungsheft (DIA-X-Lifetime); Interviewheft Querschnittsuntersuchung (DIA-X-12 Monate); Ergänzungsheft (DIA-X-12 Monate). Frankfurt: Swets & Zeitlinger; 1997.
35. Wittchen H-U, Pfister H. Diagnostisches Expertensystem für psychische Störungen. Frankfurt: Swets & Zeitlinger; 1997.
36. Bullinger M, Kirchberger I, Ware J. Der deutsche SF-36 Health Survey Übersetzung und psychometrische Testung eines krankheitsübergreifenden Instruments zur Erfassung der gesundheitsbezogenen Lebensqualität. J Public Health. 1995;3:21–36. https://doi.org/10.1007/BF02959944.
37. Beck AT, Steer RA, Brown G. Manual for the Beck depression inventory-II. San Antonio: The Psychological Corporation; 1996.
38. Bernstein DP, Stein JA, Newcomb MD, Walker E, Pogge D, Ahluvalia T, et al. Development and validation of a brief screening version of the childhood trauma questionnaire. Child Abuse Negl. 2003;27:169–90. https://doi.org/10.1016/S0145-2134(02)00541-0.
39. Wagnild GM, Young HM. Development and psychometric evaluation of the resilience scale. J Nurs Meas. 1993;1:165–78.
40. Fydrich T, Sommer G, Brähler E. Fragebogen zur Sozialen Unterstützung (F-SozU). 1st ed. Göttingen: Hogrefe; 2007.
41. Fydrich T, Sommer G, Tydecks S, Brähler E. Fragebogen zur Sozialen Unterstützung (F-SozU): Normierung der Kurzform (K-14). Z Med Psychol. 2009;18:43 8.
42. Kühner C, Bürger C, Keller F, Hautzinger M. Reliabilitat und Validitat des revidierten Beck-Depressionsinventars (BDI-II). Befunde aus deutschsprachigen Stichproben. Nervenarzt. 2007;78:651–6. https://doi.org/10.1007/s00115-006-2098-7.
43. Wingenfeld K, Spitzer C, Mensebach C, Grabe HJ, Hill A, Gast U, et al. Die deutsche Version des Childhood Trauma Questionnaire (CTQ): Erste Befunde zu den psychometrischen Kennwerten. Psychother Psychosom Med Psychol. 2010;60:442–50. https://doi.org/10.1055/s-0030-1247564.
44. Leppert K, Koch B, Brähler E, Strauß B. Die Resilienzskala (RS)–Überprüfung der Langform RS-25 und einer Kurzform RS-13. Klin Diagnostik u Evaluation. 2008;1:226–43.
45. Abramson LY, Metalsky GI, Alloy LB. Hopelessness depression: a theory-based subtype of depression. Psychol Rev. 1989;96:358–72. https://doi.org/10.1037/0033-295X.96.2.358.
46. Beevers CG. Cognitive vulnerability to depression: a dual process model. Clin Psychol Rev. 2005;25:975–1002. https://doi.org/10.1016/j.cpr.2005.03.003.
47. Mathews A, MacLeod C. Cognitive vulnerability to emotional disorders. Annu Rev Clin Psychol. 2005;1:167–95. https://doi.org/10.1146/annurev.clinpsy.1.102803.143916.
48. Friis RH, Wittchen H-U, Pfister H, Lieb R. Life events and changes in the course of depression in young adults. Eur Psychiatry. 2002;17:241–53. https://doi.org/10.1016/S0924-9338(02)00682-X.
49. Cronbach LJ. Coefficient alpha and the internal structure of tests. Psychometrika. 1951;16:297–334. https://doi.org/10.1007/BF02310555.
50. Tavakol M, Dennick R. Making sense of Cronbach's alpha. Int J Med Educ. 2011;2:53–5. https://doi.org/10.5116/ijme.4dfb.8dfd.
51. Gandek B, Ware JE, Aaronson NK, Apolone G, Bjorner JB, Brazier JE, et al. Cross-validation of item selection and scoring for the SF-12 health survey in nine countries. J Clin Epidemiol. 1998;51:1171–8. https://doi.org/10.1016/S0895-4356(98)00109-7.
52. Schumacher J, Leppert K, Gunzelrnann T, Strauß B, Brähler E. Die Resilienzskala - Ein Fragebogen zur Erfassung der psychischen Widerstandsfähigkeit als Personmerkmal. Z Klin Psychol Psychiatr Psychother. 2005;53:16–39.
53. Reichenberger J, Wiggert N, Agroskin D, Wilhelm FH, Blechert J. No praise, please: depressive symptoms, reactivity to positive social interaction, and fear of positive evaluation. J Behav Ther Exp Psychiatry. 2017;54:186–94. https://doi.org/10.1016/j.jbtep.2016.08.007.
54. Watters AJ, Williams LM. Negative biases and risk for depression; integrating self-report and emotion task markers. Depress Anxiety. 2011;28:703–18. https://doi.org/10.1002/da.20854.
55. Infurna FJ, Rivers CT, Reich J, Zautra AJ. Childhood trauma and personal mastery: their influence on emotional reactivity to everyday events in a community sample of middle-aged adults. PLoS One. 2015;10:e0121840. https://doi.org/10.1371/journal.pone.0121840.
56. Glaser J-P, van Os J, Portegijs PJM, Myin-Germeys I. Childhood trauma and emotional reactivity to daily life stress in adult frequent attenders of general practitioners. J Psychosom Res. 2006;61:229–36. https://doi.org/10.1016/j.jpsychores.2006.04.014.
57. Sansone RA, Wiederman MW, Hatic A, Flath L. Childhood trauma and emotional reactivity to hypothetical media events: a pilot study. Prim Care Companion J Clin Psychiatry. 2010; https://doi.org/10.4088/PCC.09l00898blu.
58. Tran TV, Wright R, Chatters L. Health, stress, psychological resources, and subjective well-being among older blacks. Psychol Aging. 1991;6:100–8.
59. Poole JC, Dobson KS, Pusch D. Childhood adversity and adult depression: the protective role of psychological resilience. Child Abuse Negl. 2017:89–100. https://doi.org/10.1016/j.chiabu.2016.12.012.
60. Schulz A, Becker M, Van der Auwera S, Barnow S, Appel K, Mahler J, et al. The impact of childhood trauma on depression: does resilience matter? Population-based results from the study of health in Pomerania. J Psychosom Res. 2014;77:97–103. https://doi.org/10.1016/j.jpsychores.2014.06.008.
61. von Restorff H. Ueber die Wirkung von Bereichsbildungen im Spurenfeld. Analyse von Vorgängen im Spurenfeld I. Psychol Forsch. 1933;18:299–342. https://doi.org/10.1007/BF02409636.
62. Brown GW, Harris TO. Fall-off in the reporting of life events. Soc Psychiatry. 1982;17:23–8. https://doi.org/10.1007/BF00583889
63. Brewin C, Andrews B. Recovered memories of trauma: phenomenology and cognitive mechanisms. Clin Psychol Rev. 1998;18:949–70. https://doi.org/10.1016/S0272-7358(98)00040-3

64. Appel K, Schwahn C, Mahler J, Schulz A, Spitzer C, Fenske K, et al. Moderation of adult depression by a polymorphism in the FKBP5 gene and childhood physical abuse in the general population. Neuropsychopharmacology. 2011;36:1982–91. https://doi.org/10.1038/npp.2011.81.
65. Carvalho IG, Bertolli EDS, Paiva L, Rossi LA, Dantas RAS, Pompeo DA. Anxiety, depression, resilience and self-esteem in individuals with cardiovascular diseases. Rev Lat Am Enfermagem. 2016;24:e2836. https://doi.org/10.1590/1518-8345.1405.2836.
66. Conrad R, Wegener I, Imbierowicz K, Liedtke R, Geiser F. Alexithymia, temperament and character as predictors of psychopathology in patients with major depression. Psychiatry Res. 2009;165:137–44. https://doi.org/10.1016/j.psychres.2007.10.013.
67. Di Benedetto M, Lindner H, Aucote H, Churcher J, McKenzie S, Croning N, Jenkins E. Co-morbid depression and chronic illness related to coping and physical and mental health status. Psychol Health Med. 2014;19:253–62. https://doi.org/10.1080/13548506.2013.803135.
68. Lipsanen T, Saarijärvi S, Lauerma H. Exploring the relations between depression, somatization, dissociation and alexithymia - overlapping or independent constructs? Psychopathology. 2004;37:200–6. https://doi.org/10.1159/000080132.
69. Grabe HJ, Wittfeld K, Van der Auwera S, Janowitz D, Hegenscheid K, Habes M, et al. Effect of the interaction between childhood abuse and rs1360780 of the FKBP5 gene on gray matter volume in a general population sample. Hum Brain Mapp. 2016;37:1602–13. https://doi.org/10.1002/hbm.23123.
70. Hertel J, König J, Homuth G, Van der Auwera S, Wittfeld K, Pietzner M, et al. Evidence for stress-like alterations in the HPA-Axis in women taking oral contraceptives. Sci Rep. 2017;7:14111. https://doi.org/10.1038/s41598-017-13927-7.
71. Fontana AF, Hughes LA, Marcus JL, Dowds BN. Subjective evaluation of life events. J Consult Clin Psychol. 1979;47:906–11. https://doi.org/10.1037/0022-006X.47.5.906.
72. Transferstelle für Daten- und Biomaterialienmanagement. Data Application for SHIP. https://www.fvcm.med.uni-greifswald.de/dd_service/data_use_intro.php?lang=ger. Accessed 24 Jul 2017.

14

Sleep better, feel better? Effects of a CBT-I and HT-I sleep training on mental health, quality of life and stress coping in university students

Anja Friedrich*, Merle Claßen and Angelika A. Schlarb

Abstract

Background: The SWIS sleep training for university students showed promising results regarding subjective and objective sleep parameters. As sleep disorders and impaired sleep quality are closely related to various aspects of mental health, the current study examines the effects of the SWIS sleep training on mental health in university students.

Methods: Fifty six university students (M = 25.84, SD = 5.06) participated in the study, 68% were women. Forty one were randomly assigned to the SWIS treatment (pre-post-follow-up), 15 to a Waiting List Control condition (WLC, pre-post). Besides sleep-related measures, the students completed four online questionnaires measuring mental health, quality of life and stress coping strategies. Effect sizes for the pre-post data were compared between the conditions, long-term effects were calculated with repeated measures ANOVA or Friedman ANOVA. Long-term clinical changes were analyzed with the Reliable Change Index (RCI).

Results: The pre-post comparisons between SWIS and WLC revealed lower depression scores in both conditions, a better physical state in the SWIS condition and less maladaptive stress coping strategies in the WLC students. The long-term results of SWIS provided significant improvements regarding the students' somatic complaints, reduced anxiety, an improved physical state and a better quality of life with moderate to large effect sizes. Most of the significant improvements occurred between pre- and follow-up measurement. These statistically significant results were also reflected in clinically significant changes from pre- to follow-up-test.

Conclusions: SWIS and WLC condition both improved in two mental health variables immediately after the training. These findings may be explained by unspecific treatment expectation effects in the WLC. Interestingly, most mental health outcomes showed significant improvements after 3 months, but not immediately after the training. These positive long-term effects of the SWIS training on mental health indicate that the transfer of strategies might simply need more time to affect the students' mental health.

Keywords: Sleep, Mental health, Quality of life, Stress coping strategies, CBT-I, HT-I

* Correspondence: anja.friedrich@uni-bielefeld.de
Faculty of Psychology and Sports Science, Department of Psychology, Clinical Psychology and Psychotherapy of children and adolescents, Bielefeld University, Universitätsstraße 25, 33615 Bielefeld, Germany

Background

Sleep in college and university students

Sleep problems are quite common among university students: Up to 16% need more than 30 min to fall asleep and 7.7% meet the diagnostic criteria for an insomnia disorder [1]. Aside from insomnia symptoms, more than one third (36.9%) of German college students report a poor sleep quality according to the Pittsburgh Sleep Quality Index [2]. Other studies found even higher percentages of impaired sleep quality (42.8%) in German and Luxembourgian university students [3].

Sleep and mental health

Sleep and sleep problems are closely related to various mental health variables in university students. In a sample of 1074 American college students (72% women), those with chronic insomnia according to DSM-5 (9.5%) reported significantly more fatigue, depression, anxiety, stress and stimulant use than healthy students [4]. In another study, Lund and colleagues examined the differences between good and bad sleepers according to the Pittsburgh Sleep Quality Index [5]. Of the 1125 American participants (63% women), two thirds were classified as bad sleepers. They reported delayed bed- and rise-times during the weekend, more anger, confusion, depression, fatigue and tension, more physical illness, daytime sleepiness as well as more drug and alcohol consumption [5]. In addition, Lund and colleagues showed that especially academic and emotional stress explained the students' sleep quality, while alcohol, caffeine consumption and sleep consistency were of lesser importance [5]. A recent study from Ethiopia examined 2654 college students (24% women) and found that general health (e.g. sadness, mastering daily problems, self-esteem) is significantly correlated with sleep quality and daytime sleepiness [6]. Furthermore, these correlations continued to exist even when controlling for demographic and behavioral covariates. Similar results were observed for German college student samples with impaired sleep quality that reported more mental strain, somatic complaints, as well as lower self-efficacy [2, 3]. Overall, current research shows that not only sleep disorders, but also impaired sleep is connected with mental health in university students.

Sleep and stress coping strategies

While the associations between sleep and mental health have been investigated extensively, the role of stress coping behaviors in college students remains vague. In a sample of 2892 American college students (59% women), 9.1% suffered from insomnia according to DSM-IV [7]. In this study, stress exposure was a significant predictor of insomnia onset and the relationship was mediated by the three stress coping strategies behavioral disengagement, distraction and substance abuse [7].

Sleep and quality of life

Besides mental health and stress coping strategies, the quality of life is another factor that is closely related to the students' sleep. Students with chronic insomnia reported a significantly lower quality of life, including worse physical health, more negative emotions, less leisure time activities, household duties and course work [4, 8]. Preišegolavičiūtė and colleagues examined a broader concept that included the students' work and studies, emotional status, physical health and sexual life [9]. The analysis of 405 Lithuanian students (73% women) showed that impaired sleep quality was significantly correlated with a reduced quality of life.

Sleep interventions

All in all, the current research shows that sleep in university students is associated with mental health problems, stress coping strategies and quality of life. Correspondingly, an improvement of the students' sleep quality should also improve their mental health, stress coping and quality of life. This assumption was partially confirmed in a recent review about different psychological interventions to improve sleep in university students [10]. Regarding the improvements of the students' mental health, sleep hygiene provided small effects, whereas cognitive behavior therapy (CBT) and other approaches showed medium effects, and relaxation trainings had large effects [10]. Hence, it is possible to enhance university students' mental health via sleep trainings. However, the students' stress coping and quality of life were not addressed in this review, as they were only reported in a few studies.

"Studieren wie im Schlaf"

An example of the aforementioned sleep trainings is "Studieren wie im Schlaf" (SWIS). SWIS is a group training designed to improve sleep in college and university students. It combines cognitive behavior therapy for insomnia (CBT-I) and hypnotherapy for insomnia (HT-I). With only six sessions à 100 min, SWIS is a short but effective training. In a pilot study, SWIS was a well-accepted and feasible program that improved subjective as well as objective sleep impairments [11].

Furthermore, similar sleep trainings that consist of CBT-I and HT-I proved effective in infants, children and adolescents (*infants* [12–14]; *children* [15, 16]; *adolescents* [17, 18]). These studies with younger children and adolescents showed that the improvement were largest after 3 months [16]. This incubation effect might be caused by two factors: the parents need time to transfer changed parental sleep-related behavior into daily routine, furthermore, children need to adapt newly learned self-regulated sleep strategies into autonomous behavior.

Objectives and hypotheses

As described above, sleep is closely related to a plethora of mental health aspects. Therefore, we assumed that besides the improvement of sleep, the SWIS training may result in i) a greater reduction of the students' mental health problems than the waiting list control condition (WLC) including less depression, somatic complaints, panic, anxiety, alcohol abuse, and general stress. Beyond, we hypothetized that ii) the SWIS training improves the students' stress coping strategies with a greater increase in the use of adaptive strategies and a greater reduction of maladaptive strategies in comparison to the WLC. In addition, that iii) students of the SWIS training report greater improvement of quality of life than students of the WLC. Finally and most important, iv) that the effects of the SWIS training are sustained or improved in the long-term. These long-term effects are greater for students with clinically relevant depressive symptoms.

Method

Intervention: Studieren wie im Schlaf (SWIS)

SWIS is conducted in groups with four to eight students. In six manualized weekly sessions, the students learn different strategies to cope with and improve their sleep problems and sleep behavior. These strategies include CBT-I and HT-I. The behavior therapeutic elements encompass sleep hygiene, progressive muscle relaxation, cognitive restructuring, stress management and problem solving skills. The hypnotherapeutic elements include sleep related trances, calming pictures, self-hypnosis and imagination techniques. Each session (except for the first) starts with each participants' report on their individual progress and the daily implementation of the sleep-related strategies. Afterwards follows the manualized content. Every session concludes with a trance session. A more detailed description is provided in a recent article by Schlarb, Friedrich and Claßen [11].

Procedure

An experimental pre-post-follow-up design was employed. Students were randomly assigned to the SWIS intervention condition (SWIS) or a waiting-list control condition (WLC) in a 3:1 ratio (Fig. 1). All in all, 56 participants were included. All participants provided written informed consent. The SWIS training was guided by two psychologists who were supervised by a psychotherapist. The study pertains to the Declaration of Helsinki and was approved by the ethics committee at Bielefeld University (ID: 2014–135).

The participants of SWIS completed the pre-test (T1) including a self-developed diagnostic interview to check inclusion and exclusion criteria and a 2 week sleep log. Afterwards, the SWIS training was conducted, which lasted 6 weeks, immediately followed by the post-test (T2). The follow-up test was administered after 3 months (T3). The participants in the WLC first received a 2 week pre-test (T0) and then waited for 6 weeks, after which they completed the post-test (T1). Due to ethical reasons, they received the same procedure as the intervention condition. If WLC and SWIS did not differ at T1, the WLC data were included in the long-term analyses.

Inclusion and exclusion criteria

For inclusion in the study, participants had to fulfill two criteria. First, they had to report symptoms of an insomnia disorder, a nightmare disorder or an irregular sleep-wake type according to DSM-5 criteria [19]. Secondly, based on the Pittsburgh Sleep Quality Index [20], their sleep quality was classified as poor (sum score > 5).

The inclusion and exclusion criteria were checked during the self-developed diagnostic interview. Participants with untreated organic diseases were excluded from study participation. Participants with treated organic diseases (mostly thyroid disorders) were included in the study, provided that they received continuous adequate medical treatment and that the organic disease was not the main cause of the sleep problems. Consequently, participants with reported symptoms of organic sleep disorders (such as obstructive sleep apnea) were excluded from the study. If participants presented symptoms of organic sleep disorders but were not yet diagnosed, they were referred to a sleep laboratory for further diagnosis.

Participants with previously treated psychiatric disorders were included in the current study, provided that the psychiatric disorder was not the main cause of the sleep problems and that they did not receive psychotherapy simultaneously. An exemption to this rule were participants with current psychotic episodes, trauma-related disorders, or cognitive impairments, which were excluded in general.

Sample

The sample size was computed with G*Power, version 3.1.9.2 [21]. With an alpha error of .05, a power of .95 and an estimated effect size for CBT sleep trainings in university students of $d = .59$ [10], the sample size had to exceed 33 participants for dependent t-tests.

The participants were recruited at Bielefeld University using leaflets, Email and a homepage. The sample consisted of 56 university students aged 19 to 50 years ($M = 25.84$, $SD = 5.06$) (Table 1). Sixty eight percent of the participants were women. Forty one were assigned to SWIS, 15 to the WLC. A Chi-square test and a Wilcoxon signed rank test were used to investigate group differences between SWIS and the WLC. Both tests

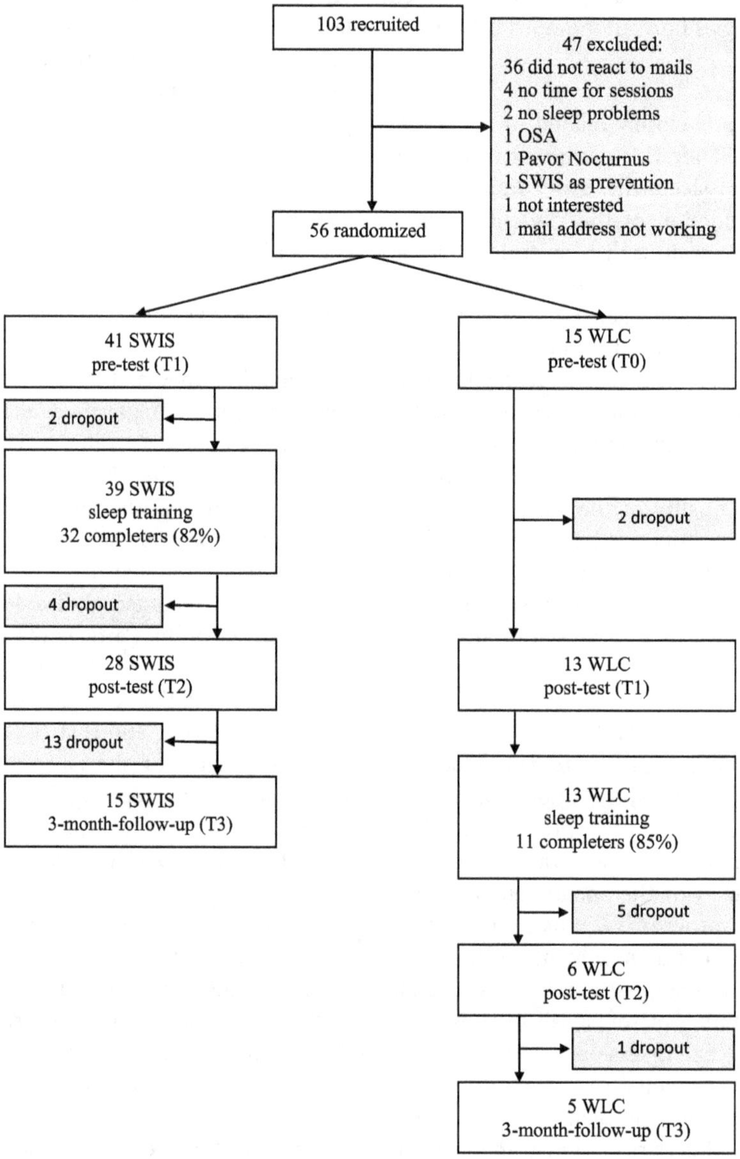

Fig. 1 Flow chart of the experimental design. One hundred three participants were recruited, 56 were randomized (SWIS: $N = 41$, WLC: $N = 15$). After the waiting period, the WLC received the SWIS sleep training. Completion rates were 82% in the SWIS condition and 85% in the WLC condition. All participants who completed at least four of the six sessions were counted as completers. Dropout rates aside from non-completers were 46% in the SWIS condition and 53% in the WLC condition

Table 1 Sample characteristics of SWIS and WLC

N	all	SWIS	WLC	SWIS vs. WLC
	56	41	15	
Gender				$X^2_{gender}(N = 56) = 1.981, p = .202$
women	38 (68%)	30 (73%)	8 (64%)	
men	18 (32%)	11 (27%)	7 (36%)	
Age				$Z_{age} = -1.471, p = .141$
mean	25.84	25.13	27.73	
SD	5.06	3.82	7.26	

provided statistical evidence that the groups did not differ regarding gender or age. One student did not complete the online questionnaires and was therefore excluded from the following analysis.

A more detailed analysis of the age range revealed that 87.3% of the sample were younger than 30 years of age. Thus, only 12.7% were older than the "usual" student sample. To ensure that the older students do not differ from the younger students, baseline differences in all dependent variables between younger (19–30, $N = 49$) and older students (31–50, $N = 7$) were examined using

Mann-Whitney-U tests for independent nonparametric samples. These analyses revealed that there were no differences between the younger and the older students (all *p*-values > .10).

Instruments

Depression

Based on the Center for Epidemiological Studies Depression Scale (CES-D), Hautzinger and Bailer generated the German *General Depression Scale* (Allgemeine Depressionsskala, ADS) [22]. It is composed of 20 items that gauge the subjects' moodiness and tendency towards depressive symptoms during the last week on a four point rating scale ranging from zero (rarely) to three (mostly). Higher values indicate a higher tendency towards depressive symptoms. The ADS showed good internal consistency (α = .89) and a reliable cut-off score of 23 [22]. The cut-off score was used to divide the participants into participants with clinically relevant depressive symptoms (ADS ≥23) and participants without clinically relevant depressive symptoms (ADS < 23) for the long-term analyses.

Somatoform complaints, panic, anxiety, alcohol abuse and general stressors

Four scales from the German version of the *Patient Health Questionnaire* (PHQ-D [23]) were used to screen for the following mental health issues: Somatic complaints (13 items, 0–26), panic (11 items, 0–11), anxiety (6 items, 0–12), alcohol abuse (5 items, 0–5) and general stressors (9 items, 0–27). The three scales panic, anxiety and alcohol abuse were only presented after a filter question was confirmed (e.g. "Do you sometimes consume alcohol (including beer and wine?")). Therefore, not all participants completed these three scales. Gräfe, Zipfel, Herzog and Löwe analyzed the psychometric qualities and confirmed construct validity, specificity, sensitivity, patient and physician acceptance as well as internal consistency (α = .79–.88) [24]. However, the authors only reported the internal consistency of some subscales (e.g. somatic complaints), as they used several subscales categorically (e.g. anxiety). Therefore, the reliabilities for the other subscales will have to be computed in this study. The test retest reliability was not provided for the subscales used in this study.

Stress

The short form of the *Stress Coping Questionnaire* (Stressverarbeitungsfragebogen, SVF-78 [25]) consists of 78 items that assess 20 different coping strategies for stressful situations, for example avoidance, aggression and relaxation. Two secondary scales, adaptive and maladaptive strategies, summarize ten and seven subscales respectively. Higher values indicate a higher probability for the application of a coping strategy. The SVF-78 shows internal consistency (α = .77–.94) and construct validity [25]. However, test retest reliability is only available for children and adolescents, not for adults.

Quality of life

The *Quality of Life Scales* (Skalen zur Erfassung der Lebensqualität, SEL [26]) contain 28 items and six scales about the subject's current mood, objective physical complaints, subjective physical condition, predominant mood, environment and general attitude towards life. These scales are combined into two global scales: Physical condition and cognitive-emotional condition. These two global scales add up to the sum score "life quality". Two global items concerning body ("How do you rate your physical condition in general?") and quality of life ("In general, how do you rate your life quality?") are added.

Participants respond on three different five point Likert scales, ranging from "never/does not apply to me at all/bad" (1) to "always/applies to me completely/very good" (5). Higher scores indicate a higher quality of life. In this study, only the two global scales physical condition, cognitive-emotional condition and the sum score were analyzed.

Although Averbeck and colleagues provide norms for healthy adults ($N = 1683$), they were not used for data analysis due to the different population characteristics. The global scales physical condition (α = .88) and cognitive emotional condition (α = .92) and the quality of life scale (α = .94) showed excellent reliabilities [26]. Test retest reliabilities were only tested in tumour patients; hence they are not applicable to the current target population. Scale intercorrelations range from .27 to .62 [26].

Data analysis

All calculations were computed with the Statistical Package for the Social Sciences version 22 [27]. First, all variables were examined for normal distribution (Shapiro-Wilk). Then, they were tested for baseline differences between SWIS and WLC with a t-test for independent samples (normally distributed), a Mann-Whitney-U test (not normally distributed), or a Chi-square test for nominal variables (depression). The missing reliability coefficients of the PHQ-D subscales anxiety and general stress were computed using Cronbach's alpha.

Pre-post comparisons between SWIS and WLC

The differences between the pre- and post-tests were tested for normal distribution (e.g. $ADS_{pre} - ADS_{post} = ADS_{diff}$). As all differences were normally distributed, only parametric tests were computed. A repeated measures ANOVA would have been the standard test for the first three hypotheses. However, the small and unequal sample sizes did not provide sufficient statistical background for an ANOVA. Instead, the two conditions (SWIS vs. WLC) were analyzed separately with dependent t-tests (pre vs. post). Then, effect sizes were calculated and compared descriptively.

Long-term effects of SWIS

For the fourth hypothesis, the pre-, post- and follow-up data were tested for normal distribution. According to normal distribution, the long-term effects of the SWIS training were examined with ANOVA or Friedman's ANOVA. The post-hoc tests were adjusted for alpha error accumulation. In this case, the ANOVA was the most feasible approach, as only one condition was examined over the course of time. If the SWIS and the WLC condition did not differ at T1, the WLC data were included in the long-term analyses.

In order to test the effect of depressive symptoms on the long-term development of the students' mental health, a between subjects factor was added that sorted the participants into two groups according to the ADS (with or without clinically relevant depressive symptoms).

Long-term clinically significant changes

Long-term clinically significant changes were examined by calculating the Reliable Change Index (RCI) for each instrument. These scores were then applied to the instruments' change scores that were calculated using the formula:

$$X_{change} = X_{pre} - X_{follow\text{-}up}$$

The RCIs were then applied to the instruments' pre- to follow-up change scores, classifying them into deterioration, no change and improvement. In the current study, the calculation of the RCIs followed Jacobson and Truax [28] with a 5% alpha error:

1) Calculate the instruments' pre-test standard error, $S_E = s_{pre}\sqrt{(1\text{-}r_{xx})}$.
   s_{pre} as the standard deviation of the instruments' pre-test score.
   r_{xx} as the instruments' internal consistency.
2) Calculate the instruments' standard deviation of the errors, $S_{Diff} = \sqrt{(2(S_E)^2)}$.
3) Calculate the RCI = $S_{Diff} * 1.96$.

Example depression (ADS):

1) Calculate the instruments' pre-test standard error, $S_E = 9.71\sqrt{(1-.89)} \approx 3.22$.
2) 2) Calculate the instruments' standard deviation of the errors, $S_{Diff} = \sqrt{(2(3.22)^2)} \approx 4.55$.
3) Calculate the RCI = $4.55 * 1.96 \approx 8.92 \approx 9$.

Interpretation:

The RCI would be 9 points on the ADS. As the change scores are computed $ADS_{pre} - ADS_{follow\text{-}up}$ and higher scores indicate more depressive symptoms, a change score of + 9 points would indicate a clinically significant improvement (as the pre-test score would be reduced by 9 points) while a change score of – 9 points would indicate a clinically significant deterioration (as the pre-test score would increase by 9 points). Change scores that lie between – 9 and + 9 would indicate no clinical change.

Completer analyses

Completer analyses were conducted to test whether post- (T2) and follow-up (T3) completers differed from non-completers at T1 (post-completers vs. non-completers) or T2 (follow-up completers vs. non-completers). Participants were compared using independent t-tests (normally distributed) or Mann-Whitney-U tests (not normally distributed). Outcome measures were the same mental health, stress coping and life quality variables as in the pre-post comparisons.

Missing data and effect sizes

Due to the small sample size and the concurrent higher variance, missing data were not imputed but excluded pairwise. The alpha level was set to $p < .05$, a tendency was detected at $p < .10$. There was no adjustment for alpha error accumulation because of the small sample size and the explorative character of the study, except for the post-hoc tests for the last hypothesis. Effect sizes were calculated for all significant results and tendencies. Cohen's d[1] was used for the parametric tests, with small ($d > .20$), medium ($d > 50$) and large effects ($d > .80$). For nonparametric tests, r [29][2] was also categorized into small ($r > .10$), medium ($r > .30$) and large effects ($r > .50$).

Results

Baseline characteristics and differences between SWIS and WLC

Table 2 displays the baseline means and standard deviations for SWIS and WLC. The reliabilities of the PHQ-D subscales anxiety ($\alpha = .69$) and general stress ($\alpha = .70$) were deemed acceptable. The scales somatic complaints, alcohol abuse, adaptive stress coping strategies and physical condition were not normally distributed and analyzed accordingly. As Table 2 demonstrates, there were no statistically significant differences between SWIS and WLC at baseline. On average, all students in both groups reported high depression scores, as 56% of the students exceeded the ADS cut-off score. 54% of the SWIS condition and 62% of the WLC condition showed clinically relevant depressive symptoms. Panic symptoms and alcohol abuse were uncommon ($N_{panic} > 0 = 1$; $N_{alcohol} > 0 = 5$).

Table 2 Baseline differences between SWIS and WLC

Variable	SWIS		WLC		Test statistic	p
	N	M / % (SD)	N	M / % (SD)		
Mental health (ADS, PHQ)						
Depression (ADS) 0–60	39	23.54 (8.84)	15	25.40 (7.51)	t(52) = .721	.474
Clinically relevant depressive symptoms (ADS ≥23)	39	21 (54%)	13	8 (62%)	$X^2(52) = .234$	.629
Somatic complaints (PHQ) 0–26	39	7.62 (4.71)	15	7.20 (4.59)	Z = –.252	.801
Panic (PHQ) 0–11	11	3.91 (3.14)	6	5.13 (2.36)	t(17) = .919	.371
Anxiety (PHQ) 0–12	38	7.58 (2.68)	14	7.57 (2.56)	t(50) = –.009	.993
Alcohol abuse (PHQ) 0–5	29	.24 (.58)	12	0 (0)	Z = –1.513	.403
General stressors (PHQ) 0–27	39	7.74 (3.40)	15	6.47 (2.89)	t(52) = – 1.284	.205
Stress coping strategies (SVF)						
Adaptive strategies	39	17.97 (2.64)	15	17.28 (3.92)	Z = –.464	.643
Maladaptive strategies	39	19.52 (3.30)	15	19.97 (4.13)	t(52) = .415	.680
Quality of life (SEL)						
Physical condition	39	2.96 (.63)	15	2.72 (.84)	Z = –1.393	.164
Cognitive emotional condition	39	2.79 (.56)	15	2.87 (.62)	t(52) = .440	.662
Quality of life	39	3.13 (.54)	15	3.03 (.50)	t(52) = –.642	.524

N varies across variables due to the fact that not all participants affirmed the filter questions for the three PHQ-scales panic, anxiety and alcohol abuse

Therefore, these two scales were excluded from further analysis.

Pre-post comparisons between SWIS and WLC

The comparisons between pre- and post-test are presented in Table 3. Students of both conditions reported significantly less depression at post-test with small (SWIS) and medium (WLC) effects. The SWIS condition additionally showed a significantly better physical condition after the training with a small effect size. WLC students reported significantly less maladaptive stress coping strategies with a small effect size. Furthermore, the participants of the SWIS condition had descriptively less anxiety and general stress after the training, while WLC students reported more anxiety and general stress.

Clinically relevant depressive symptoms

Figure 2 displays the percentage of the participants that report clinically relevant depressive symptoms (ADS ≥23) for each condition during pre- and post-test. The

Table 3 Separate pre-post comparisons with effect sizes for the two conditions

Variable	N	SWIS		t	p	d	N	WLC		t	p	d
		Pre M (SD)	Post M (SD)					Pre M (SD)	Post M (SD)			
Mental health												
Depression	28	23.43 (8.74)	20.61 (8.05)	**2.367**	**.025**	**.32**	13	24.92 (7.54)	21.46 (6.94)	**2.843**	**.015**	**.56**
Somatic complaints	28	7.75 (4.49)	7.04 (3.84)	1.285	.210		13	6.15 (3.87)	5.69 (2.02)	.496	.629	
Anxiety	28	7.96 (2.47)	7.62 (2.38)	1.104	.280		11	7.00 (2.53)	7.45 (1.97)	–.833	.424	
General stress	28	7.75 (3.05)	7.50 (3.67)	.500	.621		13	6.46 (3.13)	7.23 (4.79)	–.784	.448	
Stress coping strategies												
Adaptive strategies	27	12.32 (2.20)	12.13 (2.70)	.393	.679		13	16.91 (4.08)	16.73 (4.23)	.370	.718	
Maladaptive strategies	27	13.50 (3.47)	12.79 (3.51)	1.522	.140		13	19.23 (3.94)	16.69 (4.52)	**2.449**	**.031**	**.48**
Quality of life												
Physical condition	28	2.95 (.58)	3.27 (.57)	**–2.848**	**.008**	**.38**	13	2.78 (.89)	2.98 (.66)	–1.099	.294	
Cognitive emotional condition	28	2.82 (.58)	2.94 (.56)	–1.246	.223		13	2.89 (.66)	2.98 (.59)	–.574	.577	
Quality of life	28	3.15 (.56)	3.29 (.55)	–1.487	.149		13	3.04 (.53)	3.18 (.56)	–1.067	.307	

Bold characters indicate significant results ($p < .05$)

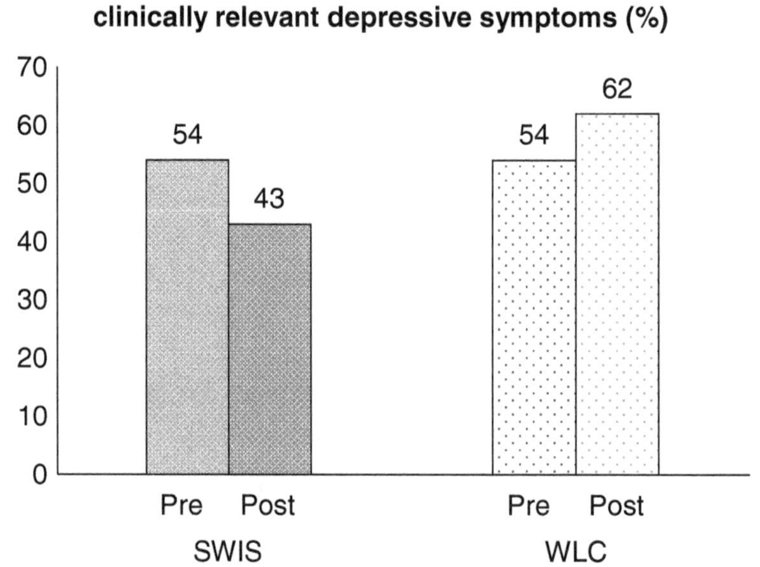

Fig. 2 Percentage of participants with clinically relevant depressive symptoms for SWIS ($N = 28$) and WLC ($N = 13$) condition during pre- and post-test. The pre-test percentages may vary from Table 2 as only participants who completed both measurements were included

percentages of participants with clinically relevant depressive symptoms did not differ between the two conditions at pre-test. However, fewer participants in the SWIS condition exceeded the cut-off score at post-test (– 11%). The WLC condition shows the opposite effect with an increase of participants with clinically relevant depressive symptoms (+ 8%). This result presents a superior effect of the SWIS condition regarding the development of clinically relevant depressive symptoms.

Long-term effects of SWIS

The long-term effects of SWIS are displayed in Table 4. Participants of the WLC were included in this analysis if they did not differ from the SWIS condition at T1. Nearly all dependent variables met this requirement, except for maladaptive stress coping strategies. Furthermore, only participants who completed all measurements from T1 to T3 of the WLC were included ($N = 5$). Using these criteria, data from five additional WLC participants were added in the remaining eight dependent variables. Again, the scales panic and alcohol abuse were excluded from the analysis due to the fact that most students did not report any impairment.

Three months after participation at the SWIS-training, the students reported fewer somatic complaints, less anxiety, an improved physical condition as well as a better quality of life with medium to large effect sizes. The significant improvements were mainly observed between pre- and follow-up measurement, indicating an improvement after the conclusion of the training. The other investigated outcome measures showed descriptive improvements, including less depressive symptoms, less stress, fewer maladaptive stress coping strategies and an improved cognitive emotional condition. The reduction of depressive symptoms remained stable under the clinical cut-off score of the ADS.

Depressive symptoms and long-term mental health development

Participants with and without clinically relevant depressive symptoms at pre-test (ADS < 23) were compared regarding their long-term mental health development. Descriptive statistics are displayed in Appendix 1. Group (depressive vs. non-depressive), time (pre- to follow-up measurement) and group x time interactions are presented in Appendix 2.

There were several group and time effects, but few group x time interaction effects. The general stress declined more rapidly in participants with clinically relevant depressive symptoms. Aside from that interaction, there were no further significant interaction effects. Hence, the presence or absence of clinically relevant depressive symptoms did not affect the development of the long-term mental health outcomes.

Clinically significant changes

The interpretation of the RCIs are provided in Appendix 3. Figure 3 provides an overview of the long-term clinical changes in the mental health variables. Approximately one fifth of the students reported clinically improved depression,

Table 4 Mental health long-term effects of SWIS

Variable	N	Pre-test $_1$ M (SD)	Post-test $_2$ M (SD)	Follow-up $_3$ M (SD)	Test statistic F / Z	p	Post-hoc	p_{adj}	Effect size d / r
Mental health									
Depression	19	21.47 (9.71)	20.32 (9.36)	17.47 (10.88)	F(2,17) = 1.212	.322	–	–	–
Somatic complaints	18	7.72 (4.44)	6.44 (3.96)	6.44 (4.02)	***F(2,16) = 3.509***	***.055***	***t_{1-2} = 2.336***	***.096***	***d = .55***
							t_{1-3} = 2.426	***.082***	***d = .57***
							t_{2-3} = n.s.	–	–
Anxiety	11	8.09 (2.02)	7.36 (2.11)	6.36 (2.25)	**F(2,9) = 1.832**	**.015**	t_{1-2} = n.s.	–	–
							t_{1-3} = 3.846	**.010**	**d = 1.16**
							t_{2-3} = 2.801	***.056***	***d = .84***
General stress	18	7.11 (3.58)	6.56 (3.89)	5.77 (2.94)	F(2,16) = 1.832	.192	–	–	–
Stress coping strategies									
Adaptive strategies	19	17.92 (2.42)	16.08 (4.01)	15.70 (5.02)	Z(2,19) = 1.425	.491	–	–	–
Maladaptive strategies	15	19.08 (3.47)	18.46 (4.23)	16.48 (5.20)	Z(2,15) = 3.138	.208	–	–	–
Quality of life									
Physical condition	19	2.97 (.73)	3.42 (.58)	3.57 (.70)	**F(2,17) = 7.401**	**.005**	**t_{1-2} = −3.000**	**.023**	**d = −.69**
							t_{1-3} = −3.903	**.003**	**d = −.89**
							t_{2-3} = n.s.	–	–
Cognitive emotional condition	19	2.94 (.59)	3.01 (.53)	3.22 (.57)	F(2,17) = 2.555	.107	–	–	–
Quality of life	19	3.25 (.61)	3.39 (.54)	3.59 (.50)	**F(2,17) = 3.670**	**.047**	t_{1-2} = n.s.	–	–
							t_{1-3} = −2.656	**.047**	**d = −.61**
							t_{2-3} = n.s.	–	–

Bold characters indicate significant results ($p < .05$). Bold italics indicate tendentially significant results ($p < .10$). – indicate statistically insignificant results. All post-hoc tests were adjusted for alpha error accumulation

anxiety and general stress. The students' somatic complaints remained stable. Only one student (5%) showed deteriorated depression scores in the long-term.

Figure 4 displays the long-term clinical changes of the students' stress coping strategies and quality of life. The students' reported divergent results regarding their stress coping strategies: While 47% showed a clinically relevant deterioration of their adaptive strategies, 53% reported a clinically relevant improvement of their maladaptive stress coping strategies.

Forty two percent of the students showed a clinically improved physical and cognitive emotional condition

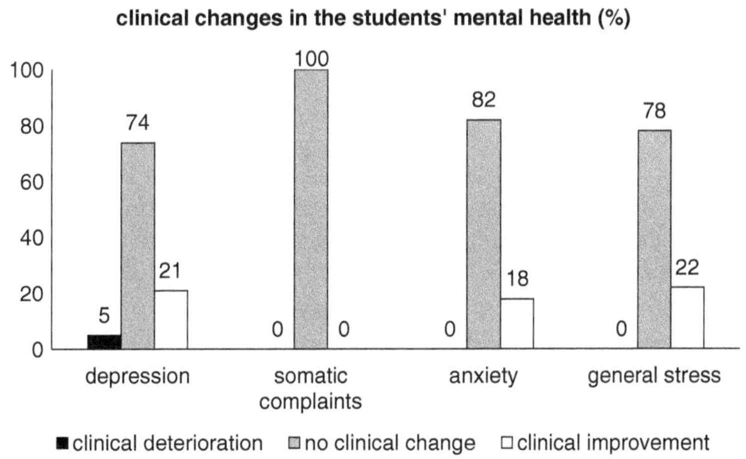

Fig. 3 Long-term clinical changes in the students' mental health

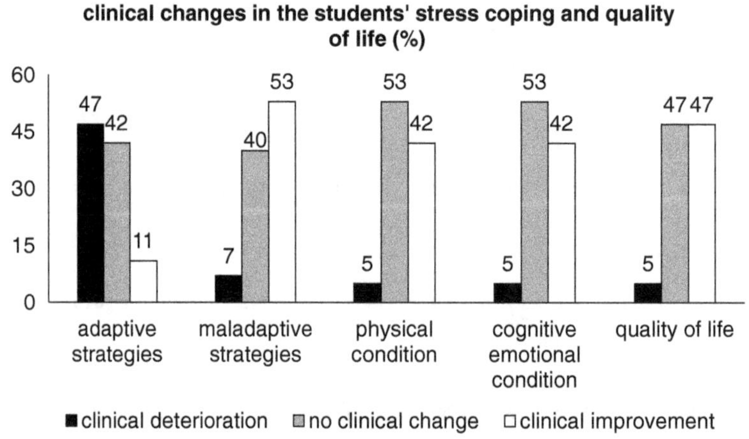

Fig. 4 Long-term clinical change in the students' stress coping strategies and quality of life

in the long-term. Regarding their general quality of life, nearly half of the sample (47%) reported clinical improvements. Again, only one student (5%) showed a clinically relevant reduction of the physical, cognitive emotional and general quality of life.

The analyses of the long-term clinical changes regarding the students' mental health, stress coping strategies and quality of life indicate moderate improvements on all scales, with the exception of the adaptive stress coping strategies.

Completer analyses

Fifteen of 56 participants were lost to attrition from pre- to post-measurement (– 27%). Of those 15 participants, 7 participants did not complete the SWIS training (– 13%) and 8 participants completed the SWIS training, but did not complete the post-measurement (– 14%). The completers did not differ from the non-completers on any dependent variable, age, or gender (all $p > .05$). Twenty two of 41 participants were lost to attrition from post- to follow-up measurement (– 54%). Again, the completers did not differ from the non-completers on any dependent variable, age, or gender (all $p > .05$).

Discussion

This randomized controlled pilot trial investigated the effects of SWIS compared with WLC concerning mental health, stress coping strategies and quality of life in university students, as well as long-term effects.

The depression scores of the students declined significantly in both conditions. Additionally, participants in the SWIS condition reported descriptively less anxiety and general stress than the WLC. Except for a significant increase in adaptive stress coping strategies in WLC students, none of the stress coping strategies changed significantly. Beyond, students had a significantly improved physical condition after the SWIS training, which was not observed in the WLC condition. However, the other two scales (cognitive emotional condition and quality of life) did not change significantly. From a clinical perspective, the SWIS condition was superior compared to the WLC condition regarding the reduction of clinically relevant depressive symptoms.

In the long-term, the students in the SWIS condition reported statistically significant fewer somatic complaints, less anxiety, an improved physical condition and a better quality of life from pre-test to follow-up with moderate to large effects. Depressive symptoms only had a statistically significant impact on general stress. Furthermore, moderate long-term clinically relevant changes occurred in most mental health variables and in the students' quality of life.

Completer analyses did not reveal any significant differences between completers and non-completers at post- or follow-up measurement. Overall, the SWIS sleep training differed only slightly from the WLC condition. However, positive long-term results support the additional benefits of SWIS on the mental health and quality of life in college and university students.

Interpretation of results

The discrepancies between the insignificant results directly after the training and the various significant long-term effects indicate that the students need more time to implement the strategies they obtained in the SWIS training. Depressive symptoms did not affect the positive long-term development of the students' mental health in nearly all variables but general stress. The moderate clinical long-term improvements concurred with the statistical analyses. This presents SWIS as a feasible and effective program for students who suffer from sleep problems as well as depressive symptoms.

These improvements were expected, as SWIS specifically targets the investigated variables. For example, sleep hygiene instructions also include rules about healthy eating, alcohol consumption, and physical activity. These aspects might reduce somatic complaints and consequently improve the students' physical condition (e.g. less stomach aches, less skin problems). Furthermore, improved sleep is connected directly with an improved physical condition. Anxiety issues are tackled with cognitive restructuring and relaxation techniques, such as progressive muscle relaxation or hypnotherapeutic elements. Finally, the stress coping strategies and the general self-care character of SWIS help to improve the students' quality of life.

The most obvious conflict regarding these results was the statistically significant improvement of the depression scores and adaptive stress coping strategies in the WLC condition. This may be explained by several artefacts including statistical regression to the mean, effects of the diagnostic sleep log and unspecific expectation effects in WLC conditions that were reported in previous publications [30]. Furthermore, the detailed analysis of ADS cut-off score revealed that more WLC participants reported clinically relevant depressive symptoms at post-test in comparison with the pre-test percentages and with the SWIS condition. Therefore, the statistically significant improvements of the WLC participants' depressive symptoms were not observed on a clinical level.

The completer analyses revealed that there were no differences between completers and non-completers at post- and follow-up measurement. This result shows that the study itself did not keep specific groups from participating, leading to the reverse conclusion that the students accepted SWIS regardless of their baseline characteristics.

Adverse effects were only inferred by a descriptive decline of the adaptive stress coping strategies in the SWIS condition. However, this reduction was not significant, rendering its interpretation negligible.

Scientific integration

Mental health

A recent review [10] provided evidence that sleep trainings improve the mental health of university students, although differences regarding the type of intervention emerged. While studies on sleep hygiene, CBT and other psychotherapeutic approaches reported small to medium effect sizes for mental health outcomes, the studies with relaxation trainings had large effect sizes. As SWIS combines CBT-I and HT-I, it also includes relaxation elements (e.g. PMR). However, comparison to other studies is impaired by a lack of mental health outcome reporting and insignificant results. Only 37% of the investigated sleep trainings showed significant improvements in mental health variables, 11% did not find significant changes and 52% did not report any mental health variables at all. Despite the small sample size, the current study revealed similar effect sizes.

In detail, two similar sleep interventions employed CBT to improve sleep in college students [31], and in students with insomnia according to DSM-5 [32]. Morris and colleagues randomized 95 healthy students into an online CBT condition (60% women) or a WLC (70% women) [31]. After the six weekly intervention sessions the students reported significantly less depression in both groups. However, the authors did not find any interaction effect. This corresponds with our results, as depression scores decreased in both conditions (SWIS and WLC) immediately after the training. The other CBT study by Taylor and colleagues investigated several mental health outcomes in 34 college students, with 17 students in each condition (59% women; CBT vs. WLC) [32]. Compared to the students in the WLC condition, those in the CBT condition reported significantly less general fatigue. Other investigated mental health aspects like quality of life, anxiety, depression, stress, alcohol and marijuana use did not change significantly after the sleep training [32]. This indicates that the SWIS training as a CBT-I and HT-I combination has a larger positive effect on the students' mental health and quality of life than similar programs that focus solely on CBT.

Stress coping

The students' stress coping strategies were not influenced by the SWIS sleep training. This conflicts with the findings of Pillai and colleagues, who reported that the relationship between stress and sleep is mediated by the three stress coping strategies behavioral disengagement, distraction and substance abuse [7]. However, these three stress coping behaviors only cover a small proportion of the stress coping behaviors that were examined in the present study. While behavioral disengagement and substance abuse can be assigned to the ten maladaptive strategies measured by the stress coping inventory, distraction belongs to the seven adaptive strategies. Thus, a more detailed examination of the different stress coping strategies, especially behavioral disengagement, substance abuse and distraction, might reveal further differences and should be analyzed in further studies.

Long-term effects

The investigation of long-term effects in the current study revealed significant improvements of the students' somatic complaints, anxiety, physical condition and quality of life. The follow-up data of Taylor and colleagues [32] did not present these mental health effects. However, the authors observed a significant improvement from post- to follow-up measurement regarding several sleep-related variables (e.g. dysfunctional beliefs, daytime impairments and general fatigue), which indicates incubation effects [32]. These effects may also be present in the current study, e.g. because the students need more time to implement the strategies that they learned in the SWIS sleep training. Beyond, studies regarding adolescents and children also reported a further enhancement 3 months after treatment [16, 18].

Completer analyses

Attrition was 27% at post-measurement and 54% at follow-up measurement. The larger attrition rate for the third assessment was not surprising, as the follow-up measurement was taken online, thus reducing the participants' feelings of obligation to comply with the procedure. This assumption is supported by similar results in the CBT-I study conducted by Taylor and colleagues [32]: There, 15% of the students did not complete the post-measurement and 56% were lost to attrition at 3 months follow-up measurement. Furthermore, a recent meta-analysis on drop-out rates in CBT-studies suggests that studies with depressed participants and outpatients had higher drop-out rates than studies with non-depressed inpatient participants [33]. As the current study contained 29 participants (56%) with clinically relevant depressive symptoms and an outpatient setting, higher drop-out rates can be expected.

Strengths and limitations

The randomized controlled design and the 3 month follow-up are important strengths of the current study. The comparison with other sleep trainings revealed the importance of long-term measurements, as the students have to implement learned strategies in daily routine. Although the general dropout rates were high, most of the students that started the training completed it (SWIS: 82%, WLC: 85%), supporting the feasibility and acceptance of SWIS. Furthermore, the investigated university students all suffered from sleep disorders or had an impaired sleep quality. The inclusion of participants with subclinical sleep impairments might result in a reduced efficacy of the SWIS sleep training due to the fact that the participants did not have severe sleep problems to begin with, creating a ceiling effect. Therefore, further studies should compare healthy participants to subclinical and clinical participants to examine sleep-related ceiling effects. Finally, the examination of statistically as well as clinically significant changes provides a better understanding of the students' long-term development.

One limitation of the current study was the small and unequal sample size. Despite the fact that the sample size exceeded the necessary 33 participants, the unequal sample sizes in the different conditions impaired statistical calculations. Another limitation is the WLC design. Recent reviews showed that WLCs may inflate intervention effect sizes [34]. Correspondingly, a review of meta-analysis found that CBT is effective compared to waiting list, but mixed results occur when comparing CBT to active control conditions or other interventions [35]. A meta-analysis investigating the effects of waiting list conditions in depression even resulted in nocebo effects, as waiting list conditions were less effective than no treatment conditions [36]. Consequently, future studies should include other control conditions. Furthermore, a long-term investigation of the WLC would have been the best design. However, such a design was not possible due to the fact that the students in the WLC received the SWIS training directly after they completed their second assessment. Due to a lack of information concerning the instruments' stabilities, real life changes in symptoms might also be attributed to a low test retest reliability. Finally, the instrument that used filter questions to investigate panic symptoms and alcohol abuse was not appropriate for such a small sample size, as only a few students confirmed that they ever had any of the aforementioned symptoms. This resulted in missing data for most of the panic and alcohol scales.

Conclusions

In the long-term, the SWIS sleep training improved not only sleep, but also different aspects of university students' mental health and quality of life. Stress coping strategies did not change significantly, although a more detailed analysis might be necessary. The positive developments between post-test and follow up in the current study again showed the importance of long-term measurements. The presence of absence of depressive symptoms at pre-measurement did not impact the long-term development of the students' mental health, leading to the conclusion that the SWIS sleep training is similarly effective for depressed and non-depressed students.

Future studies should include a larger sample size. This would allow a subdivision into impaired and non-impaired students, which facilitates the detection and avoidance of ceiling effects. Another advantage of a larger sample size would be the possibility to apply the appropriate statistical tests (e.g. repeated measures ANOVA). Furthermore, future studies should include different control conditions, e.g. alternative interventions, active control conditions, and treatment as usual. Finally, future studies should also consider alternative instruments for the measurement of panic symptoms and alcohol abuse and find ways to reduce attrition rates, e.g. by reimbursing the participants.

Endnotes

[1] $d = \frac{t}{\sqrt{N}}$

[2] $r = \frac{z}{\sqrt{N}}$

Appendix 1

Table 5 Means and standard deviations of the long-term effects in participants with clinically relevant depressive symptoms and non-clinically relevant depressive symptoms

Variable		N	Pre-test M (SD)	Post-test M (SD)	Follow-up M (SD)
Mental health					
Depression	ADS < 23	10	13.80 (5.39)	15.70 (8.59)	12.70 (6.24)
	ADS ≥23	9	30.00 (4.89)	25.44 (7.60)	22.78 (12.75)
Somatic complaints	ADS < 23	10	8.30 (3.83)	6.70 (3.89)	6.80 (4.63)
	ADS ≥23	8	7.00 (5.29)	6.12 (4.29)	6.00 (3.34)
Anxiety	ADS < 23	6	7.83 (1.94)	7.33 (2.16)	6.33 (1.97)
	ADS ≥23	5	8.40 (2.30)	7.40 (2.30)	6.40 (2.79)
General stress	ADS < 23	10	4.80 (2.86)	5.00 (3.89)	5.10 (3.14)
	ADS ≥23	8	10.00 (3.58)	8.50 (3.02)	6.63 (2.62)
Stress coping strategies					
Adaptive strategies	ADS < 23	10	17.90 (2.43)	15.86 (3.96)	16.32 (4.72)
	ADS ≥23	9	17.95 (2.55)	16.32 (4.29)	15.01 (5.54)
Maladaptive strategies	ADS < 23	8	17.13 (3.17)	16.47 (4.77)	16.56 (4.77)
	ADS ≥23	7	21.32 (2.31)	20.75 (1.95)	16.39 (6.04)
Quality of life					
Physical condition	ADS < 23	10	3.20 (.61)	3.55 (.72)	3.62 (.82)
	ADS ≥23	9	2.70 (.80)	3.27 (.35)	3.51 (.59)
Cognitive emotional condition	ADS < 23	10	3.32 (.45)	3.23 (.54)	3.43 (.57)
	ADS ≥23	9	2.52 (.41)	2.77 (.42)	2.99 (.49)
Quality of life	ADS < 23	10	3.67 (.39)	3.63 (.57)	3.76 (.53)
	ADS ≥23	9	2.79 (.44)	3.14 (.39)	3.41 (.43)

Appendix 2

Table 6 Long-term effects of SWIS in depressed and non-depressed participants: Group, time and group x time interaction effects

Variable	Group (depression)	Time	Group x time interaction
Mental health			
Depression	$F(1,19) = 20.638, p = .000$	–	–
Somatic complaints	–	$F(2,15) = 3.157, p = .072$	–
Anxiety	–	$F(2,8) = 6.377, p = .022$	–
General stress	$F(1,18) = 7.291, p = .016$	$F(2,15) = 4.121, p = .037$	$F(2,15) = 6.142, p = .011$
Stress coping strategies			
Adaptive strategies	–	–	–
Maladaptive strategies	–	$F(2,12) = 2.898, p = .094$	–
Quality of life			
Physical condition	–	$F(2,16) = 7.862, p = .004$	–
Cognitive emotional condition	$F(1,19) = 10.146, p = .005$	–	–
Quality of life	$F(1,19) = 11.200, p = .004$	$F(2,16) = 4.666, p = .025$	–

– indicate statistically insignificant results

Appendix 3

Interpretation of the RCIs

ADS depressive symptoms ➔ RCI = 9 points

≥ + 9 points = **improvement**

≤ – 9 points = **deterioration**

-9 to + 9 points = no clinical change

PHQ somatic complaints ➔ RCI = 6 points

≥ + 6 points = **improvement**

≤ – 6 points = **deterioration**

-6 to + 6 points = no clinical change

PHQ anxiety ➔ RCI = 4 points

≥ + 4 points = **improvement**

≤ – 4 points = **deterioration**

-4 to + 4 points = no clinical change

PHQ general stress ➔ RCI = 5 points

≥ + 5 points = **improvement**

≤ – 5 points = **deterioration**

-5 to + 5 points = no clinical change

SVF adaptive strategies ➔ RCI = 2.21

≥ + 2.21 points = **deterioration**, because this would indicate that the pre-test score was higher than the follow-up score, which would represent a decline in adaptive stress coping strategies

≤ – 2.21 points = **improvement**

-2.21 to + 2.21 points = no clinical change

SVF maladaptive strategies ➔ RCI = 2.16

≥ + 2.16 points = **improvement**

≤ – 2.16 points = **deterioration**

-2.16 to + 2.16 points = no clinical change

SEL physical condition ➔ RCI = .69

≥ + .69 points = **deterioration**, because higher scores indicate a better physical condition. Therefore, a positive change score (pre – follow-up) would mean that the participants had a better physical condition at pre-test compared to the follow-up measurement.

≤ – .69 points = **improvement**

-.69 to +.69 points = no clinical change

SEL cognitive-emotional condition ➔ RCI = .47

≥ + .47 points = **deterioration**

≤ – .47 points = **improvement**

-.47 to +.47 points = no clinical change

SEL quality of life ➔ RCI = .41

≥ + .41 points = **deterioration**

≤ – .41 points = **improvement**

-.41 to +.41 points = no clinical change

Abbreviations

ADS: Allgemeine Depressionsskala (general depression scale); CBT-I: Cognitive behavior therapy for insomnia; DSM: Diagnostic and Statistical Manual of Mental Disorders; HT-I: Hypnotherapy for insomnia; PHQ-D: Patient Health Questionnaire (PHQ-D = German version); PMR: Progressive muscle relaxation; RCI: Reliable change index; SEL: Skalen zur Erfassung der Lebensqualität (quality of life scales); SVF-78: Stressverarbeitungsfragebogen (Stress Coping Questionnaire); SWIS: Studieren wie im Schlaf (StudySleep); WLC: Waiting list control condition

Acknowledgements

We would like to thank Ann-Kristin Manhart for correcting the manuscript and Neele Busse for being the co-trainer.

Funding

We acknowledge support for the Article Processing Charge by the Deutsche Forschungsgemeinschaft and the Open Access Publication Fund of Bielefeld University. The funder was not involved in any part of the research or reporting of this study. There were no additional internal or external sources of support.

Authors' contributions

AF wrote this article. AF and MC designed the study, conducted the research and were the trainers. AAS had the idea, designed the study, wrote the manual, supervised the process (e.g. inclusion and exclusion criteria, supervision of the trainers, etc.), and intensely corrected the manuscript.

Consent for publication

Not applicable.

Competing interests

The authors declare that they have no competing interests.

References

1. Schlarb AA, Kulessa D, Gulewitsch MD. Sleep characteristics, sleep problems, and associations of self-efficacy among German university students. Nat Sci Sleep. 2012;9:1–7.
2. Schlarb AA, Claßen M, Hellmann S, Vögele C, Gulewitsch MD. Sleep and somatic complaints in university students. J Pain Res. 2017;10:1189–99.
3. Schlarb AA, Claßen M, Grünwald J, Vögele C. Sleep disturbances and mental strain in university students: results from an online survey in Luxembourg and Germany. Int J Ment Health Sys. 2017;11:1–10.
4. Taylor DJ, Bramoweth AD, Grieser EA, Tatum JI, Roane BM. Epidemiology of insomnia in college students: relationship with mental health, quality of life and substance use difficulties. Behav Ther. 2013;44:339–48.
5. Lund HG, Reider BD, Whiting AB, Prichard JR. Sleep patterns and predictors of disturbed sleep in a large population of college students. J Adolesc Health. 2010;46:124–32.
6. Byrd K, Gelaye B, Tadessea MG, Williams MA, Lemma S, Sleep Disturbances BY. Common mental disorders in college students. Health Behav Policy Rev. 2014;1:229–37.
7. Pillai V, Roth T, Mullins HM, Drake CL. Moderators and mediators of the relationship between stress and insomnia: stressor chronicity, cognitive intrusion, and coping. Sleep. 2014;37:1199–208.
8. Wong ML, Lau EYY, Wan JHY, Cheung SF, Hui CH, Mok DSY. The interplay between sleep and mood in predicting academic functioning, physical health and psychological health: a longitudinal study. J Psychosom Res. 2013;74:271–7.
9. Preišegolavičiūtė E, Leskauskas D, Adomaitienė V. Associations of quality of sleep with lifestyle factors and profile of studies among Lithuanian students. Medicina. 2010;46:482–9.
10. Friedrich A, Schlarb AA. Let's talk about sleep: a systematic review of psychological interventions to improve sleep in university students. J Sleep Res. 2017; https://doi.org/10.1111/jsr.12568.
11. Schlarb AA, Friedrich A, Claßen M. Sleep problems in university students - an intervention. Neuropsychiatr Dis Treat. 2017;13:1989–2001.
12. Schlarb AA, Brandhorst I, Hautzinger M. Mini-KiSS - ein multimodales Gruppentherapieprogramm für Eltern von Kleinkindern mit Schlafstörungen. Z Kinder Jugendpsychiatr Psychother. 2011;39:197–206.
13. Schlarb AA, Brandhorst I. Schlafen lernen - das Mini-KiSS-Training für verhaltensbedingte Schlafprobleme in den ersten vier Lebensjahren. Das Schlafmagazin. 2012;4:38–42.
14. Schlarb AA, Brandhorst I. Mini-KiSS online: an internet-based intervention program for parents of young children with sleep problems – influence on parental behavior and children's sleep. Nat Sci Sleep. 2012;4:41–52.
15. Schlarb AA, Velten-Schurian K, Poets C, Hautzinger M. First effects of a multicomponent treatment for sleep disorders in children. Nat Sci Sleep. 2011;3:1–11.

16. Schlarb AA, Bihlmaier I, Velten-Schurian K, Poets CF, Hautzinger M. Short- and Long-term effects of CBT-I in groups for school-age children suffering from chronic insomnia: the KiSS program. Behav Sleep Med. 2016;16:1–21.
17. Schlarb AA, Liddle CC, Hautzinger M. JuSt - a multimodal program for treatment of insomnia in adolescents: a pilot study. Nat Sci Sleep. 2011;3:13–20.
18. Roeser K, Schwerdtle B, Kübler A, Schlarb AA. Further evidence for the JuSt program as a treatment for insomnia in adolescents: results from a 1 year follow-up study. J Clin Sleep Med. 2016;12:257–62.
19. American Psychiatric Association. Diagnostic and statistical manual of mental disorders. 5th ed. Arlington: American Psychiatric Publishing; 2013.
20. Buysse DJ, Reynolds CF, Monk TH, Berman SR, Kupfer DJ. The Pittsburgh sleep quality index: a new instrument for psychiatric research and practice. Psychiatry Res. 1989;28:193–213.
21. Faul F, Erdfelder E, Lang AG, Buchner AG. Power 3: a flexible statistical power analysis program for the social, behavioral, and biomedical sciences. Behav Res Methods. 2007;39:175–91.
22. Hautzinger M, Bailer M. Allgemeine Depressions Skala: Manual. Beltz Test GmbH: Göttingen; 1993.
23. Löwe B, Spitzer RL, Zipfel S, Herzog W. PHQ-D Gesundheitsfragebogen für Patienten. 2nd ed. Karlsruhe: Pfizer; 2002.
24. Gräfe K, Zipfel S, Herzog W, Löwe B. Screening psychischer Störungen mit dem "Gesundheitsfragebogen für Patienten (PHQ-D)". Diagnostica. 2004;50:171–181.
25. Erdmann G, Stressverarbeitungsfragebogen JW. Stress, Stressverarbeitung und ihre Erfassung durch ein mehrdimensionales Testsystem. Göttingen: Hogrefe; 2008.
26. Averbeck M, Leiberich P, Grote-Kusch TM, Olbrich E, Schröder A, Brieger M, Schumacher K. Skalen zur Erfassung der Lebensqualität (SEL). Frankfurt: Swets & Zeitlinger; 1997.
27. IBM Corp. IBM SPSS Statistics for Windows, Version 22.0. Armonk: IBM Corp; 2013.
28. Jacobson NS, Truax P. Clinical significance: a statistical approach to defining meaningful change in psychotherapy research. J Consult Clin Psychol. 1991; 59:12–9.
29. Rosenthal R. Meta-analytic procedures for social research. 2nd ed. Newbury Park: Sage; 1991.
30. Kraemer HC, Wilson T, Fairburn CG, Agras S. Mediators and moderators of treatment effects in randomized clinical trials. Arch Gen Psychiatry. 2002;59: 877–83.
31. Morris J, Firkins A, Millings A, Mohr C, Redford P, Rowe A. Internet-delivered cognitive behavior therapy for anxiety and insomnia in a higher education context. Anxiety Stress Coping. 2016;29:415–31.
32. Taylor DJ, Zimmermann MR, Gardner CE, Williams JM, Grieser EA, Tatum JI, et al. A pilot randomized controlled trial of the effects of cognitive-behavioral therapy for insomnia on sleep and daytime functioning in students. Behav Ther. 2014;45:376–89.
33. Fernandez E, Salem D, Swift JK, Ramtahal N. Meta-analysis of dropout from cognitive behavioral therapy: magnitude, timing. and moderators J Consult Clin Psychol. 2015;83:1108–22.
34. Cunningham JA, Kypri K, McCambridge J. Exploratory randomized controlled trial evaluating the impact of a waiting list control design. BMC Med Res Methodol. 2013;13:150.
35. Hofmann SG, Asnaani A, Vonk IJ, Sawyer AT, Fang A. The efficacy of cognitive behavioral therapy: a review of meta-analyses. Cognitive Ther Res. 2012;36:427–40.
36. Furukawa TA, et al. Waiting list may be a nocebo condition in psychotherapy trials: a contribution from network meta-analysis. Acta Psychiat Scand. 2014;130:181–92.

15

Subtypes in clinical burnout patients enrolled in an employee rehabilitation program: differences in burnout profiles, depression, and recovery/resources-stress balance

Kathrin Bauernhofer[1*], Daniela Bassa[1], Markus Canazei[2], Paulino Jiménez[1], Manuela Paechter[1], Ilona Papousek[1], Andreas Fink[1] and Elisabeth M. Weiss[1]

Abstract

Background: Burnout is generally perceived a unified disorder with homogeneous symptomatology across people (exhaustion, cynicism, and reduced professional efficacy). However, increasing evidence points to intra-individual patterns of burnout symptoms in non-clinical samples such as students, athletes, healthy, and burned-out employees. Different burnout subtypes might therefore exist. Yet, burnout subtypes based on burnout profiles have hardly been explored in clinical patients, and the samples investigated in previous studies were rather heterogeneous including patients with various physical, psychological, and social limitations, symptoms, and disabilities. Therefore, the aim of this study is to explore burnout subtypes based on burnout profiles in clinically diagnosed burnout patients enrolled in an employee rehabilitation program, and to investigate whether the subtypes differ in depression, recovery/resources-stress balance, and sociodemographic characteristics.

Methods: One hundred three patients (66 women, 37 men) with a clinical burnout diagnosis, who were enrolled in a 5 week employee rehabilitation program in two specialized psychosomatic clinics in Austria, completed a series of questionnaires including the Maslach Burnout Inventory – General Survey (MBI-GS), the Beck Depression Inventory, and the Recovery-Stress-Questionnaire for Work. Cluster analyses with the three MBI-GS subscales as clustering variables were used to identify the burnout subtypes. Subsequent multivariate/univariate analysis of variance and Pearson chi-square tests were performed to investigate differences in depression, recovery/resources-stress balance, and sociodemographic characteristics.

Results: Three different burnout subtypes were discovered: the *exhausted* subtype, the *exhausted/cynical* subtype, and the *burned-out* subtype. The *burned-out* subtype and the *exhausted/cynical* subtype showed both more severe depression symptoms and a worse recovery/resources-stress balance than the *exhausted* subtype. Furthermore, the *burned-out* subtype was more depressed than the *exhausted/cynical* subtype, but no difference was observed between these two subtypes with regard to perceived stress, recovery, and resources. Sociodemographic characteristics were not associated with the subtypes.
(Continued on next page)

* Correspondence: kathrin.bauernhofer@uni-graz.at
[1]Department of Psychology, University of Graz, Universitätsplatz 2/DG, 8010 Graz, Austria
Full list of author information is available at the end of the article

(Continued from previous page)

Conclusions: The present study indicates that there are different subtypes in clinical burnout patients (*exhausted*, *exhausted/cynical*, and *burned-out*), which might represent patients at different developmental stages in the burnout cycle. Future studies need to replicate the current findings, investigate the stability of the symptom patterns, and examine the efficacy of rehabilitation interventions in different subtypes.

Keywords: Burnout, Burnout subtypes, Burnout profiles, Person-oriented approach, Cluster analysis, Depression, Stress-recovery

Background

During the last decade, burnout has become a public health issue affecting between 4% and 7% of the working population [1]. Nevertheless, the diagnosis is not yet included in clinical classification systems such as the Diagnostic and Statistical Manual of Mental Disorders (DSM-5) [2] or the International Statistical Classification of Diseases and Related Health Problems (ICD-10) [3]. To date, there is also no consensus on the definition of burnout and its core symptoms [4–7], and the diagnosis overlaps tremendously in symptomatology with other diagnoses, especially chronic fatigue [8] and depression [9–11].

Despite some conceptual controversies [4–7, 12], the most widely accepted definition of burnout is the one by Maslach, Schaufeli, and Leiter [6], who defined it as a work-related stress syndrome characterized by three main symptoms: exhaustion, cynicism, and reduced professional efficacy. Exhaustion refers to feelings of depletion caused by various work demands; cynicism reflects a distant attitude towards work and the people one is working with; and reduced professional efficacy represents the negative self-evaluation that one is incompetent and no longer able to perform work tasks adequately. However, past research has shown that burnout manifests in different ways. A varying number of burnout profiles [13–15] has been observed across studies, and multifaceted longitudinal trajectories of the burnout symptoms [16–21] indicate different pathways into burnout. Different burnout subtypes might therefore exist.

The person-oriented approach to burnout [15, 22] is one possibility to investigate burnout subtypes. It identifies different groups in a population that are intraindividually homogenous, but interindividually heterogeneous in various aspects such as symptomatology, psychopathology, and job- and person-related factors. In past research, the person-oriented approach has been used to identify typical burnout profiles [15], which might represent people at different developmental stages in the burnout cycle or truly different burnout subtypes [13, 23–27].

The most frequent burnout profiles that emerged in these studies [13–15], predominantly from the analysis of the three dimensions of the Maslach Burnout Inventory (MBI) [28], were the *burned-out* profile and the *healthy or engaged* profile representing people with severe or low symptomatology in all three burnout dimensions. Another common symptom profile was the *exhausted/cynical* profile characterized by high exhaustion and cynicism, but simultaneously high professional efficacy. Typical incongruent scoring patterns included the *exhausted or overextended*, the *cynical or disengaged*, and the *reduced professional efficacy* profile representing people with rather mild symptomatology where only one symptom is pronounced. However, one has to keep in mind that most previous studies have been conducted in non-clinical samples, which consist of people who report symptoms of a burnout but have not been diagnosed by a psychiatrist or clinical psychologist and who are all still working [13–15]. Therefore, the so-called healthy worker effect [29] occurred in these studies, and not all of the prior discussed burnout profiles might genuinely represent clinical burnout subtypes who need or seek treatment in specialized psychosomatic clinics or rehabilitation programs.

To date, only one study [30] has investigated subtypes based on burnout profiles in working-aged adults whose working ability was reduced or threatened by disease, disability or some other disorders, and who were therefore enrolled in an employee rehabilitation program. This study has identified four of the above mentioned subtypes: two subtypes with severe symptoms, namely the *burned-out* profile and the *exhausted/cynical* profile, one subtype with milder symptoms, namely the *reduced professional efficacy* profile, and the *healthy* profile. However, some of these profiles might have occurred because Hätinen et al. [30] explored a heterogeneous patient sample suffering from various physical, psychological, and social limitations, symptoms, and disabilities.

For that reason, the present study aims to examine whether meaningful burnout subtypes may be found in a more homogeneous group of clinically diagnosed burnout patients treated in a specialized psychosomatic clinic if the three main burnout symptoms suggested by Maslach, Schaufeli and Leiter [6] are considered and explored within a person-oriented approach [15]. Additionally, we will investigate the relationship of these subtypes to depression since an intense discussion has been going on during the last years [9–12, 31–54] whether burnout can be seen as a distinct construct or rather a new label of an already known state.

A growing body of literature has examined the overlap between burnout (subtypes) and depression-level, both in the working population [9, 12, 23, 31, 32, 39–48, 50–52] and in clinical patients [30, 54], but findings are heterogeneous and inconsistent. Several studies in the working population reported strong correlations between burnout and depression [9–11, 31, 32], especially between exhaustion and depression [10, 31, 32], while in clinically diagnosed burnout patients, the strong exhaustion-depression overlap could not be replicated [55]. Low to moderate correlations between burnout and depression were also found by others in the working population [40, 41, 47], whereas Ahola et al. [45] reported that burnout and depression overlapped particularly in severe burnout. These heterogeneous findings may partly result from using different measures of burnout and depression [11, 37] with some measures reflecting a larger concept redundancy between both disorders (for a discussion on this topic, see Maslach & Leiter [37]). Furthermore, longitudinal studies have been used to study the complex relationship between burnout and depression, but yielded inconsistent results as well. Some authors reported reciprocal relations between burnout and depression [42–44], while others found a unidirectional relationship from burnout to depression [46–50] or vice versa [51–53] or no predictive relation [36]. Studies applying a person-oriented approach to explore the burnout-depression overlap [9, 31] detected that burnout and depression were not separable from each other. Moreover, both disorders developed longitudinally in tandem supporting the hypothesis that burnout and depression may be the same disorder. In clinical burnout patients, longitudinal studies are still sparse [55]. Besides, only a few studies have explored the burnout-depression overlap by applying a person-oriented approach in clinical burnout patients [54] or burnout rehabilitation clients [30, 56], respectively. Yet, the overlap between burnout symptoms and depression might differ between burnout subtypes. Boersma and Lindblom [23] found in the working population that subtypes experiencing high exhaustion were more depressed than other burnout subtypes, and van Dam [54] could distinguish a group with mild symptoms from a group with severe symptoms on several measures (burnout, depression, anxiety, and fatigue) in clinically diagnosed burnout patients. In contrast, Hätinen et al. [30] found in working-aged rehabilitation clients that all subtypes were equally depressed, but in this study, a mixed patient sample suffering from various physiological, psychological, and social limitations, symptoms, and disabilities was explored.

Inconsistencies in organizational risk factors have been found in burnout subtypes as well. According to the job demands-resources (JD-R) model [57], burnout develops when job demands (e.g., workload, time pressure, conflict) are high, while resources (e.g., autonomy, social support, positive relationship with supervisor) are limited. Resources are therefore no longer able to buffer the negative impact of high demands on stress reactions [58]. Job demands and resources have also been linked to specific burnout symptoms: exhaustion is caused by high workload and emotional demands, whereas cynicism, reduced professional efficacy, and disengagement have been associated with a lack of resources [59–61]. Previous studies on burnout subtypes in the working population [13, 23, 27] likewise found that workload was high in subtypes experiencing high exhaustion (*burned-out, exhausted/cynical,* and *exhausted*), but resources were only low in subtypes with severe burnout symptoms (*burned-out* and *exhausted/cynical*), particularly in the *burned-out* subtype [13]. Yet, in clinical rehabilitation patients, Hätinen et al. [30] did not find any differences in job stressors and resources between three different burnout subtypes (*burned-out, exhausted/cynical,* and *low professional efficacy*), although recovery was associated with a decrease in job demands and an increase in job resources [56].

Because most prior research was conducted within the scope of the JD-R model of burnout, recovery has received comparatively less attention in relevant research. The recovery/resources-stress-balance model [62–64] is similar to the JD-R model but focusses additionally on recovery as crucial aspect to prevent burnout. According to the model, burnout develops after prolonged periods of stress without sufficient recovery and resources. More precisely, the homeostatic balance between stress and recovery is impaired because resources that were depleted during phases of stress are not adequately restored in the recovery phase [63]. The role of recovery has, however, not been systematically explored in burnout subtypes, particularly not in clinical burnout patients enrolled in an employee rehabilitation program.

Therefore, the current study aims to explore different burnout subtypes in clinical burnout patients, who are enrolled in an employee rehabilitation program in a psychosomatic clinic, by performing cluster analysis with the three subscales of the Maslach Burnout Inventory – General Survey (MBI-GS) [28] as clustering variables. Furthermore, depression levels will be compared among the subtypes, based on the expectation that the strength of the obviously existing overlap between burnout symptoms and depression might differ between burnout subtypes. Finally, differences between the burnout subtypes in the recovery/resources-stress balance and sociodemographic characteristics will be explored.

Methods

Study design and participants

This study used a person-oriented approach [15] to explore different subtypes based on burnout profiles in clinical burnout patients. A total of 103 patients (64% women) with a clinical burnout diagnosis were recruited from two specialized psychosomatic clinics in Austria. The patients were between 23 and 58 years old ($M = 44.82$ years, $SD = 8.08$) and had various educational backgrounds: 31% had a university degree or the A-level (high education), while 69% completed primary education, an apprenticeship or some other type of education or vocational training without the A-level (lower education).

Procedure

Burnout diagnosis was established by a team of psychiatrists and clinical psychologists. Since separate diagnostic codes for burnout are not yet included in clinical classification systems such as DSM-5 or ICD-10 [2, 3], the burnout diagnosis was based on the ICD-10 criteria of work-related neurasthenia, which has been proposed as the psychiatric equivalent of clinical burnout [38]. Similar to previous studies [54, 65], we included only patients that scored ≥2.20 on exhaustion and either ≥2.00 on cynicism or ≤3.67 on professional efficacy in the MBI-GS. Due to their burnout symptoms, all patients were enrolled in a 5 week employee rehabilitation program at the clinics, and they were on sick leave for at least 1 week prior to study admission ($M = 106.20$ days, $SD = 113.46$). Data were collected during the first week of the rehabilitation program and informed consent was obtained from all patients prior to participation. The study was in accordance with the 1964 Declaration of Helsinki and was approved by the ethics committee of the University of Graz, Austria.

Psychometric measures

Burnout

Burnout symptom severity was assessed with the German version [66] of the MBI-GS [28]. It has 16 items and consists of three subscales: exhaustion, cynicism, and reduced professional efficacy. The exhaustion subscale consists of five items (e.g., feeling emotionally drained from work), the cynicism subscale includes also five items (e.g., enthusiasm has decreased since work was started), and the professional efficacy subscale consists of six items (e.g., feeling that one gets done things effectively). The items are answered on a frequency rating scale ranging from 0 (never) to 6 (daily). Since all participants were on sick leave, they were instructed to respond to the items of the MBI-GS according to how they would feel if they were working at the moment.

Depression

The German version of the Beck Depression Inventory (BDI) was used to assess depression severity [67]. The BDI is a 21-item self-rating questionnaire that covers a variety of depressive symptoms along a continuum from 0 (absent or mild) to 3 (severe) symptoms. The BDI is widely used in treatment settings. A cut-off score ≥ 18 indicates a clinically relevant level of depression [68]. Additionally, all patients were screened for a past diagnosis of major depression using the Structured Clinical Interview for Axis I DSM-IV Disorders (SCID-I) [69].

Recovery/resources-stress balance

The Recovery-Stress-Questionnaire for Work (RESTQ-Work) is based on the recovery/resources-stress balance model [63] and consists overall of 92 items [62]. On a 7-point frequency rating scale ranging from 0 (never) to 6 (always), it measures the degree of stress and the extent of recovery and resources in the past 7 days/nights. The RESTQ-Work has seven subscales: *social-emotional stress* (e.g., being mentally stressed, irritated, and frequently in arguments with others), *performance (-related) stress* (e.g., time pressure, interruptions at work), *loss of meaning/burnout* (e.g., emotional exhaustion, loss of control, meaninglessness), *overall recovery* (e.g., physical recovery, relaxation, satisfying sleep), *leisure/breaks* (e.g., undisturbed leisure time without too many high-duty activities such as household chores, efficient breaks at work), *psychosocial resources* (e.g., social support from family, friends, and colleagues), and *work-related resources* (e.g., autonomy, participation, experience of personal growth). The RESTQ-Work displays good internal reliability and validity, and it has been used in burnout research before [58].

Statistical analyses

The burnout-depression overlap for the entire patient sample was analyzed using basic correlations and correlations corrected for attenuation [70] between the three MBI-GS subscales and the BDI score. To explore different burnout subtypes, cluster analyses [71] were performed. The three MBI-GS subscales (exhaustion, cynicism, and professional efficacy) served as the clustering variables and were standardized (z-score; $M = 0$, $SD = 1$) prior to the analyses. First, a hierarchical agglomerative cluster analysis with Ward's method as a linkage method and squared Euclidean distance as a similarity measure was conducted. The optimal number of clusters was determined by the dendrogram, which is a visual illustration of how the individual cases are arranged into the clusters produced by hierarchical clustering. Next, a K-means cluster analysis was conducted to improve the cluster fit [71]. To identify burnout subtypes based on burnout profiles, the same approach has been applied by others as well [23, 30].

To describe the burnout subtypes further, one-way analyses of variance (ANOVAs) with the clusters as independent variable and the three MBI-GS subscales as dependent variables were conducted. Differences in depression between the subtypes were evaluated using Pearson's chi-square tests (for BDI ≥ 18 and depression diagnosis in the past) and a one-way ANOVA. Differences between the subtypes in recovery/resources-stress balance were evaluated using a one-way MANOVA. In the ANOVAs and MANOVA, the clusters served as the independent variable, while the BDI and the seven RESTQ-Work subscales were the dependent variables, respectively. Sociodemographic differences between the subtypes were investigated with one-way ANOVAs (for age and days on sick leave) and Pearson's chi-square tests (for gender, education, and rehabilitation clinic). In case of homogeneous variances, post-hoc comparisons were made with the Bonferroni test; in case of inhomogeneous variances, the Games-Howell test was used. Effect sizes are reported as partial eta-square (η_p^2) indicating small ($0.01 \leq \eta_p^2 < 0.06$), medium ($0.06 \leq \eta_p^2 < 0.14$), and large ($\eta_p^2 \geq 0.14$) effects, respectively [72]. All statistical procedures were calculated in SPSS 24 and were performed with $\alpha = 0.05$ (two-tailed).

Results

Burnout-depression overlap in the entire patient sample

To explore the burnout-depression overlap in the entire patient sample, basic correlations and correlations corrected for attenuation [70] between the MBI-GS subscales and the BDI were inspected (see Table 1). The three burnout subscales correlated moderately with depression. The highest correlation emerged between cynicism and depression ($r = 0.41$; $p < 0.01$), the lowest correlation occurred between exhaustion and depression ($r = 0.30$; $p < 0.01$). Regarding the correlations between the three MBI-GS subscales, both exhaustion and cynicism ($r = 0.53$; $p < 0.01$) and cynicism and professional efficacy ($r = -0.51$; $p < 0.01$) correlated strongly with each other, whereas a low correlation emerged between exhaustion and professional efficacy ($r = -0.16$; $p = 0.10$).

Table 1 Cronbach's alpha (α) and correlations (correlations corrected for attenuation are in italics) between the MBI-GS subscales and the BDI

	1.	2.	3.	4.	α
1. MBI – exhaustion	1	0.53**	−0.16	0.30**	0.86
2. MBI – cynicism	*0.65***	1	−0.51**	0.41**	0.77
3. MBI – professional efficacy	*−0.20**	*−0.66***	1	−0.35**	0.78
4. BDI	*0.35***	*0.51***	*−0.42***	1	0.88

*$p < 0.05$; **$p < 0.01$

Burnout subtypes in clinically diagnosed burnout patients

Cluster analysis with the three MBI-GS subscales indicated two to four burnout subtypes in the present sample. In the two-cluster solution, cluster 1 and cluster 2 grouped together although the patients of cluster 2 had more severe burnout symptoms than the patients of cluster 1 (see Table 2). In the four-cluster solution, a cluster of patients with elevated burnout symptoms emerged that lay in between cluster 1 and cluster 2. However, since the four-cluster solution did not provide more conceptual clarity than the three-cluster solution, we considered the three-cluster solution representing three different burnout subtypes the best. Subsequent ANOVAs showed how the three subtypes differed in burnout symptomatology (see Table 2).

Figure 1 displays the symptom profile of the burnout subtypes graphically, both in z-scores and in mean scores. Each burnout subtype was described based on its mean score profile and based on which symptoms were most pronounced within the subtype. The three subtypes were labeled as follows: *burned-out* (subtype 3), *exhausted/cynical* (subtype 2), and *exhausted* (subtype 1). The *burned-out* subtype ($n = 30$) had the most severe burnout symptomatology. It displayed high exhaustion, high cynicism, and low professional efficacy. The *exhausted/cynical* subtype ($n = 39$) had severe burnout symptoms as well. It was characterized by high exhaustion, elevated levels of cynicism, but simultaneously high professional efficacy. Finally, the *exhausted* subtype ($n = 34$) showed the least severe burnout symptoms. It displayed elevated levels of exhaustion, the lowest scores on cynicism, and high professional efficacy.

Based on the z-score profile, the three subtypes could have been labeled as *burned-out* (subtype 3), *exhausted* (subtype 2), and *healthy* (subtype 1). However, we decided to label the subtypes based on the means score profile because of the general higher symptom severity in clinical burnout patients. Based on the z-score profile, particularly the label *healthy* for subtype 1 and the label *exhausted* for subtype 2 would have been misleading because both subtypes had elevated levels of exhaustion and subtype 2 had additionally elevated levels of cynicism. Hence, subtype 1 did not seem to be healthy and subtype 2 did not seem to be solely exhausted.

Level of depression in the burnout subtypes

Depression score was highest in the *burned-out* subtype, followed by the *exhausted/cynical* subtype, and the *exhausted* subtype (see Table 2; Bonferroni-corrected post-hoc tests: *burned-out* subtype vs. *exhausted/cynical* subtype, $p = 0.02$; *burned-out* subtype vs. *exhausted* subtype, $p < 0.01$; *exhausted/cynical* subtype vs. *exhausted* subtype, $p = 0.05$). Moreover, there were significant differences between the subtypes with regard to how many

Table 2 Differences between the burnout subtypes in burnout, depression, and recovery/resources-stress balance

			subtype 1		subtype 2		subtype 3				
	overall (*N* = 103)		exhausted (*N* = 34)		exhausted/ cynical (*N* = 39)		burned-out (*N* = 30)				
	M	*SD*	*M*	*SD*	*M*	*SD*	*M*	*SD*	*F*(2,100)	η_p^2	contrasts
MBI											
exhaustion	5.06	0.84	4.13	0.62	5.60	0.37	5.43	0.54	84.51**	0.63	3,2 > 1
cynicism	4.13	1.01	3.28	0.71	4.17	0.85	5.03	0.63	43.84**	0.47	3 > 2 > 1
professional efficacy	4.56	0.80	4.83	0.55	5.05	0.43	3.60	0.54	77.73**	0.61	1,2 > 3
BDI											
depression	21.46	9.65	16.41	8.68	21.31	8.74	27.39	8.69	12.70**	0.20	3 > 2 > 1
RESTQ-Work											
social-emotional stress	2.58	1.12	1.88	0.79	2.69	1.18	3.22	0.95	14.85**	0.23	3,2 > 1
performance (−related) stress	3.08	1.10	2.32	0.92	3.32	0.94	3.63	1.03	16.96**	0.25	3,2 > 1
loss of meaning/burnout	3.04	1.20	2.04	0.83	3.47	0.94	3.62	1.18	26.63**	0.35	3,2 > 1
overall recovery	2.12	0.81	2.65	0.77	1.98	0.74	1.70	0.61	15.27**	0.23	1 > 2,3
leisure/breaks	2.95	1.21	3.56	1.13	2.72	1.12	2.56	1.18	7.39**	0.13	1 > 2,3
psychosocial resources	2.88	1.28	3.34	0.98	2.75	1.37	2.51	1.34	3.84*	0.07	1 > 3
work-related resources	2.70	0.90	3.02	0.86	2.73	0.86	2.31	0.85	5.39**	0.10	1 > 3

$^*p < 0.05$; $^{**}p < 0.01$

patients scored above the BDI cut-off score ≥ 18 for clinical depression (*burned-out* subtype: 27 patients (90%); *exhausted/cynical* subtype: 27 patients (69%); *exhausted* subtype: 14 patients (41%); χ^2 (2, $N = 103$) = 17.22, $p < 0.01$). Concerning previous depression diagnosis, no significant difference was observed between the subtypes, χ^2 (2, $N = 103$) = 0.77, $p = 0.68$, (see Table 3).

Level of recovery/resources-stress balance in the burnout subtypes

The MANOVA showed significant differences in recovery/resources-stress balance between the three subtypes (using Pillai's trace, $V = 0.48$, $F(14, 190) = 4.33$, $p < 0.01$, $\eta_p^2 = 0.24$). Subsequent ANOVAs indicated significant differences in all seven RESTQ-Work subscales (see Table 2). Post-hoc analyses further revealed that both the *burned-out* and the *exhausted/cynical* subtype experienced significantly more social-emotional stress ($p < 0.01$), performance(−related) stress ($p < 0.01$), and loss of meaning/burnout ($p < 0.01$) as well as significantly less overall recovery ($p < 0.01$) and less leisure/breaks during work ($p < 0.01$) than the *exhausted* subtype. Furthermore, the *burned-out* subtype had significantly less psychosocial resources ($p = 0.02$) and less work-related

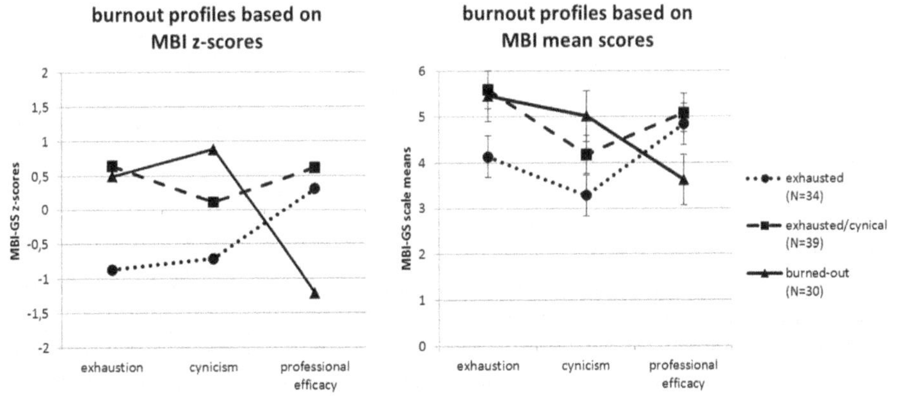

Fig. 1 Burnout profiles based on MBI z-scores and based on MBI mean scores. [a] subtype 1 = *exhausted*; subtype 2 = *exhausted/cynical*; subtype 3 = *burned-out*. [b] post-hoc tests MBI-GS: exhaustion (*burned-out subtype* vs. *exhausted subtype*, $p < 0.01$; *exhausted/cynical* subtype vs. *exhausted* subtype, $p < 0.01$; *burned-out* subtype vs. *exhausted/cynical* subtype, $p = 0.30$); cynicism (*burned-out subtype* vs. *exhausted subtype*, $p < 0.01$; *exhausted/cynical* subtype vs. *exhausted* subtype, $p < 0.01$; *burned-out* subtype vs. *exhausted/cynical*, $p < 0.01$); professional efficacy (*burned-out subtype* vs. *exhausted subtype*, $p < 0.01$; *exhausted/cynical* subtype vs. *exhausted* subtype, $p = 0.20$; *burned-out* subtype vs. *exhausted/cynical*, $p < 0.01$).

Table 3 Sociodemographic characteristics of the burnout subtypes

		overall ($N = 103$)	subtype 1 exhausted ($N = 34$)	subtype 2 exhausted/ cynical ($N = 39$)	subtype 3 burned-out ($N = 30$)
gender	female	66 (64%)	21 (32%)	24 (36%)	21 (32%)
	male	37 (36%)	13 (35%)	15 (41%)	09 (24%)
education	high	32 (31%)	08 (25%)	12 (38%)	12 (38%)
	lower	71 (69%)	26 (37%)	27 (38%)	18 (25%)
BDI ≥ 18	yes	68 (66%)	14 (21%)	27 (40%)	27 (40%)
	no	35 (34%)	20 (57%)	12 (34%)	03 (9%)
depression diagnosis in the past	yes	70 (68%)	25 (36%)	25 (36%)	20 (29%)
	no	33 (32%)	09 (27%)	14 (42%)	10 (30%)
rehabilitation clinic[a]	A	51 (49%)	15 (29%)	21 (41%)	15 (29%)
	B	52 (51%)	19 (37%)	18 (35%)	15 (29%)
age	*M (SD)*	44.82 (8.08)	44.96 (9.72)	45.76 (6.26)	43.43 (8.22)
days sick leave	*M (SD)*	106.20 (113.46)	73.65 (94.66)	115.56 (104.04)	130.93 (137.13)

[a]data from two different rehabilitation clinics

resources ($p < 0.01$) than the *exhausted* subtype, while the *burned-out* and the *exhausted/cynical* subtype did not differ from each other in any of the RESTQ-Work subscales.

Sociodemographic characteristics of the burnout subtypes

Sociodemographic data for the burnout subtypes are presented in Table 3. There were no significant differences between the three subtypes with regard to sociodemographic characteristics. Men and women were equally distributed across the three clusters, χ^2 (2, $N = 103$) = 0.65, $p = 0.72$, and the subtypes did not differ in age, $F(2, 100) = 0.71$, $p = 0.50$, and education, χ^2 (2, $N = 103$) = 2.02, $p = 0.36$, respectively. The rehabilitation clinic was not significantly associated with the burnout subtype, χ^2 (2, $N = 103$) = 0.69, $p = 0.71$, and there was no significant difference between the subtypes in how many days the patients had already been on sick leave prior to study admission, $F(2, 100) = 2.30$, $p = 0.10$.

Discussion

Burnout subtypes in clinical burnout patients

The present study explored different burnout subtypes based on MBI profiles in clinical burnout patients enrolled in an employee rehabilitation program in a psychosomatic clinic. As increasing evidence points to intra-individual patterns of burnout symptoms in non-clinical samples such as students, athletes, healthy and burned-out employees [13, 15], this study addressed the specific research question of whether different burnout subtypes can also be identified in clinically diagnosed burnout patients and whether these burnout subtypes differ in depression, recovery/resources-stress balance, and sociodemographic characteristics. Previously, van Dam [54] investigated subgroups in clinically diagnosed burnout patients by means of cluster analysis using fatigue (CIS), depression (SCL-90-D), and anxiety (SCL-90-A) as clustering variables and found two clusters that differed from one another in terms of symptom-severity on the three aforementioned measures. To date, only Hätinen et al. [30] have explored MBI burnout profiles in a mixed sample of working-aged rehabilitation clients, in which four different symptom patterns occurred: the *burned-out* profile, the *exhausted/cynical* profile, the *reduced professional efficacy* profile, and the *healthy* profile. However, some of these profiles might have occurred because Hätinen et al. [30] explored a heterogeneous patient sample suffering from various physical, psychological, and social limitations, symptoms, and disabilities. A study analyzing burnout subtypes in a group of clinically diagnosed burnout patients with the three MBI-GS dimensions (exhaustion, cynicism, professional efficacy) as clustering variables, is to the very best of our knowledge not available yet. Cluster analysis with the three MBI-GS subscales as clustering variables revealed three distinct burnout subtypes in the present study.

In line with Hätinen et al. [30], we found two subtypes with severe burnout symptoms, namely the *burned-out* and the *exhausted/cynical* subtype, whereas the *reduced professional efficacy* subtype and the healthy burnout profile could not be replicated in the present study. Instead, we identified an *exhausted* subtype representing patients with milder symptomatology. Sociodemographic characteristics were not systematically associated with the subtypes in the present study, but all groups differed in depression severity. The *burned-out* subtype showed overall the highest level of depression, while the *exhausted* subtype was the least depressed. Moreover, the *burned-out* and the *exhausted/cynical* subtype had a worse recovery/resources-stress balance compared to the *exhausted* subtype, but they did not differ from each in perceived stress, recovery, and resources. Since neither the depression scale, nor the RESTQ-Work subscales were used for clustering, these differences further support the validity of the cluster solution. Taken together our findings suggest that different burnout subtypes can be identified in clinical patients who were diagnosed with burnout by a professional team of psychiatrists and clinical psychologists working in a specialized psychosomatic clinic.

In line with past research [30, 54], our study indicates that the three subtypes represent patients at different stages in the burnout cycle. The subtypes correspond well with the process model of burnout [18], according to which burnout starts with exhaustion due to prolonged periods of stress, followed by cynicism as an attempt to cope with the intense emotional strain, before finally reduced professional efficacy occurs because a negative attitude towards one's job precludes achieving work goals. Yet, it cannot be ruled out that the *burned-out* and the *exhausted/cynical* subtype might be truly different burnout subtypes, each characterizing the final stage in the burnout cycle. Several researchers have shown that professional efficacy develops rather independently of the other two burnout symptoms [21, 60], and both burnout profiles seem to be relatively stable over time [23]. Moreover, an alternative longitudinal trajectory of the burnout symptoms starting with reduced professional efficacy, followed by cynicism, and ending in emotional exhaustion, has been found as well [21]. The *reduced professional efficacy* subtype is a common subtype in the general working population [15], and two different pathways into burnout—one starting with exhaustion, the other one starting with reduced professional efficacy—have been addressed [13, 15, 24].

Truly different burnout subtypes might also explain why Hätinen et al. [30] found the *reduced professional efficacy* subtype, while the present study found the *exhausted* subtype representing patients with milder symptomatology, although the same methodology was applied in both studies, namely cluster analysis with the three MBI-GS subscales. Nevertheless, one has to keep in mind that our study sample markedly differed from the rehabilitation clients analyzed in the study by Hätinen et al. [30]. The present study solely included clinical burnout patients diagnosed with the ICD-10 criteria of work-related neurasthenia, which has been proposed as the psychiatric equivalent of clinical burnout [38]. In addition, all patients scored high on exhaustion (≥ 2.20) and either high on cynicism (≥ 2.00) or low on professional efficacy (≤ 3.67) in the MBI-GS [54, 65]. In contrast, Hätinen et al. [30] explored a mixed patient sample from an employee rehabilitation clinic suffering from various physical, psychological, and social limitations, symptoms, and disabilities. Patients with physical impairments displayed particularly the *healthy* burnout profile in their study, but physical impairments can lead to the experience of reduced professional efficacy as well, when one is no longer able to conduct one's job properly.

Regarding the possible antecedents of burnout, we revealed that the three burnout subtypes in our study differed in their recovery/resources-stress balance. The two subtypes with severe burnout symptoms, namely the *burned-out* subtype and the *exhausted/cynical* subtype, experienced more social-emotional stress, performance(-related) stress, and loss of meaning in their job than the *exhausted* subtype. Both subtypes reported also the lowest overall recovery, leisure, and breaks during work. Furthermore, the *burned-out* subtype tended to have less psychosocial and work-related resources than the *exhausted* subtype. According to the JD-R model [57] and the recovery/resources-stress balance model [62–64], burnout develops due to high job demands and simultaneously low resources and recovery. Both would be necessary to buffer the negative effects of high job demands on stress reactions [58]. Our findings are in line with these assumptions, which have also received support in burnout subtypes in the working population [13, 23, 27] and in longitudinal studies in clinical rehabilitation clients [56]. Yet, the *burned-out* and the *exhausted/cynical* subtype did not differ in recovery/resources-stress balance from each other in the present study. This is in line with some previous studies [23, 30] but not with others [13] reporting that the *burned-out* subtype had even less organizational resources than the *exhausted/cynical* subtype. To clarify, whether the *exhausted/cynical* subtype and the *burned-out* subtype represent people at different developmental stages in the burnout cycle or truly different burnout subtypes, future studies should explore longitudinally which characteristics differentiate between these two subtypes.

Burnout-depression overlap

During the last years, an intense discussion has been going on whether burnout can be seen as a distinct construct or rather a new label of an already known state, and much of this debate has focused around the burnout-depression overlap [9–12, 31–54]. Until now, a vast majority of studies confirms that burnout and depression are not independent and especially in severe burnout, both disorders strongly overlap [11, 32, 45, 54]. This was also demonstrated in our own data. In the present study, 90% of the patients in the *burned-out* subtype scored above the BDI cut-off score ≥ 18 for clinical depression [68], whereas only 69% / 41% of the patients reached this threshold in the *exhausted/cynical* subtype and the *exhausted* subtype, respectively. Similarly, Ahola et al. [45] showed that 90% of people with severe burnout reported a physical or mental disease; more specifically, pain and depression. In contrast, Hätinen et al. [30] could not replicate these findings; the authors found that several burnout subtypes in rehabilitation clients were equally depressed. Yet, in their study, a mixed sample of rehabilitation clients suffering from various physiological, psychological, and social limitations, symptoms, and disorders was explored, while other studies [23, 54] using a person-oriented approach to explore burnout subtypes found that subtypes with severe burnout symptoms had higher depression scores than subtypes with milder burnout symptoms, which is in line with our study.

Interestingly, our results differed also from previous findings with regard to the burnout-depression overlap when the correlations between the three MBI-GS subscales and the BDI score were considered [9, 10, 31, 32]. For example, Bianchi et al. [10] found a high correlation between the MBI sum score and the BDI ($r = 0.68$) in the working population. Importantly, in their study, the correlation between emotional exhaustion and depression was much stronger ($r = 0.74$) than the correlations between the three dimensions of the MBI. Similar to the study of van Dam [54], the present study could not replicate such a strong correlation between exhaustion and depression ($r = 0.30$) in clinical burnout patients. For more than half a century [73], researchers have debated about the utility of using non-clinical samples such as students as analogues for patients with clinical diagnosis. Generalizing findings from non-clinical burnout samples to clinical burnout patients might therefore be problematic. However, another explanation for the lower correlation between exhaustion and depression in the present study and in the study of van Dam [54] might be that the range of exhaustion and depression scores is limited in clinical burnout patients, which might have flattened the correlation between both constructs. Furthermore, some of the heterogeneity in study results concerning the burnout-depression overlap may result from using different measures of burnout and depression [11, 12, 31, 32, 37, 40, 41, 47]. Hence, the high correlations between burnout and depression, especially with the burnout dimension emotional exhaustion in some studies, might partly reflect a large level of concept redundancy between specific burnout and depression measures (for a discussion on this topic, please see Maslach & Leiter [37]).

Especially longitudinal studies provide the opportunity to study the complex relationship between burnout and depression. Longitudinal studies focusing on the question whether burnout predicted depression or vice versa, revealed inconsistent results. Some authors [42–44] found a reciprocal relation between burnout and depression, with each predicting subsequent developments in the other, while other authors [46–50] reported a predictive relation from burnout to depression. Furthermore, three longitudinal studies showed a unidirectional relationship from depression to burnout [51–53] and one study failed to find any predictive relation [36]. Bianchi, Schonfeld and Laurent [31] focused on how burnout and depressive symptoms clustered at baseline and follow-up by applying a person-oriented approach. In this study, burnout was measured with a global burnout index (the combination of the MBI subscales emotional exhaustion and cynicism); depression was assessed with the Patient Health Questionnaire (PHQ-9). A similar person-oriented approach by using cluster analysis to study the relationship between burnout and depressive symptoms at baseline and over 7 years in dentists was applied by Ahola et al. [9]. Again, burnout was measured with a global index (more specifically, a weighted sum score of the MBI dimensions was calculated, so that emotional exhaustion, depersonalization, and diminished personal accomplishment had different weights in the syndrome); depressive symptoms were assessed using the short form of the Beck Depression Inventory (BDI-SF). In both studies, similar findings were obtained as both studies could show that the participants formed three clusters with low, intermediate, or high levels of burnout and depressive symptoms at baseline. Additionally, in both studies long-term development occurred in tandem, either remaining stable or changing in synchrony. Therefore, both studies support the hypothesis that burnout and depression overlap or may even be the same disorder.

Up to now, longitudinal studies in clinical burnout patients are still sparse. Oosterholt et al. [55] examined the course of cognitive performance and cortisol level in clinical burnout patients and non-clinical burnout individuals over a time period of 1.5 years. After 1.5 years, clinical burnout patients showed improvement of burnout symptoms and general physical and psychological complaints, but the patients still reported subjective cognitive impairments that were also evident in a cognitive test. In contrast, the non-clinical burnout group expressed the same elevated level of burnout symptoms, general physical and psychological complaints, and cognitive problems, but did not show objective cognitive deficits after 1.5 years.

Hätinen et al. [30] used a person-oriented approach to explore MBI burnout profiles and the changes in burnout 4 months after a rehabilitation intervention in a mixed sample of working-aged rehabilitation clients. In this study, four different burnout profiles (*burned-out* profile, *exhausted/cynical* profile, *reduced professional efficacy* profile, and *healthy* profile) were found and the burnout changes observed 4-month after the intervention depended on the burnout profile membership. While exhaustion showed a decreasing trend in the *burned-out* and *exhausted/cynical* profile, the decreasing trend in cynicism was only evident in the *burned-out* profile compared to the other profiles. Furthermore, reduced professional efficacy showed an increasing trend in the *exhausted/cynical* profile, whereas in the *reduced professional efficacy* profile the trend was decreasing. In a subsequent study, Hätinen et al. [56] investigated burnout trajectories in a one-year rehabilitation program with a six-month follow-up and found inter-individual changes in how clients reacted to the interventions and how these reactions were manifested in burnout symptoms during follow-up. The authors found three burnout patterns: two patterns with high levels of burnout and one pattern with low levels of burnout. However, only in one group with high burnout levels, exhaustion and cynicism were decreased at follow-up. This group was labeled as "high burnout-benefited trajectory" by the authors. For the "low burnout trajectory" and the "high burnout-benefited trajectory", positive changes were detected in job-related antecedents (e.g., time pressure at work, job control, workplace climate) and consequences (e.g. depressive symptoms, job satisfaction). Thus, preliminary results suggest that in clinical burnout samples distinct symptom profiles exist and that not all burnout profiles benefit equally from rehabilitation in terms of reduction in burnout symptoms, job-related antecedents, and consequences [30, 56].

Practical implications

Burnout prevention/intervention programs in non-clinical burnout employees are either person-directed (individual level interventions), organization-directed or a combination of both [74]. Person-directed interventions usually consist of different kinds of relaxation exercises and/or cognitive behavioral techniques to enhance social support, job competence, and personal coping skills. Organization-directed interventions target on poor workplace climate, dissatisfaction with supervision, and changes in work procedures such as task restructuring. Furthermore, organization-directed interventions aim at decreasing job demand, increasing job control and expanding the level of participation in decision-making. Several reviews in non-clinical populations [74–77] concluded that burnout intervention programs had a beneficial effect on burnout outcome measures, especially when person-directed and organization-directed interventions were combined. Nonetheless, a recent meta-analysis [78] on the effectiveness of controlled interventions to reduce burnout indicated statistically significant effects of interventions only on general burnout scales ($d = 0.224$) and exhaustion ($d = 0.172$); no effect was observed on cynicism or professional inefficacy. Moreover, the reported effect sizes were overall rather small. Yet, most studies included in this meta-analysis investigated non-clinical burnout employees who do not necessarily possess a high level of burnout, since the interventions were aimed at decreasing the level of stress.

Studies assessing the efficacy of interventions in burnout patients who are treated in clinical settings are rare [30, 55, 56]. Preliminary results suggest that in clinical burnout samples distinct symptom profiles exist and that not all burnout profiles benefit equally from rehabilitation in terms of reduction in burnout symptoms, job-related antecedents, and consequences [30, 56]. For the burnout subtypes with severe symptomatology such as the *exhausted/cynical* and the *burned-out* subtype, the first step in rehabilitation should lie on the alleviation of the burnout and depression symptoms (e.g., psychotherapy and if indicated antidepressants). Additionally, rehabilitation should focus on organization-directed intervention activities in these subtypes, since burnout patients with severe symptomatology reported worse interpersonal relations, poor workplace climate, and dissatisfaction with supervision in previous studies [30]. Similarly, in our own study, the *burned-out* and the *exhausted/cynical* subtype experienced high social-emotional stress, performance-related stress and limited (work-related) resources. There is still an ongoing debate about the efficacy of antidepressants and psychotherapies in the treatment of subclinical depression, which is defined as a level of clinically relevant depressive symptoms in the absence of a major depressive disorder [79, 80]. Therefore, the *exhausted* subtype might profit from a person-directed approach focusing on factors contributing to exhaustion and recovery (e.g., interventions targeting workload, relaxation, and work-life balance [27]. In sum, identifying different subtypes of clinical burnout patients and analyzing the relationship of these subtypes to depression will enable psychiatrists and clinical psychologists to focus their intervention activities more effectively.

Study limitations

Several limitations of the current study need to be addressed. Similar to previous studies [54, 65], in the current paper the term clinical burnout is used to distinguish our study population of clinically diagnosed patients treated in a specialized psychosomatic clinic from non-clinical burnout groups who report symptoms of a burnout but are neither diagnosed by a psychiatrist or clinical psychologist as such and who are all still working. To date, there are no consensual diagnostic criteria for the burnout syndrome and the disorder is not yet included in clinical classification systems such as

DSM-5 or ICD-10 [2, 3]. Therefore, in the current study, the burnout diagnosis was based on the ICD-10 criteria of work-related neurasthenia, which has been proposed as the psychiatric equivalent of clinical burnout [38]. Additionally, we included only patients who scored ≥2.20 on exhaustion and either ≥2.00 on cynicism or ≤3.67 on professional efficacy in the MBI-GS. Hence, the findings of our study might not be generalizable to clinical burnout patients who are diagnosed differently. An extensive discussion about the problem of simplification burnout to ICD-10/DSM-5 codes such as neurasthenia, somatic symptom disorder or exhaustion, can be found in a current review by Maslach and Leiter [37].

Furthermore, the patients in the present study were on average three and a half months on sick leave, and hence, a recall bias may have occurred; especially in patients who had been longer on sick leave. However, the burnout subtypes did not differ in how many days the patients had been on sick leave; thus, the distortion bias was at least equally distributed between the subtypes. Additionally, data were collected during the first week of the rehabilitation program. Therefore, it cannot be ruled out that the burnout profiles we found occurred because some patients already started benefiting from the positive effects of the rehabilitation program before they filled in the questionnaires. A further limitation of the present study is that the patients were not screened for comorbid psychiatric disorders using the Structured Clinical Interview for Axis I DSM-IV Disorders (SCID-I) [69] or the Mini-International Neuropsychiatric Interview (MINI) [81]. Therefore, we cannot ensure that comorbid disorder are equally divided over the burnout types. Finally, the analyses were based on cross-sectional report questionnaires. Hence, we were not able to investigate whether the *exhausted/cynical* and the *burned-out* subtype represent people at different developmental stages in the burnout cycle or truly different burnout subtypes. Due to the rather small sample size and different interventions in the two rehabilitation clinics, we were also not able to investigate if the three burnout subtypes responded differently to therapy.

Conclusions

In recent years, different burnout subtypes or profiles, based on cluster/profile analysis with the three MBI subscales, have been proposed by several research groups [13, 15]. However, until now, intra-individual patterns of burnout symptoms have primarily been investigated in non-clinical samples such as students, athletes, healthy, and burned-out employees. Therefore, the current study aimed to investigate whether different burnout subtypes can also be identified in a more homogeneous group of clinically diagnosed burnout patients enrolled in an employee rehabilitation program in a psychosomatic clinic. Our results provide evidence that in clinical burnout patients three different burnout subtypes can be revealed: the *exhausted* subtype, the *exhausted/cynical* subtype, and the *burned-out* subtype, which might represent patients at different developmental stages in the burnout cycle. Furthermore, the *exhausted* subtype displayed the lowest depression level and the best recovery/resources-stress balance, while the *burned-out* subtype exhibited the most severe depression symptoms and a worse recovery/resources-stress balance than the *exhausted* subtype. Clearly, the current findings need to be replicated in future studies involving larger, ideally longitudinal data sets to investigate the efficacy of rehabilitation interventions in different burnout subtypes and to track the stability and change patterns between the burnout subtypes over time.

Abbreviations

ANOVA: Analysis of variance; BDI: Beck depression inventory; BDI-SF: Beck depression inventory – short form; CIS: Checklist individual strength; DSM-5: Diagnostic and statistical manual of mental disorders; ICD-10: International statistical classification of diseases and related health problems; JD-R: Job demands-resources; MANOVA: Multivariate analysis of variance; MBI: Maslach burnout inventory; MBI-GS: Maslach burnout inventory – general survey; MINI: Mini-international neuropsychiatric interview; PHQ-9: Patient health questionnaire; RESTQ-Work: Recovery-stress-questionnaire for work; SCID-I: Structured clinical interview for Axis I DSM-IV disorders; SCL-90-A: Symptom checklist – anxiety subscale; SCL-90-D: Symptom checklist – depression subscale

Acknowledgements

We would like to thank two rehabilitation clinics in Austria for support in this research by permitting access to their burnout patients.

Funding

This work was supported by the Austrian Research Promotion Agency (Grant No. 827511/BULT).

Authors' contributions

KB, EW, MC and DB contributed in the conceptualization of the study. DB participated in collecting the data. KB conducted the statistical analyses, supported by MP and IP. KB drafted the manuscript, and EW, PJ, IP and AF contributed to the interpretation of the data. All authors revised the manuscript and gave final approval of the version to be published.

Consent for publication

Not applicable

Competing interests

The authors declare that they have no competing interests.

Author details

[1]Department of Psychology, University of Graz, Universitätsplatz 2/DG, 8010 Graz, Austria. [2]Department of Psychology, University of Innsbruck, Bruno-Sander-Haus Innrain 52f, 6020 Innsbruck, Austria.

References

1. Schaufeli W. Past performance and future perspectives of burnout research. SA J Ind Psychol. 2003;29:1 15.

2. American Psychiatric Association. Diagnostic and statistical manual of mental disorders. 5th ed. Arlington, VA: American Psychiatric Publishing; 2013.
3. World Health Organization. The ICD-10 classification of mental and Behavioural disorders: diagnostic criteria for research. Geneva: World Health Organization; 1993.
4. Demerouti E, Bakker AB. The Oldenburg burnout inventory: a good alternative to measure burnout and engagement. In: Halbesleben JRB, editor. Handbook of stress and burnout in health care. Hauppauge, NY: Nova Science Publishers; 2008. p. 65–78.
5. Kristensen TS, Borritz M, Villadsen E, Christensen KB. The Copenhagen burnout inventory: a new tool for the assessment of burnout. Work Stress. 2005;19:192–207.
6. Maslach C, Schaufeli WB, Leiter MP. Job burnout. Annu Rev Psychol. 2001;52:397–422.
7. Shirom A, Melamed S. A comparison of the construct validity of two burnout measures in two groups of professionals. Int J Stress Manag. 2006; 13:176–200.
8. Huibers MJ, Beurskens AJ, Prins JB, Kant IJ, Bazelmans E, van Schayck CP, Knottnerus JA, Bleijenberg G. Fatigue, burnout, and chronic fatigue syndrome among employees on sick leave: do attributions make the difference? Occup Environ Med. 2003;60:26–31.
9. Ahola K, Hakanen J, Perhoniemi R, Mutanen P. Relationship between burnout and depressive symptoms: a study using the person-centred approach. Burnout Res. 2014;1:29–37.
10. Bianchi R, Boffy C, Hingray C, Truchot D, Laurent E. Comparative symptomatology of burnout and depression. J Health Psychol. 2013;18:782–7.
11. Bianchi R, Schonfeld IS, Laurent E. Burnout-depression overlap: a review. Clin Psychol Rev. 2015;36:28–41.
12. Bianchi R, Schonfeld IS, Laurent E. Is burnout a depressive disorder? A reexamination with special focus on atypical depression. Int J Stress Manag. 2014;21:307–24.
13. Leiter MP, Maslach C. Latent burnout profiles: a new approach to understanding the burnout experience. Burnout Res. 2016;3:89–100.
14. Maslach C, Leiter M. Early predictors of job burnout and engagement. J Appl Psychol. 2008;93:498–512.
15. Mäkikangas A, Kinnunen U. The person-oriented approach to burnout: a systematic review. Burnout Res. 2016;3:11–23.
16. Golembiewski RT, Munzenrider RF, Stevenson JG. Phases of burnout: developments in concepts and applications. New York: Praeger; 1986.
17. Friedman IA. Multiple pathways to burnout: cognitive and emotional scenarios in teacher burnout. Anxiety Stress Coping. 1996;9:245–59.
18. Leiter MP, Maslach C. The impact of interpersonal environment of burnout and organizational commitment. J Organ Behav. 1988;9:297–308.
19. Taris TW, Le Blanc PM, Schaufeli WB, Schreurs PJ. Are there causal relationships between the dimensions of the Maslach burnout inventory? A review and two longitudinal studies. Work Stress. 2005;19:238–55.
20. Te Brake H, Smits N, Wicherts JM, Gorter RC, Hoogstraten J. Burnout development among dentists: a longitudinal study. Eur J Oral Sci. 2008;116:545–51.
21. van Dierendonck R, Schaufeli WB, Buunk BP. Toward a process model of burnout: results from a secondary analysis. Eur J Work Organ Psy. 2001;10:41–52.
22. Bergman LR, Trost K. The person-oriented versus the variable-oriented approach: are they complementary, opposites, or exploring different worlds? Merrill Palmer Q. 2006;52:601–32.
23. Boersma K, Lindblom K. Stability and change in burnout profiles over time: a prospective study in the working population. Work Stress. 2009;23:264–83.
24. Demerouti E, Verbeke WJ, Bakker AB. Exploring the relationship between a multidimensional and multifaceted burnout concept and self-rated performance. J Manage. 2005;31:186–209.
25. Innanen H, Tolvanen A, Salmela-Aro K. Burnout, work engagement and workaholism among highly educated employees: profiles, antecedents and outcomes. Burnout Res. 2014;1:38–49.
26. Lee SM, Cho SH, Kissinger D, Ogle NT. A typology of burnout in professional counselors. J Couns Dev. 2010;88:131–8.
27. Timms C, Brough P, Graham D. Burnt-out but engaged: the co-existence of psychological burnout and engagement. J Educ Adm. 2012;50:327–45.
28. Maslach C, Jackson SE, Leiter M. Maslach burnout inventory. Manual. 3rd ed. Palo Alto, CA: Consulting Psychologists Press; 1996.
29. Karasek R, Theorell T. Healthy work: stress, productivity and the reconstruction of working life. New York: Basic Books; 1990.
30. Hätinen M, Kinnunen U, Pekkonen M, Aro A. Burnout patterns in rehabilitation: short-term changes in job conditions, personal resources, and health. J Occup Health Psychol. 2004;9:220–37.
31. Bianchi R, Schonfeld IS, Laurent E. Is burnout separable from depression in cluster analysis? A longitudinal study. Soc Psychiatry Psychiatr Epidemiol. 2015;50:1005–11.
32. Schonfeld IS, Bianchi R. Burnout and depression: two entities or one? J Clin Psychol. 2016;72:22–37.
33. Bianchi R, Schonfeld IS, Laurent E. Physician burnout is better conceptualised as depression. Lancet. 2017;389:1397–8.
34. Bianchi R, Schonfeld IS, Laurent E. Burnout or depression: both individual and social issue. Lancet. 2017;390:230.
35. Bianchi R, Schonfeld IS, Vandel P, Laurent E. On the depressive nature of the "burnout syndrome": a clarification. Eur Psychiatry. 2017;41:109–10.
36. Bianchi R, Schonfeld IS, Laurent E. Burnout does not help predict depression among French schoolteachers. Scand J Work Environ Health. 2015b;41:565–8. https://doi.org/10.5271/sjweh.3522.
37. Maslach C, Leiter MP. Understanding the burnout experience: recent research and its implications for psychiatry. World Psychiatry. 2016;15:103–11.
38. Schaufeli WB, Bakker AB, Hoogduin K, Schaap C, Kladler A. On the clinical validity of the Maslach burnout inventory and the burnout measure. Psychol Health. 2001;16:565–82.
39. Schaufeli WB, Enzmann D. The burnout companion to study and practice: a critical analysis. London: Taylor and Francis; 1998.
40. Leiter MP, Durup J. The discriminant validity of burnout and depression: a confirmatory factor analytic study. Anxiety Stress Coping. 1994;7:357–73.
41. Raedeke TD, Arce C, De Francisco C, Seoane G, Ferraces MJ. The construct validity of the Spanish version of the ABQ using a multi-trait/multi-method approach. Anales de Psi-cologia. 2012;29:693–700.
42. Ahola K, Hakanen J. Job strain, burnout, and depressive symptoms: a prospective study among dentists. J Affect Disord. 2007;104:103–10.
43. McKnight JD, Glass DC. Perceptions of control, burnout, and depressive symptomatology: a replication and extension. J Consult Clin Psychol. 1995;63:490–4.
44. Toker S, Biron M. Job burnout and depression: unraveling their temporal relationship and considering the role of physical activity. J Appl Psychol. 2012;97:699–710.
45. Ahola K, Honkonen T, Isometsä E, Kalimo R, Nykyri E, Aromaa A, Lönnqvist J. The relationship between job-related burnout and depressive disorders—results from the Finnish health 2000 study. J Affect Disord. 2005;88:55–62.
46. Armon G, Melamed S, Toker S, Berliner S, Shapira I. Joint effect of chronic medical illness and burnout on depressive symptoms among employed adults. Health Psychol. 2014;33:264–72.
47. Hakanen JJ, Schaufeli WB. Do burnout and work engagement predict depressive symptoms and life satisfaction? A three-wave seven-year prospective study. J Affect Disord. 2012;141:415–24.
48. Hakanen JJ, Schaufeli WB, Ahola K. The job demands–resources model: a three-year cross-lagged study of burnout, depression, commitment, and work engagement. Work Stress. 2008;22:224–41.
49. Salmela-Aro K, Savolainen H, Holopainen L. Depressive symptoms and school burnout during adolescence: evidence from two cross-lagged longitudinal studies. J Youth Adolesc. 2009;38:1316–27.
50. Shin H, Noh H, Jang Y, Park YM, Lee SM. A longitudinal examination of the relationship between teacher burnout and depression. J Employ Couns. 2013;50:124–37.
51. Armon G, Shirom A, Melamed S. The big five personality factors as predictors of changes across time in burnout and its facets. J Pers. 2012;80:403–27.
52. Campbell J, Prochazka AV, Yamashita T, Gopal R. Predictors of persistent burnout in internal medicine residents: a prospective cohort study. Acad Med. 2010;85:1630–4.
53. Salmela-Aro K, Aunola K, Nurmi JE. Trajectories of depressive symptoms during emerging adulthood: antecedents and consequences. Eur J Dev Psychol. 2008;5:439–65.
54. van Dam A. Subgroup analysis in burnout: relations between fatigue, anxiety, and depression. Front Psychol. 2016; doi: https://doi.org/10.3389/fpsyg.2016.00090.
55. Oosterholt BG, Maes JH, van der Linden D, Verbraak MJ, Kompier MA. Getting better, but not well: a 1.5 year follow-up of cognitive performance and cortisol levels in clinical and non-clinical burnout. Biol Psychol. 2016;117:89–99.

56. Hätinen M, Kinnunen U, Mäkikangas A, Kalimo R, Tolvanen A, Pekkonen M. Burnout during a long-term rehabilitation: comparing low burnout, high burnout – benefited and high burnout – not benefited trajectories. Anxiety Stress Coping. 2009;22:341–60.
57. Demerouti E, Bakker AB, Nachreiner F, Schaufeli WB. The job demands-resources model of burnout. J Appl Psychol. 2001;86:499–512.
58. Jiménez P, Dunkl A. The buffering effect of workplace resources on the relationship between the areas of worklife and burnout. Front Psychol. 2017; doi:https://doi.org/10.3389/fpsyg.2017.00012.
59. Bakker AB, Demerouti E, Taris T, Schaufeli WB, Schreurs PJ. A multigroup analysis of the job demands-resources model in four home care organizations. Int J Stress Manag. 2003;10:16–38.
60. Lee RT, Ashforth BE. A meta-analytic examination of the correlates of the three dimensions of job burnout. J Appl Psychol. 1996;2:123–33.
61. Schaufeli WB, Bakker AB. Job demands, job resources, and their relationship with burnout and engagement: a multi-sample study. J Organ Behav. 2004;25:293–315.
62. Jiménez P, Dunkl A, Kallus KW. Recovery-stress questionnaire for work. In: Kallus KW, Kellmann M, editors. The recovery-stress questionnaire. User manual. Frankfurt/Main: Pearson; 2016. p. 158–87.
63. Kallus KW. Stress and recovery: an overview. In: Kallus KW, Kellmann M, editors. The recovery-stress questionnaire. User manual. Frankfurt/Main: Pearson; 2016. p. 27–48.
64. Kallus KW, Kellmann M. The recovery-stress questionnaire. User manual. Frankfurt/Main: Pearson; 2016.
65. Oosterholt BG, van der Linden D, Maes JH, Verbraak MJ, Kompier MA. Burned out cognition – cognitive functioning of burnout patients before and after a period with psychological treatment. Scand J Work Environ Health. 2012;38:358–69.
66. Büssing A, Glaser J. Managerial stress und burnout. A collaborative international study (CISMS). Die deutsche Untersuchung. [managerial stress and burnout. The German study]. Bericht nr. 44 aus dem Lehrstuhl für Psychologie. München: Technische Universität, Lehrstuhl für Psychologie; 1998.
67. Hautzinger M, Bailer M, Worall H, Keller F. Beck-Depressions-Inventar (BDI). Bearbeitung der deutschen Ausgabe. Testhandbuch. Bern, Göttingen, Toronto, Seattle: Huber; 1994.
68. Beck AT, Steer RA, Carbin MG. Psychometric properties of the Beck depression inventory: twenty-five years of evaluation. Clin Psychol Rev. 1988;8:77–100.
69. First MB, Spitzer RL, Gibbon M, Williams JB. User's guide for the structured clinical inter-view for DSM-IV interview for DSM-IV Axis I disorders. Washington, DC: Ameri-can Psychiatric Press; 1997.
70. Cohen J, Cohen P, West SG, Aiken LS. Applied multiple regression/correlation analysis for the behavioral sciences. 3rd ed. Mahwah, NJ: Earlbaum; 2003.
71. Everitt BS, Landau S, Leese M, Stahl D. Cluster analysis. 5th ed. Chichester, West Sussex: Wiley; 2011.
72. Cohen J. Statistical power analysis for the behavioral sciences. 2nd ed. Hillsdale, NJ: Lawrence Erlbaum; 1988.
73. Endler NS, Deisoff E, Rutherford A. Anxiety and depression: evidence for the differentiation of commonly cooccurring constructs. J Psychopathol Behav Assess. 1998;20:149–71.
74. Awa WL, Plaumann M, Walter U. Burnout prevention: a review of intervention programs. Patient Educ Couns. 2010;78:184–90.
75. Ruotsalainen J, Serra C, Marine A, Verbeek J. Systematic review of interventions for reducing occupational stress in health care workers. Scand J Work Environ Health. 2008;34:169–78.
76. Walter U, Krugmann CS, Plaumann M. Preventing burnout? A systematic review of effectiveness of individual and comorbid approaches [German]. Bundesgesundheitsblatt Gesundheitsforschung Gesundheitsschutz. 2012;55: 172–82. https://doi.org/10.1007/s00103-011-1412-0.
77. Westermann C, Kozak A, Harling M, Nienhaus A. Burnout intervention studies for inpatient elderly care nursing staff: systematic literature review. Int J Nurs Stud. 2014;51:63–71.
78. Maricutoiu LP, Sava FA, Butta O. The effectiveness of controlled interventions on employees' burnout: a meta-analysis. J Occup Organ Psychol. 2016;89:1–27.
79. Cameron IM, Reid IC, MacGillivray SA. Efficacy and tolerability of antidepressants for sub-threshold depression and for mild major depressive disorder. J Affect Disord. 2014;166:48–58.
80. Cuijpers P, Koole SL, van Dijke A, Roca M, Li J, Reynolds CF. Psychotherapy for subclinical depression: meta-analysis. Br J Psychiatry. 2014;205:268–74.
81. Sheehan DV, Lecrubier Y, Sheehan KH, Amorim P, Janavs J, Weiller E, Herqueta T, Baker R, Dunbar GC. The Mini-international neuropsychiatric interview (M.I.N.I.): the development and validation of a structured diagnostic psychiatric interview for DSM-IV and ICD-10. J Clin Psychiatry. 1998;59:22–33.

16

A research study review of effectiveness of treatments for psychiatric conditions common to end-stage cancer patients: needs assessment for future research and an impassioned plea

Ralph J. Johnson III

Abstract

Background: Rates of psychiatric conditions common to end-stage cancer patients (delirium, depression, anxiety disorders) remain unchanged. However, patient numbers have increased as the population has aged; indeed, cancer is a chief cause of mortality and morbidity in older populations. Effectiveness of psychiatric interventions and research to evaluate, inform, and improve interventions is critical to these patients' care. This article's intent is to report results from a recent review study on the effectiveness of interventions for psychiatric conditions common to end-stage cancer patients; the review study assessed the state of research regarding treatment effectiveness. Unlike previous review studies, this one included non-traditional/alternative therapies and spirituality interventions that have undergone scientific inquiry.

Methods: A five-phase systematic strategy and a theoretic grounded iterative methodology were used to identify studies for inclusion and to craft an integrated, synthesized, comprehensive, and reasonably current end-product.

Results: Psychiatric medication therapies undoubtedly are the most powerful treatments. Among them, the most effective (i.e., "best practices benchmarks") are: (1) for delirium, typical antipsychotics—though there is no difference between typical vs. atypical and other antipsychotics, except for different side-effect profiles, (2) for depression, if patient life expectancy is ≥4–6 weeks, then a selective serotonin reuptake inhibitor (SSRI), and if < 3 weeks, then psychostimulants or ketamine, and these generally are useful anytime in the cancer disease course, and (3) for anxiety disorders, bio-diazepams (BDZs) are most used and most effective. A universal consensus suggests that psychosocial (i.e., talk) therapy and spirituality interventions fortify the therapeutic alliance and psychiatric medication protocols. However, trial studies have had mixed results regarding effectiveness in reducing psychiatric symptoms, even for touted psychotherapies.

(Continued on next page)

Correspondence: rjjohnson@mdanderson.org; ralph.j.johnson16.mil@mail.mil
Departments of Myeloma, TMC Catholic Chaplain's Corps, and Houston Hospice, University of Texas—MD Anderson Cancer Center, Unit 439, 1515 Holcombe Blvd, Houston, Texas 77030, USA

(Continued from previous page)

Conclusions: This study's findings prompted a testable linear conceptual model of co-factors and their importance for providing effective psychiatric care for end-stage cancer patients. The complicated and tricky part is negotiating patients' diagnoses while articulating internal intricacies within and between each of the model's co-factors. There is a relative absence of scientifically derived information and need for more large-scale, diverse scientific inquiry. Thus, this article is an impassioned plea for accelerated study and better care for end-stage cancer patients' psychiatric conditions.

Keywords: Psychiatry, Psycho-oncology, End stage cancer care, Depression, Delirium, Anxiety, Adjustment disorder, Literature review, Research needs assessment

Background

Not surprisingly, psychiatric symptoms, disorders, and emotional distress are relatively common among cancer patients, in particular those with end-stage cancer ([1], also see [2]; see Fig. 1), which is the terminal phase of cancer—including hospice and the latter part of palliative care [1–29]).

The psychiatric symptoms and disorders in end-stage cancer patients have remained unchanged over time and include delirium at 20–65%, depression at 21%, and anxiety and adjustment disorder at 14% ([30–42], also see [4, 5, 7–9, 16, 19]). Note that this includes approximately 3% of end-stage cancer patients who also suffer from severe and persistent mental illnesses (e.g., schizophrenia, bi-polar disease, major depressive disorder) ([43], also see [4]). Though the rates have been consistent over time, the actual volume has increased due to the growing number of older adults in the general population and cancer within these populations being a chief cause of morbidity and mortality ([44, 45], also see [7]). Patients 65 years old and older are the fastest growing segment of the population and the incidence and prevalence of cancer and related psychiatric disorders among them is consequently expanding. [45] This is evidenced by the substantial and statistically significant increments in dispensing all classes of psychotropic medications in recent years among end-stage cancer patients. [46–49]

Psychiatric symptoms and disorders not only cause extreme suffering in their own right but can also exacerbate physical ailments and substantially degrade the quality of life, which end-stage cancer care aims to ameliorate ([50–52], also see [28]). In response to this growing need, psychiatric therapeutic interventions including psychopharmacology and psychosocial therapy alone or in combination have been used with end-stage cancer patients to treat commonly occurring psychiatric disorders (cf. [53], see [54], cf. [55], see [56], cf. [57], see [58], also see [6, 19, 23]).

Thus, treating psychiatric conditions in end-stage cancer patients is reaching a watershed in terms of both practice and research opportunities to assess treatment effectiveness (cf [46]). Key to addressing end-stage patients' psychiatric symptoms and disorders, especially going forward, is the effectiveness of psychiatric interventions and the state of research assessing that effectiveness (cf [4, 18, 19, 23, 29]). Past literature reviews ([4], also see [7, 19]) on end-stage cancer patients'

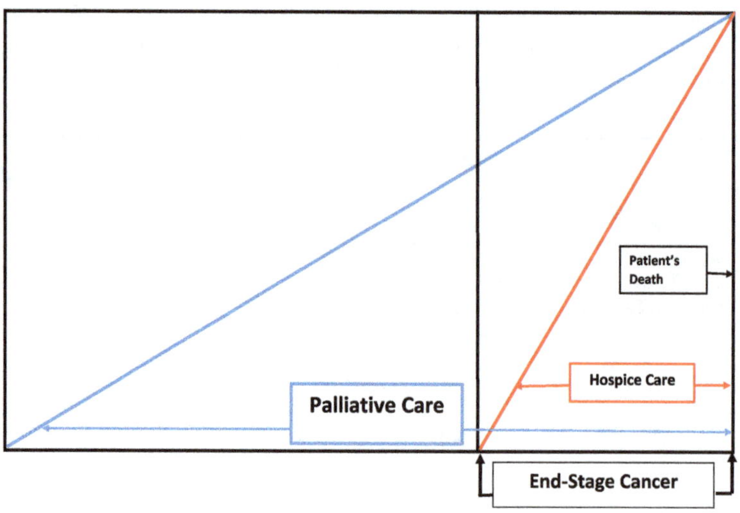

Fig. 1 End stage cancer in relation to palliative and hospice care

psychiatric symptoms and disorders have included particular aspects of psychiatric treatment effectivenes-s—one of which is an ongoing and expanding internet compilation solely on depression [23]. Few, if any, studies provide a reasonably current comprehensive overview regarding the effectiveness of various psychiatric treatments with an assessment of the state of research and the need for further research. The intent of this article is to report on a recent systematic literature review study regarding the effectiveness of interventions for psychiatric conditions commonly prevalent among end-stage cancer patients; the review study assessed the state of the research into treatment effectiveness. Furthermore, the review study attempted to include non-traditional (i.e., alternative) therapies that have undergone scientific study regarding their effectiveness in treating end-stage cancer patients' psychiatric symptoms and disorders. This has not been done previously. This article is intended to provide a well-integrated compendium of "pearls" (i.e., a psychiatric pharmacopeia). The goal is to inform oncologists and mental health practitioners regarding how to reduce end-stage cancer patients' emotional distress and psychiatric discomfort and improve their quality of life—the ultimate goal of end-stage cancer care [1, 2, 11, 49].

Methods

A five-phase systematic strategy was used to derive the articles for this literature review, as illustrated in Fig. 2.

An initial PubMed search was undertaken to identify related articles. This also was used to identify and expand the keywords and keyword combinations (i.e., Booleans) in a second and more comprehensive search of the PubMed, Medscape, Cochranes, and Oxford databases. Studies that did not refer to psychiatry, end-stage cancer, or effectiveness of treatment were excluded. All studies, abstracts, reviews, raw reports, observational studies, and (random) controlled clinical trials found relevant have been included. A grounded [59–61] qualitative methodology was used to iteratively generate and assign themes to research study articles (i.e., code) until thematic saturation, an exhaustion of themes, was achieved. The inherent risk in this process is that some studies or themes will be missed, but the assumption is that a general and credible assessment will be produced [61]. The ultimate aim of this process was to produce an integrated, synthesized end-product consisting of brief descriptive accounts of the effectiveness of psychiatric interventions and a needs assessment on the state-of-effectiveness research.

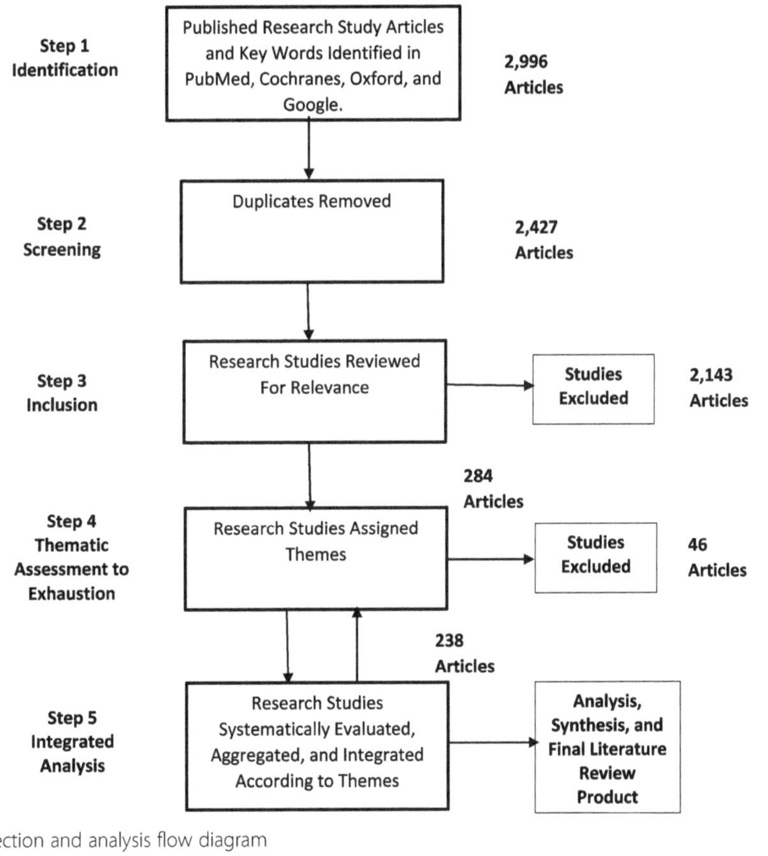

Fig. 2 Research article collection and analysis flow diagram

Results

Findings are organized in accordance with the prevalence of common psychiatric disorders found among end-stage cancer patients, the most employed treatments (i.e., the "best practices benchmarks") (cf. [4, 18, 19, 23, 27, 43, 52]) followed by other treatments, and the state of research on their effectiveness, with recommendations for future inquiry.

Delirium

Delirium is the most prevalent neuropsychiatric disorder in end-stage cancer patients ([62–64], also [7, 13, 25, 46, 62]). Antipsychotics (e.g., haloperidol, clorapromazide, methotrimeprazine, olanzapine, risperidone, quentiapine) are the mainstays for effective psychiatric symptom management of delirium ([65–69], also see [7, 13, 18]).

Typical (traditional) antipsychotics

Haloperidol has been and continues to be the psychiatric medication of choice and the best practices benchmark for end-stage cancer delirium symptom relief ([70–72], also see [7, 18, 19, 25, 46, 73]) It has low dose tolerance, flexibility in route administration (e.g., by mouth, intravenous, intramuscular, subcutaneous), relative safety, and high efficacy ([74–78], also see [7, 13, 18, 62, 65–67, 70]). Haloperidol and other typical antipsychotics (e.g., methotrine, epramazine) have also been reported to have additional analgesic properties. Evidence also suggests they are adjuncts to pain management or have anti-nausea/emetic effects [79–83]—especially for intractable nausea [84]. In addition, they have a controversial and ethically questionable role in terminal sedation, namely, rendering unconscious the end-stage patient who has truly distressing, hyper-aroused, and refractory delirium symptoms ([85, 86], also see [13]). Note that there are no official guidelines for practitioners and only limited data on the use of antipsychotics for terminal sedation [13, 87]. Antipsychotics may also be used in combination with lorazepam for rapid onset and augmentation of sedative effects in pronounced hyper-aroused delirious patients [7]. Reports have suggested that aripiprazole is effective with hypoactive delirium; however, it is ineffective with hyperactive delirium and may even trigger it. Chlopromazine has calmative effects in agitated or combative delirium patients [88], also see [19, 73].

Atypical (new-generation) antipsychotics

In studies and case reports, risperidone, clozapine, quetiapine, and levomepromazine have proven effective in low doses compared to traditional/typical antipsychotics but with reduced extra pyramidal symptom side-effects, which is the case in end-stage cancer patients ([89–92], also see [13, 14, 18, 65, 67, 88]). They also may have hypotensive and cardiac side-effects (e.g., arrhythmias), which must be monitored ([93–98], also see [7, 13, 18, 19, 36]). Like haloperidol, new-generation anti-psychotics can be used parenterally, which is advantageous with patients in end-stage cancer where oral medications are not possible [7, 18, 54, 72, 94]. These agents may have other side-effects such as hyperglycemia, hyperlipidemia, and weight gain, which must be reasonably balanced in light of the state of advancement in the end-stage cancer and symptom relief.([99–101], also see [7, 18, 19]).

Antipsychotics, whether traditional/typical or atypical/new-generation, are the approved psychiatric medications for patients with severe mental disorders who suffer from schizophrenia and in some cases bi-polar disorders and who also have end-stage cancer [29, 43].

State of antipsychotic scientific research for delirium symptom relief for end-stage cancer patients

To date, except for treating hyper-aroused/distressed delirium and particular medication side-effect profiles, reports in the literature have shown no difference between typical/traditional vs. atypical/new-generation antipsychotics in terms of effectiveness for delirium symptom reduction in end-stage cancer patients ([102], also see [7, 18, 19, 69, 96]). Thekdi, Trinidad, and Roth [19] noted that a small study found that advanced prophylactic use of antipsychotic medications in patients at risk for delirium reduced symptom occurrence later on in 50% of the cases. They further argued for early and aggressive use of low-dose antipsychotics with cancer populations with an anticipated trajectory toward end-stage disease. They also noted the absence of and, thus, called for definitive trial studies on the effectiveness of the newer generation of antipsychotic agents for cancer patients experiencing delirium, in particular end-stage cancer patients (e.g., asenapine, iloperidone, lorasidone, paliperidone) and others in the pipeline—about which for end-stage cancer patients almost nothing is known.

Masman ([103–106], also see [74]) reported that far more studies have been conducted on the traditional/typical as opposed to the atypical/new generation as the former have been around longer. Nevertheless, most studies are retrospective studies, overviews, or case reports and few have been prospective, large-scale trials, much less randomized controlled trials, regardless of old or new generation [106]. Also there is a tendency to echo shaky previous findings. Thus, critics of the research on antipsychotic treatments for delirium in end-stage cancer patients contend that most of it is the consequence of extrapolation and expert opinion (cf. [74, 103–106]). Given that one antipsychotic is as effective as any other except for side-effect profiles, there is definitely a need for solid large-scale prospective studies that also take into account patient type and type of delirium (e.g., hypo- vs. hyper-aroused) [18, 102]. Also, more research is needed to support and advance effective therapies for prevention and management of delirium, especially prospective random controlled clinical trials, that account for persistent, refractory symptoms and cumulative antipsychotic use in end-stage cancer patients. In sum, it appears that no large-scale prospective random controlled clinical trials have focused on antipsychotic treatments of delirium in end-stage disease, much less end-stage cancer [52].

Clinical depressive disorder

Among end-stage cancer patients, depression is the second most common psychiatric disorder encountered ([107–109], also see [4, 9, 13, 18, 19, 23, 47, 53]).

Selective serotonin reuptake inhibitors (SSRIs)

The approach to treatment of depression depends on the patient's life expectancy ([109], also see [110, 111]). If the patient's life expectancy is 4–6 weeks or longer, then serotonin reuptake inhibitor (SSRI) antidepressants (e.g., escitalopram, citalopram, sertraline, fluoxetine, paroxetine, mirtazapine ([112, 113], also see [114]) are the medication of choice and the best practices benchmarks for effective treatment ([115], also see [4, 7, 18, 23, 25, 53, 73]). For end-stage cancer patients, these medications are relatively safe, inexpensive, and useful with co-morbid conditions like anxiety and irritability; they also serve as possible analgesic synergists ([116], also see [13, 18, 19]). One downside is that they take 4–6 weeks or more to titrate to a normal response dose to achieve a beneficial effect ([117, 118], also see [7, 13, 18, 19, 23, 114]). Reports have suggested that they have some side-effects (e.g., restlessness, agitation, insomnia, sedation, parkinsonianism) that can be problematic with end-stage cancer patients, especially with co-morbid delirium [7, 23]. On the other hand, compared to other classes of antidepressants, they have few interactions with other drugs [7, 13, 18, 19, 23, 119], which is an important consideration with end-stage cancer patients ([117, 118, 120], cf. [72], also see [21]). (Note: Kiener, Weixler, Massel, Gartner, et al. [121] revealed that end-stage cancer patients were taking an average of 4–6 different prescription medications and up to 11 at the point of death.)

Serotonin–norepinephrine reuptake inhibitors (SNRIs)

Serotonin–norepinephrine reuptake inhibitors (SNRIs; e.g., veralfaxine, duloxetine) like SSRIs are well tolerated and have similar side-effects, except that SNRIs lead to hypertension and have been reported to cause bleeding in rare cases [13]. In addition to the side-effects, their downside is that they may take substantially longer than SSRIs to achieve optimal effect (e.g., > 4–6 weeks) and end-stage cancer patients may not have that much time left. [4, 13, 18, 19, 23, 53, 114, 122].

Tricyclic antidepressants

Tricyclic antidepressants (TCAs; e.g., amoxapine, desipramine, imipramine, doxepin, clomipramine, amitriptyline, nortriptyline) are not well tolerated by end-stage cancer patients and have major anti-histaminic and anti-cholonergic side-effects (e.g., delirium, confusion, hallucinations); they also have the potential for serious drug-drug interactions—though some reports suggest they have analgesic effects ([4, 7, 13, 18, 53, 114, 122], cf. [19, 23, 25, 73]).

Bupropione

Bupropione is a well-tolerated antidepressant in end-stage cancer patients, and it triggers mild stimulation as a side-benefit in patients with chronic fatigue ([123], also see [13, 18, 19, 53]). However, for the same beneficial reasons, it is counter-indicated for patients prone to seizure disorders ([13, 19, 123], also see [53, 114]). Also, it might increase anxiousness, restlessness, and angina [123].

Mitrazapine

Mitrazapine was shown to be statistically significantly effective in that it not only improved depression symptoms over other available antidepressants but it also helped with anorexia, anxiety, and insomnia, though it led to constipation ([124, 125] also see [4, 19, 53]). In a small random controlled clinical trial, Cankurtaran, Ozalp, Soygur, Akbiyik, et al. [126] found that mirtazapine was more effective than imipramine in cancer patients in reducing depressive and adjunct symptoms.

Trazadone

Trazadone is considered too sedating and needs extremely high and potentially risky doses to be effective with end-stage cancer patients [7].

Monoamine oxidase inhibitors

Monoamine oxidase inhibitors (MAOs) are considered the least effective of antidepression medications for cancer patients in general, much less end-stage cancer patients [7, 23]. Thus, MAOs have been abandoned in favor of SSRIs [7]. MAOs also have a high number of drug-drug interactions and may lead to hypertensive crises with the wrong foods or medications [7, 23].

Ketamine

If the patient's life expectancy is < 2–3 weeks, then an atypical psychiatric medication option to very effectively treat depression might be ketamine [127]. Ketamine has been studied in limited Phase I trials to treat refractory depression with a statistically significant 93% improvement rate within 0–3 days and an 80% post-dose improvement rate [127–129]. A statistically significant number of subjects showed few or no side-effects related to the medication

[129]. A meta-analytic study of ketamine use in general palliative care found that it can be extremely effective in patients with refractory depression, especially those with chronic pain ([130–139], also see [5, 23]). However, it is unclear exactly for which patients ketamine is optimal or what the best modes for administration are.

State of antidepressant scientific research for clinical depression symptoms relief for end-stage cancer patients

Except for the trial for mitrazapine, ketamine, and fluxoetine [23, 140, 122, 126], few large-scale, prospective, systematic, rigorous, scientific randomized controlled clinical trials are reported in the literature on medication effectiveness in end-stage cancer patients ([141–145] also see [58, 140, 122, 126]). Much of what is known or suspected is based heavily on expert opinion extrapolated from case reports and/or small non-end-stage cancer patient studies [58, 114]. What has been clearly established regarding the efficacy of antidepressants in treating cancer patients, including end-stage cancer patients, is that an antidepressant—any antidepressant—is better than none at all—provided the patient has sufficient life expectancy ([146–148], also see [5, 7, 13, 18, 19, 23, 25, 53, 58, 73, 135, 141, 145]). That is, any antidepressant is as effective as another, except when considering their different side-effect profiles, potential for overdose, and concomitant drug-drug interactions.

End-stage cancer patient guidelines for antidepressants based on practitioners' experience, expert opinion, case reports, the few small trials, and extrapolation appear to have been codified as scientific fact through a process of successive repetition and echoing in medical practice journals and then translated into best practices ([146–159, 160], also see [18, 19, 25, 114, 74]). Given that the discipline has recognized a paucity of solid scientific research, researchers have called for closer, more thorough, and more comprehensive examinations of the effectiveness of antidepressants for end-stage cancer patients suffering depressive symptoms ([152, 153], also see [52]). This is especially the case in the context of ethical considerations surrounding end-stage cancer patients' refusal of medical care [52]. These calls have included the desperate need for large-scale, prospective, multi-site studies of end-stage histolologically similar cases [58]. Unfortunately, yet ultimately, the use of particular antidepressants with end-stage cancer patients suffering depression depends on practitioners' preferences and individual preferences (e.g., side-effects, tolerance, poly pharmacy, reactions). As Fitzgerald, Lo, Li, Gagliese, et al. [154] noted, vital research is desperately needed to better understand treatment effectiveness in terms of the phenomenology of "subthreshold" depression as well as all aspects of depression in end-stage cancer patients to strengthen the evidence-based effectiveness of psychiatric best practice guidelines.

Psychostimulants

The other treatment option for depressive symptoms in end-stage cancer patients with a short (e.g., 2–3 weeks) life expectancy is low-dose psychostimulants (e.g., methylphenidate, dextro-amphetamine, modofinil) ([156, 157], also see [4, 5, 7, 13, 18, 19, 23, 25, 53, 73]). Low-dose psychostimulants have almost immediate benefit—-peaking within 3–8 h ([158–174], also see [7, 13, 19, 23, 53]). Patients experience a marked elevation in mood, self-esteem, alertness, focus, cognitive function, and regulation of appetite [7, 13, 18, 19, 23, 53, 158]. A study of patients taking 10 mg methylphenidate twice a day, limited to 80 mg per day or adequate response, found that 23 out of 30 (77%) end-stage cancer patients treated had moderate to marked improvement in depressive symptoms ([167], also see [166]). Only two patients withdrew due to intractable side-effects ([167], also see [53]). In a similar study, 30 out of 41 patients (73%) showed improvement in 7 days [167].

Psychostimulants also are particularly effective in combating opiate sedation and synergizing analgesics [7]. Due to the immediacy of onset, there is no question regarding effectiveness and, thus, they are the treatment of choice and the best practices benchmarks for short-term care of end-stage cancer patients' depression; they are often combined with SSRIs [4]. Note that there is a black box warning about methylphenidate causing cardiac arrest and mandating consent to use ([168], also see [13, 114]). Methylphenidate is also associated with side-effects such as headaches, anxiety, hypertension, and cardiac arrhythmias [23]. Additionally, modofinil has sympathomimetic effects and, thus, is a good choice for older end-stage cancer patients [7, 13, 114, 166, 168].

State of psychostimulant scientific research for clinical depression symptom relief for end-stage cancer patients

The effectiveness of psychostimulants in treatment of depression symptoms in cancer patients in general and (in the short term) end-stage cancer patients is fairly well established based on a series of scientifically sound randomized controlled clinical trials, the "gold standard" in research [4, 13, 18, 19, 74]. Nevertheless, and ironically, the use of these medications, though common in this population, may still be off-label (cf. [4, 74]).

Non-traditional/alternative psychiatric therapies

Electroconvulsive treatment

Electroconvulsive treatment (ECT) is extremely effective in ameliorating depression and is remarkably safe in elderly cancer patients except those prone to seizures and cardiac problems ([54], also see [7]). ECT is especially effective in depression refractory to antidepressant medications. It does cause short-term memory loss, but cognitive effects are lower with unilateral as opposed to bilateral ECT. However, Winnell and Roth [7] noted ethical questions about the image of electrically shocking terminal cancer patients, especially elderly patients.

Herbal remedies

In a double-blind, cross-over randomized controlled clinical trial examining the effectiveness of guariana (paullina aipana) on 36 patients with breast cancer, despite guariana's psychostimulant properties, no difference was detected between those receiving it versus those receiving a placebo [169, 160]. A review of studies on visum album L (European mistletoe) used in cancer patients who also suffered from depression and anxiety found that the treatment was effective for both depression and anxiety; [170, 172] mistletoe treatments were well tolerated with fewer side-effects than conventional treatments.

State of non-standard/alternative psychiatric therapy scientific research for clinical depression symptom relief for end-stage cancer patients

Notably, Breitbart and Dickerman [23] claimed that of all the psychiatric therapies that treat depression, ECT's effectiveness has received the most definitive, extensive, solid, and generalizable scientific examination. Non-standard/alternative herbal studies, though few, seem to be well designed or account for drug-drug interactions well. They are proliferating outside the United States, with the particular herb studied indigenous to the cultural locality and region where found.

Adjustment disorder/anxiety

Adjustment disorder and anxiety are the third most common psychiatric conditions encountered with end-stage cancer patients. Moivic [4] reported that "according to the DSM-V ([175], also see [15, 57]). Adjustment Disorders are emotional/behavioral symptoms in excess of what would be normal response to a given stressor in excess of a mere diagnosis of depression" ([176], also see [4]). Since psychiatric medication interventions are similar to those for anxiety, they are included with anxiety, though the symptoms dictate treatment, and these interventions may also have depressive features [4].

End-stage cancer patients naturally experience anxiety and anxiety-related psychiatric symptoms and disorders, especially at crisis points ([7], cf. [15]). This can be considered normal people reacting normally to extremely abnormal circumstances. Determining the point at which anxiety becomes abnormal and pathological is tricky, making exactly when a therapeutic intervention is necessary problematic ([177–179], also see [7, 15, 25, 56]), cf. [180]. Also, anxiety can be a component of delirium or depression, as well as a pathological feature of the cancer itself or its treatment [179]. For example, dexamethasone and metocloprapromide can cause anxiety and restlessness along with emotional distress and hyperactivity [25].

Nevertheless, biodiazepines (BDZs—temazepam, midazolam, alopazalam, lorazepam, oxezapam, diazepam, clonazepam) are the most effective and powerful drugs in treating anxiety and related adjustment disorders, though they do cause sedation, confusion, motor confusion, and un-coordination, build up over time, inordinately affect elderly patients, pose a risk for renal dysfunction, and are associated with drug-drug reactions ([181, 182], also see [4, 7, 13, 18, 19, 74]). Also, there is an exception to their use with lung cancer patients in that the disease is associated with respiratory distress (i.e., air hunger) in patients and BDZs' depressive effects can exacerbate this condition and increase related anxiety [183]. Similarly, caution must be used with BDZs as they are synergists with opiates, which can lead to deadly pulmonary depression [7, 13, 18, 19, 74]. Nevertheless, several studies have found that BDZs are effective and powerful in relieving anxiety and are adjuncts to relieving the pain, nausea, and emesis that end-stage cancer patients commonly suffer; BDZs can even help with end-stage sedation ([175, 184–192], also see [13, 85]) (Note: In lieu of BDZs, other medications that can be employed but are less effective are antidepressants, bupropione, and low-dose antipsychotics [7]). Whatever the case, Dauchy, Dolbeault, and Reich [114] cautioned that BDZs should not be prescribed indiscriminately for anxiety or depression because they might further complicate an already complicated clinical picture.

Nabalone

Maida, Ennis, Irani, Corbo, et al. [193], in a prospective study of nabalone (Casamet)—a cannabinoid—therapy in managing pain found a statistically significant ($P = .0284$) reduction in anxiety post-nabalone administration; nabalone also lowered or eliminated the use of anti-inflammatories.

Homeopathy

In a study on homeopathy and anxiety and anxiety disorders, Pilkington, Kirkwood, Rampes, Fisher, et al. [194] found that homeopathy was frequently and preferably used by a range of cancer patients suffering anxiety. Homeopathy was shown to be effective without side-effects, but the exact degree of effectiveness was questionable and needs further study.

Herbal remedies

Su, Wang, Grant, and Liu's [195] comprehensive review of Chinese herbal medication trials with a range of cancer patients found that Chinese herbal remedies were ineffective in relieving anxiety. The exact herbal medicines were unclear. Also, though adverse events were related to the medicines, no serious adverse events were reported. A review of studies on visum album L (European mistletoe) found that herbal medicine was effective for both psychiatric disorders (cf. [196], also see [171, 172, 180]) and the treatments were well tolerated with fewer side-effects than conventional treatments.

State of psychiatric therapy scientific research for adjustment disorder/anxiety relief for end-stage cancer patients

Research studies on BDZ interventions with end-stage cancer patients appear relatively robust and comprehensive. One reason offered for this is the overlap between BDZs and anxiety and the proliferation of post-traumatic stress disorder (PTSD) studies, extensions and extrapolations of those PTSD case and observational studies, meta-analytic reviews, and trials [4, 197–199]. Nevertheless, appearances might be deceiving in that Masman, van Dijk, Tibboel, Baar, et al. ([74], also see [200–202]), in their study on midozolam—one of the most prescribed BDZs in hospice settings—found that only case studies and small outdated trials were available to justify this practice in best practices guidelines (cf. [49]). Whatever the case, at a minimum, more and larger trials are needed on BDZs' effectiveness to establish best practices guidelines, especially in conforming prescription of these drugs to the particular needs of end-stage cancer patients [74].

Psychosocial therapy

Many reports in the literature address psychosocial (i.e., talk) therapy interventions with communicative and cognizant end-stage cancer patients in terms of relieving psychiatric symptoms and emotional distress, including but not limited to individual counseling, hypnotherapy, group therapy, psychotherapy, cognitive behavioral therapy (e.g., relaxation training, biofeedback), dignity therapy, and existential therapy ([203–209], also see [4, 5, 17, 23–25, 52, 73, 114, 90]). The general consensus in the discipline is that psychosocial interventions can reduce psychiatric disorders in communicative and cognizant end-stage cancer patients. ([210, 211], also see [4, 17, 23, 114]).

Meaning-centered and dignity therapy

Both meaning-centered and dignity therapy have been tested in Phase I, multi-site, randomized controlled clinical trials with promising but mixed results in terms of efficacy with end-stage cancer patients ([210–219], also see [5, 17, 23, 52, 63, 203, 204]). Dignity therapy (i.e., therapy intended to enhance diminished dignity and achieve a sense of purpose) was related to higher levels of helpfulness, quality of life, and sense of dignity in end-stage cancer patients [52, 215]. However, the patients did not experience a reduction in emotional distress [219].

Meaning-centered psychotherapy refers to the brief psychotherapeutic intervention predicated in Victor Frankl's logotherapy ([220], also see [52]). It aims to enhance psychosocial well-being in end-stage patients through individual and group applications [52, 203]. In a Phase I randomized controlled clinical trial, end-stage cancer patient study participants received group and individual psychotherapy; in a follow-up trial, individual psychotherapy was compared with a placebo intervention [220]. In both trials, participants receiving individual psychotherapy reported improvements in well-being and quality of life. However, the half-life of the intervention was brief in that differences in treatment outcomes were completely absent 2 months later (also see [52]).

Hypnotherapy

A small trial examining a hypnotherapy intervention designed to reduce anxiety for patients at an inpatient hospice facility found a statistically significant reduction in anxiety by the fourth treatment session ([221, 222], also see [52]).

Self-help

In a random controlled clinical trial, a brief guided self-help intervention was conducted with hospice inpatients targeting their depression symptoms ([223], also [52], cf. [114]). The intervention consisted of a trainer training participants to break cyclic cognitions of worry followed by practice sessions over a four-week period; in contrast, the control group received no intervention but crossed over in 4 weeks to the training intervention to receive treatment ([223], also see [52]). Participants experienced statistically significant reductions in anxiety but no reductions in depression ([223], also see [52]).

Orientation and cognitive behavioral therapy

Two other trials assessed the effectiveness of psychosocial interventions in cancer patients suffering from major depression. Both trials were enhanced orientation programs with the control group receiving the standard of care and both found reductions in depression symptoms ([224–226], also see [58], cf. [114]). Two other studies comparing the effectiveness of classic psychotherapy and cognitive behavioral therapy (CBT) found no reductions in depressive symptoms [58]. In a trial with cancer patients, Chen, Chen, and Zhi [227] found no difference between CBT and busprione and sertraline in terms of reducing depression and anxiety. They inferred that CBT was just as effective as psychiatric medication in treating anxiety and depression.

Psychosocial education

Between 1999 and 2002, a series of meta-analytic studies was conducted on previous studies (1970–1990) that examined the effectiveness of psychosocial education on emotional distress in cancer patients with respect to reducing depression and anxiety ([150], also see [114]). The studies universally found substantial evidence of a positive benefit on depression and anxiety in end-stage adult cancer patients but no difference in treatment effectiveness, especially in advanced disease cancer patients—even when delivered by experienced practitioners ([228–230], also see [59], cf. [114]). Notably, the investigators concluded that the interventions were beneficially effective in reducing emotional distress (also see [151]). Put differently, end-stage cancer patients appreciate one-to-one therapeutically delivered management of expectations and this type of intervention may be supportive of other interventions (also see [231]).

State of psychosocial therapy scientific research for end-stage cancer patients' psychiatric disorders

Other than the trials previously mentioned, no other reports were found that approximated large-scale, prospective, rigorous scientific inquiry regarding the effectiveness of psychosocial intervention with end-stage cancer patients' psychiatric disorders. Nevertheless, the fact that psychosocial (i.e., talk) therapy is venturing into clinical trials to scientifically verify interventions' effectiveness must be commended and encouraged. Dauchy, Dolbeault, and Reich [114] argued that a specific fit between types of psychosocial therapies that are effective with patients' expressive capacities, psychosocial situations, and timing in their process of oncological care must be identified.

Despite a seemingly solid universal consensus among experts that psychosocial therapies synergistically augment psychiatric medication interventions' effectiveness and the two are mutually supportive, the shortage of empirical evidence means that the jury is still out ([232, 233], also see [4, 17, 23, 114, 211, 213, 230], cf. [25]). Solid, large-scale, prospective trials are needed to investigate whether the therapeutic alliance is supported by psychosocial interventions and augments psychiatric medication interventions with end-stage cancer patients (also see [23, 150, 234], cf. [17, 25, 211]). This research should establish what aspects of psychotherapy are more or less beneficial, such as mutual trust, respect, sensitivity, coping, mechanisms/tools, and decreasing/eliminating maladaptive thinking. The literature contains increasing calls to use less intensive and less invasive data sources, including secondary administrative and medical records [235]. Regarding psychosocial education interventions, after a spate of studies culminating in a series of meta-analytic studies, research on this aspect of psychiatric interventions has dissipated—and this should not be where it ends as there is always more to learn.

Spirituality

Though spirituality and religion (religiosity) were not the province of this study, they may have positive influences on psychiatric interventions and end-stage cancer care that are worthy of informed commentary. Patients in end-stage cancer naturally experience multi-layered and inter-connected physical problems and emotional stressors, such as deterioration in quality of life, pain and increased sensitivity to pain, difficulty communicating, loss of control, physical disfiguration, burdens placed on others, costs of care, self-demoralization, feelings of worthlessness, helplessness, guilt, indifference, loss of interest and pleasure, and pathological pessimism ([73], also see [25, 114], cf. [236]). End-stage cancer patients often confront existential questions such as: Why? Why me? What have I done to deserve this? They often need to find meaning in their suffering, death, and the afterlife, and their illness may cause them to draw on or seek refuge in their faith or religion as a way of coping. Recently, small yet promising trials testing the effectiveness of interventions designed to boost spirituality have found that spirituality can positively affect end-stage cancer patients' mood and quality of life [237–241]. Not surprisingly, these studies found that spirituality interventions increased spirituality among the participants receiving these interventions. The good news is that some of the studies [212] are in the process of being replicated at several sites worldwide.

Discussion

In sum, at the risk of over-simplification, this review of the literature revealed a testable linear model of a combination of psychiatric treatments for communicative and cognizant end-stage cancer patients, as shown in Fig. 3.

This model has correlative models that emerged through rigorous scientific retrospective study of the cost-effectiveness of treatments on other psychiatric patient populations [242] (Note: The weight or importance of co-factors is displayed by their order of precedence, left to right.) First, consistent with best practice guidelines, the goal of psychiatric treatments with end-stage cancer patients is reduction in their psychiatric symptoms and enhancement of their quality of life ([243], also see, [1, 2, 11, 49, 52, 152, 153]). Second, depending on symptoms, medications are the most powerful tools in the psychiatric arsenal and this armory is expanding and extending with new editions and off-label combinations (cf. [74]). Third, some form of psychological counseling/intervention appears to support and augment psychiatric medication interventions. Though their effectiveness might be mixed, common sense dictates that the potential harm is relatively minimal, and they can serve as vehicles for fortifying the therapeutic alliance. Fourth, though a connection between psychosocial education and psychiatric therapeutic

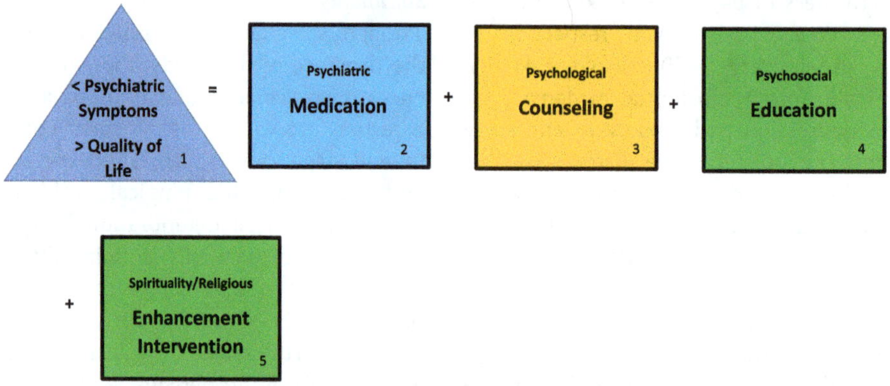

Fig. 3 End-stage cancer patient psychiatric treatment effectiveness linear model—the therapeutic alliance

effectiveness has yet to be established, such education has some beneficial or helpful effects for patients in crisis and research on it should not be abandoned entirely. Fifth, studies on interventions designed to enhance spirituality have shown substantially promising results in terms of quality of life and should be considered for inclusion in the constellation of future psychiatric treatment planning.

Of course, these recommendations take into account that the first priority is always treating physical medical conditions ([243], also see [7, 17, 27, 58, 74, 183, 211], cf. [22, 53, 114]). In terms of end-stage cancer patients who are cognitively impaired or unable to communicate (e.g., advanced delirium), psychiatric medication is probably the only appropriate therapeutic choice [74], but counseling, psychosocial education, and spirituality interventions may be appropriate interventions for family members and caregivers (cf. [25, 27, 73, 114]). Nevertheless, "the devil is in the details." Specifically, the complicated and tricky part of each component in the model is negotiating, balancing, conforming, and/or fitting the right treatment with the right patient, diagnosis (cf. [5, 7, 27, 56, 58]), dose for response, titration and tapering, drug-drug interactions, route of administration, and context and doing so decisively and quickly. Though varying amounts of quality scientific evidence exists in terms of components in the model, the review reported herein noted that some studies lack supporting evidence, or worse offer pseudo-evidence, and that much more rigorous and larger scale scientific studies must be conducted. This is particularly true for research on end-stage cancer patients in general and newly developed treatments and off-label combinations in particular—and of course effectiveness studies that include psychiatric intervention costs (cf. [74, 242]).

As cancer treatments become more aggressive and successful, and as the populations of older adults and, by extension, the populations with end-stage cancer, grow, patients' quality of life is of paramount importance. Delirium, clinical depression, and anxiety/adjustment disorder are complex and multi-faceted disorders and the psychotherapeutic and psychopharmacological interventions for their treatment require further study to inform more precise and powerful cancer care and best practices, especially in end-stage cancer. Thus, quality of life can be improved for patients dying of cancer. Universally endorsed care principles for end-stage cancer care affirm the importance of psychological health and access to the best mental health care that can be rendered to improve patients' quality of life at life's end ([244], also see [49, 52, 152, 153]). The wide dissemination of findings should alert clinicians and patients and their families as developments emerge. If anything, this article serves as an impassioned plea for further, better, and accelerated study of treatment effectiveness and care improvement for end-stage cancer patients' psychiatric conditions, if only because these patients cannot wait.

Conclusion

This article reported on a systematic, comprehensive, integrated review that investigated the effectiveness of interventions employed to treat psychiatric conditions common to end-stage cancer patients. The aim of this effort was to provide empirical findings to mental health practitioners so that they can hone their expertise in reducing emotional distress and psychiatric discomfort common to actively dying cancer patients and help these patients cope and improve their overall quality of life. Also, this work attempted to achieve an understanding of the state of the research on which best practices is predicated and to shed light on avenues for further inquiry. Undoubtedly, based on this review, more effective interventions are needed for psychiatric conditions/disorders; also needed are rapid and effective treatments to relieve psychiatric symptoms and disorders as well as strategies and tools to reduce or prevent them in advance [27].

Abbreviations

<: Less than; >: Greater than; BDZ: Bio-diazepam; CBT: Cognitive behavioral therapy; ECT: Electroconvulsive shock therapy; LTC: Lieutenant colonel; MAO: Monoamine oxidase inhibitor; PTSD: Post traumatic stress disorder; SNRI: Serotonin–norepinephrine reuptake inhibitors; SSRI: Selective serotonin reuptake inhibitors; TCA: Tricyclic antidepressants; TMC: Texas medical center; UT-MDACC: University of Texas MD Anderson cancer center

Acknowledgements

The Author wishes to acknowledge Ms. Lore Lagrone for materials and encouragement. The Author also gratefully recognizes Ms. Carla Miller research study nurse and Ms. Liliana Vallejo research coordinator for the review of the diagrams and proof of concept. The Author also thanks Ms. Jacqueline Ramey freelance copy-editor for proofing and copyediting.

Funding

Support has been provided by the U.S. Army and University of Texas-MD Anderson Cancer Center. The funding bodies had no involvement with the design of the study and collection, analysis, and interpretation of data and in writing the manuscript.

Author's contributions

RJJ is the sole author and accepts sole responsibility for content. The author read and approved the final manuscript.

Consent for publication

Not applicable

Competing interests

The author declare that they have no competing interests.

References

1. Hospice. https://www.cancer.gov/publications/dictionaries/cancer-terms/def/hospice.
2. Palliative. https://www.cancer.gov/publications/dictionaries/cancer-terms/search?contains=false&q=palliative.
3. Roy-Byrne PP. Diagnosis of psychiatric disorders in patients with cancer. https://www.uptodate.com/contents/diagnosis-of-psychiatric-disorders-in-patients-with-cancer?search=diagnosis-of-psychiatricdisorders-in-patients-with-cancerAQ13&source=search_result&selectedTitle=1~150&usage_type=default&display_rank=1
4. Miovic M, Block S. Psychiatric disorders in advanced cancer. Cancer. 2007; 110(8):1665–73. https://doi.org/10.1002/cncr.22980. PMID: 17847017
5. Marks S, Heinreich T. Assessing and treating depression in palliative care patients. Curr Psychol. 2013;12(8):37–40. https://doi.org/10.1089/jpm.2010.0530. PMID: 21815815
6. Irwin SA, Rao S, Bower K, Palica J, et al. Psychiatric issues in palliative care recognition of depression in patients enrolled in hospice care. J Palliat Med. 2008;11(2):158–63. https://doi.org/10.1089/jpm.2007.0140. PMID: 18333728
7. Winell J, Roth AJ. Psychiatric assessment and symptom management in elderly cancer patients. Cancer Network. 2005:1–14. PMID: 16370448
8. Massie MJ. The prevalence of depression in patients with cancer. J Natl Cancer Inst Monogr. 2004;32:57–71. PMID: 15263042
9. Fitzgerald P, Miller K, Li M, Rodin G. Depressive disorders: chapter 3. In psycho-oncology. New York: Oxford University Press; 2015. https://doi.org/10.1093/med/9780199363315.003.0037.
10. Kim S-H, Shin DW, Kim S-Y, Suh BS, et al. Terminal vs. advanced cancer: do the general population and health care professionals share a common language? Cancer Res Treat. 2016;48(2):759–67. https://doi.org/10.4143/crt2015:124
11. American Cancer Society. Advance directives: why do you need an advance directive? . Mobile: American Cancer Society; 2015. Available from: http://www.cancer.org/treatment/findingandpayingfortreatment/understandingfinancialandlegalmatters/advancedirectives/advance-directives-why-do-we-need-advancedirectives. [Cited 2015 Aug 1].
12. Levy MH, Back A, Benedetti C, Billings JA, et al. NCCN clinical practice guidelines in oncology: palliative care. J Natl Compr Cancer Netw. 2009; 7:436–73. PMID: 19406043
13. Garcia C, Lynn R, Breitbart W. Psychotropic medications in palliative care. Primary Psychiatry. 2009;16(5):25–32.
14. Breitbart W, Alici-Evcimen Y, Ruenda-Lara M. Psycho-oncology. In: Sandock BJ, Sandack VA, editors. Kaplan and Sandock's comprehensive Texbook of psychiatry. 8th ed. New York: Lippicott, Wilkins and Williams; 2008.
15. Wilson KG, Chochinov HM, Skirko MG, Allard P, et al. Depression and anxiety disorders in palliative Cancer care. J Pain Symptom Mang. 2007;33(2):118–28. https://doi.org/10.1016/j.jpainsymman.2006.07.016. PMID: 17280918
16. Hotopf M, Chidgey J, Addington-Hall J, Ly Kl. Depression in advanced disease: a systematic review, part 1. Prevalence and case finding. Palliat Med. 2002;16: 81–97. https://doi.org/10.1191/0269216302pm507oa. PMID: 11969152
17. Wilson KG, Chochinov HM, de Faye BJ, Breitbart W. Diagnosis management in depression in pailliative care. In: Chochinov HM, Breitbart W, editors. Handbook of psychiatry and palliative medicine. New York: Oxford University Press; 2000. p. 25–49.
18. Mehta RD, Roth AJ. Psychiatric considerations in the oncology setting. CA Cancer J Clin. 2015;65(4):300–14. https://doi.org/10.3322/Caac.21285. PMID: 26012508
19. Thekdi SM, Trinidad A, Roth A. Psychopharmacology in cancer. Curr Psyhiatry Rep. 2015;17(529):1–10. https://doi.org/10.1007/s11920-0529-x. PMID: 25417593
20. Mitchell AJ, Chan M, Bhatti H, Halton M, et al. Prevalence of depression, anxiety, and adjustment disorder in oncological, hematological, and palliative-care settings: a meta-analysis of 94 interview-based studies. Lancet Oncol. 2011;12(2):160–74. https://doi.org/10.1016/S1470-2045(11)70002-X. Epub 2011 Jan 19. PMID: 21251875
21. Pirl WF, Roth AJ. Diagnosis and treatment of depression in cancer patients. Oncology (Williston Park). 1999;13(9):1293–301. PMID: 10509324
22. Maixner S, Vitale CA, Stoltz AM, Wisely M, et al. Poster Number: NR 38 Geriatric Psychiatry Consultations in the Hospice Setting: A Case Series. 2012 AAGP Annual Meeting. http://www.ajgponline.org/article/S1064-7481(12)61556-5/pdf.
23. F W and Dickerman AL. Assessment and management of depression in palliative care. Section Eds Roy-Byrne PR and block AD, deputy Eds Savarese DMF and Solomon D: 2017: https://www.uptodate.com/contents/assessment-and-management-of-depression-in-palliative-care.
24. Muriel AC, Hwang VS, Kornblith A, Greer J, et al. Management of psychosocial distress by oncologists. Psychiatr Serv. 60(8):1132–4. https://doi.org/10.1176/appi.ps 60.8.1132.
25. Dein S. Psychiatric liaison in palliative care. Adv in Psychiatr Treat. 2003;9: 241–8. http://apircpsych.org
26. Blum B, Duane D, Ferris D, Herbst L, et al. Let's talk about hospice and palliative care. San Diego: San Diego Hospice and Palliative Care; 2004. http://www.chpca.net/media/238224/hpc-first-pritnable_booklet-english.pdf.
27. Irwin SA, Ferris FD. The opportunity for psychiatry in palliative care. Can J Psychiatr. 2008;53 https://doi.org/10.1177/070674370805301103. PMID: 19087465
28. Ferris FD, Balfour HM, Bowen K, Farley J, et al. A model to guide patient and family care: based on nationally accepted principles and norms of practice. J Pain Symptom Manag. 2002;24(2):106–23. PMID: 1223112
29. Trachsel M, Irwin SA, Biller-Adorno N, Hoff P, et al. Palliative psychiatry for severe persistent mental illness as a new approach to psychiatry? Definition, scope, benefits, and risks. BMC Psychiatry. 2016;16(260):1-1-6. https://doi.org/10.1186/s12888-016-0970-y. PMID: 27450328 PMCID: PMC4957930
30. Van der Lee MI, Sware NB, Van der Nom JG, Den Bout V, et al. Positive feelings among terminally ill cancer patients. Eur J Cancer Care (Engl). 2006; 15:51–5. https://doi.org/10.1111/j.1365-2354.2005.00619.x. PMID: 16441677
31. Grabsch B, Clarke DM, Love A, McKenzie DP, et al. Psychological morbidity and quality of life in women with advanced breast cancer: a cross-sectional survey. Palliat Support Care. 2006;4:47–56. PMID: 16889323
32. Wilson KG, Chocchinov HM, Skirko MG, Allard P, et al. Depression and anxiety disorders in palliative cancer care. J Pain Symptom Manag. 2007;33: 118–29. https://doi.org/10.1016/j.jpainsymman.2006.07.016. PMID: 17280918
33. Kirsh KL, McGrew JH, Dugan M, Passik SD. Difficulties in screening for adjustment disorders, part 1: use of existing screening instruments in cancer patients undergoing bone marrow transplantation. Palliat Support Care. 2004;2:23–31. PMID: 16594232

34. Kadan-Lottick NS, Vanderwerker LC, Block SD, Zhang B, et al. Psychiatric disorders and mental health service use in patients with advanced cancer: a report from the coping with cancer study. Cancer. 2005;104:2872–81. https://doi.org/10.1002/cncr.21532. PMID: 16284994 PMCID: PMC1459283
35. Prieto JM, Blanch J, Atala J, Carerreras E, et al. Psychiatric morbidity and impact on hospital length of stay among hematologic cancer patients receiving stem-cell transplantation. J Clin Oncol. 2002;20:1907–17. https://doi.org/10.1200/JCO.2002.07.101. PMID: 11919251
36. Akechi T, Okamura H, Nishiwaki Y, Uchitomi Y. Psychiatric disorders and associated and predictive factors in patients with unresectable nonsmall cell lung carcinoma: a longitudinal study. Cancer. 2001;92:2609–22.
37. Roth AJ, Modi R. Psychiatric issues in older cancer patients. Oncol Hematol. 2003;48:185–97. PMID: 14607382
38. Blazer DG. Epidemiology of late life depression. In: Schneider LS, Reynolds CF, Lebowitz BD, et al., editors. Diagnosis and treatment of depression in late life. Washington, D.C: American Psychiatric Press; 1994. p. 9–19.
39. Dewey M, de la Camara CJRM, Lobo A, et al. Cross-cultural comparison of depression and depressive symptoms in older people. Acta Psych. 2005;162: 184–6. PMID: 8356886
40. Bergquist H, Ruth M, Hammerlid E. Psychiatric morbidity among patients with cancer of the esophagus or the gastro-esophageal junction: a prospective, longitudinal evaluation. Dis Esophagus. 2007;20(6):523–9. https://doi.org/10.1111/j.1442-2050.2007.00741.x. PMID: 17958729
41. Teunissen SCCM, Wesker W, Kruiwagen C, de Haes HCJM, et al. Symptom prevalence in patients with incurable cancer: a systematic review. J Pain Symptom Manag. 2007;34:94–104. https://doi.org/10.1016/j.jpainsymman.2006.10.015. PMID: 17509812
42. Caraceri A, Nanni O, Maltoni M, Piva L, et al. Impact of delirium on the short term prognosis of advanced cancer patients. Italian multicenter study group on palliative care. Cancer. 2000;89(5):1145–9. PMID: 10964345
43. Ellison N. Mental health and palliative care: a literature review. UK: The Mental Health Foundation; 2008. https://www.mentalhealth.org.uk/publications/mental-health-and-palliative-care-literature-review.
44. Rao A, Cohen HJ. Symptom management in the elderly cancer patient: fatigue, pain, and depression. J Natl Cancer Inst. 2004;32:150–7. https://doi.org/10.1093/jncimonographs/lgh031. PMID: 15263059
45. Yanick R, Reis LA. Cancer in older persons: an international issue in an aging world. Semin Oncol. 2004;31:125–296. PMID: 15112144
46. Farriols C, Ferrandez O, Planas J, Pere O, et al. Changes in the prescription of psychotropic drugs in the palliative care of advanced cancer patients over a 7 year period. J Pain Symptom Manag. 2012;43(5):945–52. https://doi.org/10.1016/j.jpainsymman.2011.05.010. PMID: 22436835
47. Wilson KG, Chochinov HM, McPherson CJ, LeMay K, et al. Suffering with advanced cancer. J Clin Oncol. 2007;25:1691. https://doi.org/10.1200/JCO.2006.08.6801. PMID: 17470861
48. Spitzer RI, Kroenke K, Linzar M, Hahn SR, et al. Health-related quality of life in primary care patients with mental disorders: results from the PRIME-MD 1000 study. JAMA. 1995;274:1511–7. PMID: 7474219
49. Tan WW. Palliative Cancer care guidelines. http://emedicine.medscape.com/article/2500043-overview
50. Greer JA, Jackson VA, Meier DE, Temel JS. Early integration of palliative care services with standard oncology care for patients with advanced cancer. CA Cancer J Clin. 2013;63(5):349–63. https://doi.org/10.3322/caac.21192. PMID: 23856954
51. Ferrell BR, Temel JS, Temin S, Alesi ER, et al. Integration of palliative care into standard oncology care: American Cancer Society of clinical oncology clinical practice guideline update. J of Clin Oncol. 2017;35(1):96–112. https://doi.org/10.1200/JCO.2016.70.1474. PMID: 28034065
52. Fairman N, Irwin SA. Palliative care psychiatry: update on an emerging dimension of psychiatric practice. Curr Psychiatry Rep. 2013;15(7):374. https://doi.org/10.1007/s11920-0374-3.
53. Ginsburg A. Cancer-related depression and potential pharmacologic therapies. Proc (Bay Univ Med Cent). 2008;21(4):439–41. PMID: 18982092 PMCID: PMC2566922
54. Franco-Bronson K. The management of treatment-resistant depression in the medically ill. Psychiatr Clin North Am. 1996;19(2):329–50. PMID: 8827193
55. Check DV, Rosenmstein DL, Dusetzina SB. Early supportive medication use and end-of-life care among Medicare beneficiaries with advanced breast cancer. Support Care Cancer. 2016;24:346–3472. https://doi.org/10.1007/s00520-016-3174-6.
56. Barnhill JW, Dickerman AL. DSM-5 and psycho-oncology. New York: Oxford University Press; 2015. https://doi.org/10.1093/med/9780199363315.003.0083.
57. Hoge M, Roth AJ. Training psychiatrists and psychologists in psycho-oncology. New York: Oxford University Press; 2015. https://doi.org/10.1093/med/9780199363315.003.0093.
58. Rodin G, Katz M, Lloyd N, Green E, et al. Treatment of depression in cancer patients. Curr Onc. 2007;14(5):180–8. PMID: 17938701 PMCID: PMC2002483
59. Glaser BG and Strauss AL. The Discovery of Grounded Theory: Strategies for Qualitative Research. Aldine Transaction; New Brunswick, 1967 (Reprinted 2006).
60. Strauss A, Corbin J. Basics of qualitative research – techniques and procedures for developing grounded theory, second edition. London: Sage Publications; 1998.
61. Ramalho R, Adams P, Huggard P, Hoare K. Literature review and constructivist grounded theory methodology. Forum Qual Soc Res. 2015;16(3):19. http://www.qualitative-research.net/index.php/fqs/article/view/2313/3876
62. Fang C, Chen H, Liu S, Lin C, et al. Prevalence, detection, and treatment of delirium in terminal cancer inpatients: a prospective survey. Jpn J Clin Oncol. 2008;38(1):56–63. https://doi.org/10.1093/jjco/hym155. PMID: 18238881
63. Pereira J, Hanson J, Bruera E. The frequency in clinical course of cognitive impairment in patients with terminal cancer. Cancer. 1997;79:835–41. PMID: 9024722
64. Lipowski J. Transient cognitive disorders, delirium, acute confusional states in the elderly. AJP. 1983;140:1426–36. https://doi.org/10.1176/ajp.140.11.1426. PMID: 6624987
65. Gangon PR. Treatment of delirium in supportive and palliative care settings. Curr Opin Support Palliat Care. 2008;2(1):60–6. https://doi.org/10.1097/SPC.0b013e3282f4ce05. PMID: 18685397
66. Leonard M, Agar M, Mason C, Lawlor P. Delirium issues in palliative care settings. J Psychosom Res. 2008;65(3):289–98. https://doi.org/10.1016/j.jpsychores.2008.05.018. PMID: 18707953
67. Breitbart W, Freidlander M, Lawlor P. Delirium issues in the terminally ill. In: Chuchinov H, Breitbart W, editors. Handbook of psychiatry and palliative medicine. 2nd ed. New York: Oxford University Press; 2010.
68. Tune L. The role of anti-psychotics in treating delirium. Curr Psychiatry Rep. 2002;4(3):209–12. PMID: 12003684
69. Yuppa DP, Braun IM. Psychotropic medications in Cancer care. New York: Oxford University Press; 2015. https://doi.org/10.1093/med/9780199363315.0052.
70. Breitbart W, Alici Y. Evidence-based treatment of delirium in patients with cancer. J Clin Oncol. 2012;30(11):1206–14. https://doi.org/10.1200/JCO.2011.39.8784. PMID: 22412123 PMCID: PMC3646320
71. Maldonando JR. Delirium in the acute care setting: characteristics, diagnosis and treatment. Crit Care Clin. 2011;9(4):657–722. https://doi.org/10.1016/j.ccc.2008.05.008. PMID: 18929939
72. Akechi T, Uchtomi Y, Oamura H, Fukue M, et al. Usage of haloperidol for delirium in cancer patients. Support Care Cancer. 1996;4:390–2. PMID: 8883234
73. Dein S. Transcultural psychiatry. Br J Psychiatry. 2002;181:535–6. PMID: 12456530
74. Masman AD, van Dijk M, Tibboel D, Baar FPM, et al. Medication use during end-of-life care in a palliative care Centre. Int J Clin Pharm. 2015;37:767–75. https://doi.org/10.1007/s11096-015-0094-3. PMID: 25854310 PMCID: PMC4594093
75. Nauck F, Ostgathe C, Klaschick E, Bausewein C, et al. Drugs in palliative care: results from a representative survey in Germany. Palliat Med. 2004;18:100–7. https://doi.org/10.1191/0269216304pm852oa. PMID: 15046406
76. Lawlor PG, Gangnon B, Mancini IL, Pereira JL, et al. Occurrence, causes, and outcome of delirium in patients with advanced cancer: a prospective study. Arch Intern Med. 2000;160:786–94. PMID: 10737278
77. Del Fabbro E, Dalal S, Bruera E. Symptom control in palliative care–part III: dyspnea and delirium. J Palliat Med. 2006;9:422–36. https://doi.org/10.1089/jpm.2006.9.409. PMID: 16629571
78. Michaud L, Burnand B, Stiefel F. Taking care of the terminally ill cancer patient: Delerium as a symptom of terminal disease. Am Oncol. 2004;15(suppl 4):iv 199–203. https://doi.org/10.1093/annonc/mdh927. PMID: 15477308
79. Seidel S, Aigner M, Ossege M, Pernicka E, et al. Antipsychotics for acute and chronic pain in adults. Cochrane Data Base Sys Rev. 2013;(4):CD004844. https://doi.org/10.1002/14651858.pub3. PMID: 23990266
80. Langohr HD, Stohr M, Petruch F. An open and double-blind cross-over study on the efficacy of clomipramine (Anafranil) in patients with painful mono- and polyneuropathies. Eur Neurol. 1982;21(5):309–17. PMID: 6126361
81. Plotkin DA, Plotkin D, Okun R. Halperidol in the treatment of nausea and vomiting due to sytoxic drug administration. Curr Ther Res Clin Exp. 1973; 15(9):599–602. PMID: 4201543

82. Kelly SL, Braun TJ, Meyer TJ, Rempel P, et al. Trial of droperidol as an anti-emetic in cisplatin chemotherapy. Cancer Treat Rep. 1986;70(4):469–72. PMID: 3698040
83. Mason BA, Dambra J, Grissman B, Catalam RB. Effective control of cisplatin-induced nausea using high-dosed steroids and droperidol. Cancer Ther Rep. 1982;66(2):243–5. PMID: 7198937
84. Baymaster FP, Falcone JF, Bauzon D, Kennedy S, et al. Patient antagonism of S-HT (3) and 5-HT (6) receptors by olanzapine. Eur J Pharamcil. 2003;430(20–3):341–9. PMID: 11711053
85. Cowan JD, Palmer TW. Practical guide to palliative sedation. Curr Ocol Rep. 2002;4(3):242–9. PMID: 11937015
86. Morita T. Palliative sedation to relieve psycho-existential suffering of terminally ill cancer patients. J Pain Sympt Manag. 2004;28(2):445–50. https://doi.org/10.1016/j.jpainsymman.2004.02.017. PMID: 15504621
87. Sipahinamalani A, Masand PS. Use of risperidone in delirium case reports. Ann Clin Psychiatry. 1997;2:105–7.
88. Boettger S, Breitbart W. An open trial of aripiprazole for the treatment of delirium in hospitalized cancer patients. Palliat Supp Care. 2011;9(4):351–7. https://doi.org/10.1017/S1478951511000368. PMID: 22104410
89. Liu CY, Juang YY, Liang HY, Lin NC, et al. Efficacy of risperidone in treating the hyperactive symptoms of delirium. Int Clin Psychopharmcol. 2004;19(3):165–8. PMID: 15107660
90. Paellada E, Baeza I, de Pablo I, Martinez G. Risperidone in the treatment of patients with delirium. Psychiatry. 2004;65(3):348–53. PMID: 15096074
91. Han CS, Kim YK. A double-blind trial of risperidone and halperidol in the treatment of delirium. Psychosomatics. 2004;45(4):297–301. https://doi.org/10.1016/S0033-3182(04)70170-X. PMID: 15232043
92. Dietz I, Schmitz A, Lampey I, Schulz C. Evidence for the use of Levomepromazine for symptom control in the palliative care setting: a systematic review. BMC Palliat Care. 2013;12:2. https://doi.org/10.1186/1472-684X-12-2.
93. Stiefel F, Rasavi D. Common psychiatric disorders in cancer patients. II. Anxiety and acute confusional states. Supp Care Cancer. 1994;2:223–37. PMID: 8087441
94. Murray GB. Confusion, delirium, and demetia. In: Hackett TP, Cassem NH, editors. Massachusetts general hospital handbook of general hospital psychiatry, 2nd ed, vol. 84. Littleton: PSG Publishing; 1987.
95. Stiefel F, Holland J. Int Psychogeriatr. 1991;3:333–6. PMID: 1811785
96. Yoon HK, Kim YK, Han C, Ko YH, et al. Paliperidone in the treatment of delirium: results of a prospective open-label pilot trial. Acta Neuropsychiatr. 2011;23(4):179–83. https://doi.org/10.1111/j.1601-5215.2011.00568. PMID: 25379796
97. Pae CU, Lee SJ, Lee CU, Palik IH. A pilot trial of quetiapine. Prim Care Companion J Clin Psychiatry. 2000;2(1):10–2. https://doi.org/10.1002/hup.559. PMID: 14994323
98. Leso L, Schwartz TL. Ziprazadone treatment of delirium. Psychosomatics. 2002;43(1):61–2. https://doi.org/10.1176/appi.psy.43.1.61. PMID: 11927760
99. Breitbart W, Tremblay A, Gibson C. An open trial of olanzapine for the treatment of delirium in hospitalized cancer patients. Psychosomatics. 2002;43:175–82.
100. Wang HR, Woo YS, Bahk WM. Atypical antipsychotics in the treatment of delirium. Psychiatry Clin Neurosci. 2013;67(5):657–722. https://doi.org/10.1111/pcn.12066. PMID: 23859663
101. Ganzani L, Gross AF. Cancer Care for Patients with schizophrenia. New York: Oxford University Press; 2015. https://doi.org/10.1093/med/9780199363315.003.0044.
102. Agar MR, Rowett D, McCaffey NM. Efficacy of oral risperidone, haloperidol, or placebo for symptoms of delirium among patients in palliative care: a randomized clinical trial. JAMA Intern Med. 2017;177(1):34–42. https://doi.org/10.1001/jamainternmed.2016.7491. PMID: 27918778
103. Stiefel F, Fainsinger R, Bruera E. Acute confusional states in patients with advanced cancer. J Pain Symp Manag. 1992;7:94–8. PMID: 157329
104. Olofsson SM, Weitzner MA, Valentine AD, Baile WF, et al. A retropspective study of the psychiatric management and outcome of delirium in the cancer patient. Supp Care Cancer. 1996;4:351–94. PMID: 8883228
105. LeGrand SB. Delirium in palliative medicine: a review. J Pain Symp Manag. 2012; 44:583–94. https://doi.org/10.1016/j.jpainsymman.2011.10.013. PMID: 22682074
106. Caraceni A, Simonetti F. Palliating delirium in patients with cancer. Lancet Oncol. 2009;10:164–72. https://doi.org/10.1016/S1470-2045(09)70018-X. PMID: 19185834
107. McDaniel IS, Musselman DL, Porter MR, Reed DA, et al. Depression in patients with cancer: diagnosis, biology, and treatment. Arch Gen Psychiatry. 1995;52:89–99. PMID: 7848055
108. Potash M, Breitbart W. Affective disorders in advanced cancer. Hematol Oncol North Am. 2002;16:671–700. PMID: 12170575
109. Chochinov HM, Tataryn D, Clinch JJ, Dudgeon D. Will to live in the terminally ill. Lancet. 1999;354:816. https://doi.org/10.1016/S0140-6736(99)80011-7. PMID: 10485723
110. Hinton J. Which patients with terminal cancer are admitted from home care? Palliat Med. 1994;8:197. https://doi.org/10.1177/026921639400800303. PMID: 7952370
111. Tiernan E, Casey P, O'Boyle C, Birkbeck G, et al. Relations between desire for early death, depressive symptoms and antidepressant prescribing in terminally ill patients with cancer. JRS Med. 2002;95(8):386-390. PMID: 12151487 PMCID:PMC1279962
112. Cipriani A, Furukawa TA, Salanti G, Geddes JR, et al. Comparative efficacy and acceptability of 12 new-generation antidepressants: a multiple-treatments meta-analysis. Lancet. 2009;373(9665):746–58. https://doi.org/10.1016/S0140-6736(09)60046-5.
113. Theobald DE, Kish KL, Holtsclaw E, Donaghy K, et al. A open label pilot study of citalopram for depression and boredom in ambulatory cancer patients. Palliat Support Care. 2003;1:71–7. PMID: 16594290
114. Dauchy S, Dolbeault S, Reich M. Depression in cancer patients. EJC Suppl. 2013:205–15. https://doi.org/10.1016/j.ejcsup.2013.07.006
115. Lyons KS, Bennett JA, Nail LM, Fromme EK, et al. The role of patient pain and physical function on depressive symptoms in couples with lung cancer: a longitudinal dyadic analysis. J Fam Psychol. 2014;28(5):692–700. https://doi.org/10.1037/fam0000017. Epub 2014 Aug 4
116. Fisch MJ, Loehrer PJ, Kristeller PS, et al. Fluoxetine versus placebo in advanced cancer outpatients: a double-blinded trial of the Hoosier oncology group. J Clin Ocolo. 2003;21(10):1937–43. https://doi.org/10.1200/JCO.2003.08.025. PMID: 12743146
117. McClean S, Sheehy-Skeffington B, O'Leary N, O'Gorman A. Pharamacological management of co-morbid conditions at the end of life: is less more? Ir J Med Sci. 2013;182:107–12. https://doi.org/10.1007/s11845-012-0841-6. PMID: 22843427
118. Richelmann RP, Kryzanowski MK, O'Carroll A, Zimmermann C. Symptom and medication profiles among cancer patients attending a palliative care clinic. Support Care Cancer. 2007;15:1407–12. https://doi.org/10.1007/s00520-007-0253-8. PMID: 17429699
119. Ellershaw J. Care for the dying: what a difference an LCP makes! Palliat Med. 2007;21:365–8. https://doi.org/10.1177/0269216307081117. PMID: 17901095
120. Currow DC, Stevenson JP, Abernathy AP, Plummer J, et al. Prescribing in palliative care as death approaches. J Am Geriatr Soc. 2007;55:590–5. https://doi.org/10.1111/j.1532-5415.2007.01124.x. PMID: 17397439
121. Kierner KA, Weixler D, Masel EK, Gartner V, et al. Polypharmacy in the terminal stage of cancer. Supp Care Cancer. 2016;24(5):2067–74. https://doi.org/10.1007/s00520-015-3007-z. Epub 2015 Nov 5. PMID: 26542274 DOI: 10.1007/s00520-015-3007-z
122. Holland RC, Romano SI, Hollingstein JH, Tepner RG, et al. A controlled trial of fluoxetine and desipramine in depressed women with advanced cancer. Psychopharmacology. 1998;7(4):291–300. https://doi.org/10.1002/(SICI)1099-1611(199807/08)7:4<291::AID-PON361>3.0.CO;2-U. PMID: 9741068
123. Moss EL, Simpson JS, Pelletier G, Forsyth P. An open-label study of the effects of bupropion SR on fatigue, depression and quality of life of mixed-site cancer patients and their partners. Psycho-Oncology. 2006;15(3):259–67. https://doi.org/10.1002/pon.952. PMID: 16041840
124. Theobald DE, Ki K, Holtsclaw E, Doughy F, et al. An open-label, cross-over trial of mirtazapine [15 & 230 mg.] in cancer patients with pain and other distressing symptoms. J Pain Sympt Manage. 2002;23:442–7. PMID: 12007762
125. Kim SW, Shin IS, Kim JM, Kim YC, et al. Effectiveness of mirtazapine for nausea and insomnia in cancer patients with depression. Psychiatry Clin Neurosci. 2008 ;62(1):75–83. doi: https://doi.org/10.1111/j.1440-1819.2007.01778.x. PMID: 18289144 DOI: 10.1111/j.1440-1819.2007.01778.x.
126. Cankurtaran ES, Ozalp E, Soygur H, Akbiyik DI, et al. Mirtazapine improves sleep and lowers anxiety and depression in cancer patients: superiority over imipramine. *Supp Care Cancer.* 2008;16(11):1291–8. https://doi.org/10.1007/s00520-008-0425-1. Epub 2008 Feb 26. PMID: 18299900 DOI: 10.1007/s00520-008-0425-
127. Inglewicz A, Morrison K, Nelesen RA, Tingting Z, et al. Ketamine for the treatment of depression in patients receiving hospice care: a retrospective chart review of thirty-one cases. Psychosomatics. 2015; 56(4):329–37. https://doi.org/10.1016/j.psym.2014.05.005. PMID: 25616995 PMCID: PMC4308579

128. Murrough JW, Iosifescu DV, Chang LC, Al Jurdi RK, et al. Antidepressant efficacy of ketamine in treatment-resistant major depression: a two-site randomized controlled trial. Am J Psychiatry. 2013;170(10):1134–42. https://doi.org/10.1176/appi.ajp.2013.13030392. PMID: 23982301 PMCID: PMC3992936
129. Murrough JW, Perez AM, Pillemer S, Stern J, et al. Rapid and longer-term anti-depressant effects of repeated ketamine infusions in treatment-resistant major depression. Biol Psychiatry. 2013;74(4):250–6. https://doi.org/10.1016/j.biopsych.2012.06.022. PMID: 22840761 PMCID: PMC3725185
130. Zanicotti CG, Perez D, Glue P. Mood and pain response to repeat dose intramuscular ketamine in a depressed patient with advanced cancer. J Palliat Med. 2012;15:400. https://doi.org/10.1089/jpm.2011.0314. PMID: 22468772
131. Stefanczyk-sapieha L, Oneschuk D, Demas M. Intravenous ketamine "burst" for refractory deression in a patient with advanced cancer. J Palliat Med. 2008;11:1268. https://doi.org/10.1089/jpm.2008.9828. PMID: 19021495
132. Yang C, Zhou ZQ, Yang JJ. Be prudent of ketamine in treating resistent depression in patients with cancer. J Palliat Med. 2011;14:537. https://doi.org/10.1089/jpm.2010.0525. PMID: 21592028
133. Thangathural D, Roby J, Roffey P. Treatment of resistent depression in patients with cancer with low doses of ketamine and desiprimine. J Palliat Med. 2010;13:235. https://doi.org/10.1089/jpm.2009.0312. PMID: 20178430
134. Kollmar R, Markovic K, Thurauf SH, et al. Ketamine followed by memantine for the treatment of major depression. Aust N Psychiatry. 2008;42:170. https://doi.org/10.1080/00048670701787628. PMID: 18197514
135. Irwin SA, Inglewicz A, Nelesen RA, Lo JY, et al.. Daily oral ketamine for the treatment of depression and anxiety in patients receiving hospice care: a 28-day open-label proof-of-concept trial. J Palliat Med. 2013;16(8):958–65. doi: https://doi.org/10.1089/jpm.2012.0617. Epub 2013 Jun 27. PMID: 23805864 PMCID: PMC3717203 DOI: 10.1089/jpm.2012.0617.
136. Jafarinia M, Afarideh M, Tafakhori A, Arbabi M, et al. Efficacy and safety of oral ketamine versus diciofenac to alleviate mild to moderate depression in chronic pain patients: a double-blind, randomized, controlled trial. J Affect Disord. 2016;204:1. https://doi.org/10.1016/j.jad.2016.05.076. PMID: 27317968
137. Singh JB, Fedgchin M, Daly EJ, DeBoer P, et al. A double-blind, randomized, placebo-controlled, dose-frequency study of intravenous ketamine in patients with treatment-resistant depression. Am J Psychiatry. 2016;173:816. https://doi.org/10.1176/appi.ajp.2016.16010037. PMID: 27056608
138. Berman RM, Pereira J, Cappiello A, Anand A, et al. Anti-depressant effects of ketamine and anxiety in patients needing hospice care. Biol Psychiatry. 2000;47(4):351–4. PMID: 10686270
139. Irwin SA, Inglewicz A. Oral ketamine for the rapid treatment of depression and anxiety patients receiving hospice care. J Palliat Med. 2010;24(4):903–8. https://doi.org/10.1089/jpm.2010.9808. PMID: 20636166 PMCID: PMC3120058
140. Miller AH, Maletic V, Raison CL. Inflammation and its discontents: the role of cytokins in the pathophysiology of major depression. Biol Psychiatry. 2008; 65(9):732–41. https://doi.org/10.1016/j.biopsych.2008.11.029. PMID: 19150053 PMCID: PMC2680424
141. Costa D, Magos I, Toma T. Efficacy and safety of mianserin in the treatment of depression in women with cancer. Acta Psychiatr Scand Suppl. 1985;320: 85–92. PMID: 3901675
142. Holland RC, Morrow GR, Schmale A, et al. A randomized clinical trial of alprazolam versus progressive muscle realization in cancer patients with anxiety and drepressive symptoms. J Clin Oncol. 1991;9:1004–11. https://doi.org/10.1200/JCO.1991.9.6.1004. PMID: 2033413
143. Pezella G, Moslinger-Gehmayr R, Contu A. Treatment of depression in patients with breast cancer: a comparison between paroxetine and amitriptyline. Breast Cancer Res Treat. 2001;701:1–10. PMID: 11766999
144. Razavi D, Allilaire JF, Smith M, et al. The effect of fluoxetine on anxiety and depressive symptoms in cancer patients. Acta Psychiatr Scand. 1996;94:205–10. PMID: 8891089
145. van Heeringen K, Zivkov M. Pharmacological treatment of depression in cancer patients. A placebo-controlled study of mianserin. Br J Psychiatry. 1996;169:440–3. PMID: 8894194
146. Murlow CD, William JW Jr, Chiquette E, Aquilar C, et al. Efficacy of newer medications for treating depression in primary care patients. Am J Med. 2000;108:54. PMID: 11059441
147. Hansen RA, Gartlehner G, Lohr KN, Gaynes BN, et al. Efficacy and safety of second-generation antidepressants in the treatment of major depressive disorder. Ann Intern Med. 2005;143:415. PMID: 16172440
148. Attard A, Ranjith G, Taylor D. Alternative route to oral antidepressant therapy: case vignettes and literature review. Psychopharmacol. 2010;24(4): 449–54. https://doi.org/10.1177/0269881109102545. PMID: 19264816
149. Callari A, Mauri M, Miniati M, Mancino M, et al. Treatment of depression in patients with breast cancer: a critical review. Tumori. 2013;99(5):623–33. https://doi.org/10.1700/1377.15313.
150. Jacobsen PB, Donovan KA, Swaine ZN, Watson IS. Management of Anxiety and Depression in adult Cancer patients: toward an evidenced-based approach #89. Oncology:1561–88. https://link.springer.com/chapter/10.1007%2F0-387-31056-8_89.
151. Carr D, Goudas L, Lawrence D, et al. Management of cancer symptoms, pain, depression, and fatigue. Evidenced report/technology assessment no. 61. AHRQ publication no 02-E032. Rockville: Agency for Health Care Research and Quality; 2002. PMID: 12187571 PMCID: PMC4781249
152. Kissane DW. The contribution of demoralization to end of life decision making. Hast Cent Rep. 2004;34(4):21–31. PMID: 15379099
153. Schuman-Olivier Z, Bendel DH, Forstein M, Price BH. The use of palliative sedation for existential distress: a psychiatric perspective. Harv Rev Psychiatry. 2008;16(6):339–51. https://doi.org/10.1080/10673220802576917. PMID: 19085388
154. Fitzgerald P, Lo C, Li M, Gagliese L, et al. The relationship between depression and physical symptom burden in advanced cancer. BMJ Supp Palliat Care. 2015;5(4):381–8. https://doi.org/10.1136/bmjspcare-2012-000380. Epub 2013 Aug 6. PMID: 24644172 DOI: 10.1136/bmjspcare-2012-000380
155. Jackson V, Block S. Use of psycho-stimulants in palliative care. 2nd ed: End of Life/Palliative Education Resource Center. Medical College of Wisconcin. https://www.capc.org/fast-facts/.
156. Rozans M, Dreisbach A, Lertora JJ, Kahn MJ. Palliative uses of methylphenidate in patients with cancer: a review. J Clin Oncol. 2002;20(1): 335–99. https://doi.org/10.1200/JCO.2002.20.1.335. PMID: 11773187
157. Dean S, George R. A place for psychostimulants in palliative care. J Palliat Care. 2002;18:196–9. PMID: 12418371
158. Mansand PS, Tesar GE. Use of stimulants in the medically ill. Psychitr Clin North Am. 1996;19(3):515–47. PMID: 8856815
159. Macleod AD. Methylphenidate in terminal depression. J Pain Symptom Manag. 1998;16(3):193–8. PMID: 9769622
160. de Oliveira Campos MP, Riechelmann R, Martins LC, Hassan BJ, et al. Guarana (Paullinia cupana) improves fatigue in breast cancer patients undergoing systemic chemotherapy. J Altern Complement Med. 2011; 17(6):505–12. https://doi.org/10.1089/acm.2010.0571. Epub 2011 May 25. PMID: 21612429
161. Olin J, Masand P. Psychostimulants for depression in hospitalized cancer patients. Psychossomatics. 1996;37(1):57–62. https://doi.org/10.1016/S0033-3182(96)71599-2. PMID: 1381072 PMID: 8600496
162. Bruera E, Fainsinger R, MacEachern T, Hanson J. The use of methylphenidate in patients with incident cancer pain receiving regular opiates. A preliminary report. Pain. 1992;50(1):75–7. PMID: 1381072
163. Gagnon B, Low G, Schreier G. Methylphenidate hydrochloride improves cognitive function in patients with advanced cancer and hypoactive delirium: a prospective clinical study. J Psychiatry Neurosci. 2005;30(2):100–7. PMID: 15798785 PMCID: PMC551162
164. Prommer E. Methylphenidate: established and expanding roles in symptom management. Am J Hosp Palliat Care. 2012;29(6):483–90. https://doi.org/10.1177/1049909111427029. Epub 2011 Dec 4. PMID: 22144657 DOI: 10.1177/1049909111427029
165. Rifkin A, Reardon G, Siris S, Karagji B, et al. Trimipramine in physical illness with depression. J Clin Psychiatry. 1985;46(2 Pt 2):4–8. PMID: 3881418
166. Centeno C, Sanz A, Cuervo MA, Ramos D, et al. Multicentre, double-blind, randomized placebo-controlled clinical trial on the efficacy of methylphenidate on depressive symptoms in advanced cancer patients. BMJ Support Palliat Care. 2012;2(4):328–33. https://doi.org/10.1136/bmjspcare-2011-000093. Epub 2012 Jun 1. PMID: 24654216 DOI: 10.1136/bmjspcare-2011-000093
167. Homsi J, Walsh D, Nelson KA, LeGrand S, et al. Methylphenidate for depression in hospice practice: a case series. Am J Hosp Palliat Care. 2000; 17(6):393–8. https://doi.org/10.1177/104990910001700610. PMID: 11886041
168. Breitbart W, Alici Y. Pharmacologic treatment options for cancer-related fatigue: current state of clinical research. Clin J Oncol Nursing. 2008; 1215(Suppl 1):27–36. https://doi.org/10.1188/08.CJON.S2.27-36. PMID: 18842522
169. deCosta MV, Trufelli DC, Santos J, Campos MP, et al. Effectiveness of guaraná (Paullinia cupana) for postradiation fatigue and depression: results of a pilot double-blind randomized study. J Altern Complement Med. 2009; 15(4):431–3. https://doi.org/10.1089/acm.2008.0324. PMID: 19388866

170. Kienle GS, Kiene H. Complementary cancer therapy: a systematic review of prospective clinical trials on anthroposophic mistletoe extracts. Eur J Med Res. 2007;12(3):103–19. PMID: 17507307
171. Kienle GS, Kiene H. Review article: influence of Viscum album L (European mistletoe) extracts on quality of life in cancer patients: a systematic review of controlled clinical studies. Integr Cancer Ther. 2010;9(2):142–57. https://doi.org/10.1177/1534735410369673. Epub 2010 May 18. PMID: 20483874
172. Kienle GS, Glockmann A, Schink M, Kiene H. Viscum album L. extracts in breast and gynaecological cancers: a systematic review of clinical and preclinical research. J Exp Clin Cancer Res. 2009;28:79. https://doi.org/10.1186/1756-9966-28-79. PMID: 19519890 PMCID: PMC2711058
173. American Psychiatric Association. Diagnostic and statistical manual of mental disorders. Fifth ed. Lake St. Louis: APA Publishing; 2013. http://dsm.psychiatryonline.org/doi/book/10.1176/appi.books.9780890425596
174. Clarke DM, Kissane DW. Demoralization its phenomenology and importance. Aust N Z Psychiatry. 2002;36:733–42. https://doi.org/10.1046/j.1440-1614.2002.01086.x. PMID: 12406115
175. Coda BA, Mackie A, Jill HF. Influence of alprazolam on opiod analgesics and steady state during morphione infusion. Pain. 1992;50(3):309–16.
176. Mangelli L, Fava GA, Grandi GL, et al. Assessing demoralization and depression in the setting of medical disease. J Clin Psychiatry. 2005;66:391–4. PMID: 15766307
177. Maguire P, Lee E, Bevington D, et al. Psychiatric problems in the first year after mastectomy. BMJ. 1978;1:963–5. PMID: 565239 PMCID: PMC1603831
178. Peck A, Bowland J. Emotional reactions to radiation treatment. Cancer. 1977;40:180–4. PMID: 880549
179. Alter C, Pelovitz D, Axelrod A, Goldenberg B, et al. The identification of PTSD in cancer survivors. Psychosomatics. 1996;37:137–43. https://doi.org/10.1016/S0033-3182(96)71580-3. PMID: 8742542
180. Sykes N, Thorns A. Sedative use in the last week of life and the implications for end-of-life decision making. Arch Intern Med. 2003;163(3):341–4. PMID: 12578515
181. Good PD, Ravenscroft PJ, Cavenagh J. Effects of opioids and sedatives on survival in an Australian inpatient palliative care population. Intern Med J. 2005;35(9):512–7. https://doi.org/10.1111/j.1445-5994.2005.00888.x. PMID: 16105151
182. Good PD, Cavenagh JD, Currow DC, Woods DA, et al. What are the essential medications in pallative care? - a survey of Australian palliative care doctors. Aust Fam Physician. 2006;35(4):261–4. PMID: 16642246
183. Key RG. Psychiatric care of lung cancer patients. Oncology (Williston Park). 2015;29(3):195–7. PMID: 25772455
184. Fernandez F, Adams F, Holmes VF. Analgesic effect of alprozolam in patients with chronic, organic pain of malignant origin. J Clin Psychopharmacol. 1987;7(3):167–9. PMID: 3597802
185. National Cancer Institute. Nausea and vomiting PDQ. Health professional. www.cancer.gov/cancertopics/pdq/supportivecare/nausea/HealthProfessional.
186. Greenberg DB, Surman OS, Clarke J, Baer L. Alprazolam for phobic nausea and vomiting related to cancer chemotherapy. Cancer Treat Rep. 1987;71(3):549–50. PMID: 3567983
187. Mori K, Saito Y, Tominaga K. Antiemetic efficacy of alprazolam in the combination of metoclopramide plus methylprednisone. Double-blind randomized crossover study with patinets with cisplatic-induced emisis. Am J Clin Oncol. 1993;16(4):338–41. PMID: 8392288
188. Potanovich LM, Pisters KM, Kris MG, Tyson LB, et al. Midazolam in patients receiving anticancer chemotherapy and anti-emetics. J Pain Symptom Manag. 1993;8(8):519–24. PMID: 7963777
189. Bishop JF, Oliver IN, Wolf MM, Matthews JP, et al. Lorazepam: a randomized double-blind crossover study of a new antiemetic in patients receiving cytoxin chemotherapy and prochlorpersine. J Clin Oncol. 1984;2(6):691–5. https://doi.org/10.1200/JCO.1984.2.6.691. PMID: 6374058
190. Hasselaar JG, Reuzel RP, Verhagen SC, de Graff A, et al. Improving prescription in palliative sedation: compliance with Dutch guidelines. Arch Intern Med. 2007;167(11):1166–71. https://doi.org/10.1001/archinte.167.11.1166. PMID: 17563025
191. Reuzel RP, Hasselaar GJ, Vissers KC, der Wilt V, et al. Inappropriateness of using opiods for end-stage palliative sedation: a Dutch study. Palliat Med. 2008;22(5):641–6. https://doi.org/10.1177/0269216308091867. PMID: 18612030
192. Cowan JD, Palmer TW. Terminal sedation in palliative medicine–definition and review of the literature. Am J Hosp Palliat Care. 2008;22(5):403–7. PMID: 11585266
193. Maida V, Ennis M, Irani S, Corbo M, et al. Adjunctive nabilone in cancer pain and symptom management: a prospective observational study using propensity scoring. J Support Oncol. 2008;6(3):119–24.
194. Pilkington K, Kirkwood G, Rampes H, Fisher P, et al. Homeopathy for anxiety and anxiety disorders: a systematic review of the research. Homeopathy. 2006;95(3):151–62.
195. Su CX, Wang LQ, Grant SJ, Liu JP. Chinese herbal medicine for cancer-related fatigue: a systematic review of randomized clinical trials. Complement Ther Med. 2014;22(3):567–79. https://doi.org/10.1016/j.ctim.2014.04.007. Epub 2014 May 5
196. Kienle GS, Glockmann A, Schink M, Kiene H. Viscum album L. extracts in breast and gynaecological cancers: a systematic review of clinical and preclinical research. J Exp Clin Cancer Res. 2009;28:79. PMID: 17507307
197. Gurevich M, Devins GM, Rodin GM. Stress response syndromes and cancer: conceptual and assessment issues. Psychosomatics. 2002;43:259–81. https://doi.org/10.1176/appi.psy.43.4.259. PMID: 12189252
198. Pitman RK, Lanes DM, Williams SK, Guillaume JL, et al. Psychophysiologic assessment of post-traumatic stress disorder in breast cancer patients. Psychosomatics. 2001;42:133–40. https://doi.org/10.1176/appi.psy.42.2.133. PMID: 11239126
199. Stark D, Kiely M, Smith A, Morley S, et al. Reassurance and the anxious cancer patient. Br J Cancer. 2004;91:893–9. https://doi.org/10.1038/sj.bjc.6602077. PMID: 15292934 PMCID: PMC2409992
200. Bottomley DM, Hanks GW. Subsuctaneous, idazolam infusion in palliative care. J Pain Symptom Manag. 1990;5:259–61. PMID: 2384705
201. de Souza E, Jepson BA. Midazolam in terminal care. Lancet. 1988;1:67–8. PMID: 2891939
202. Bleasel MD, Peterson GM, Dunne PF. Plasma concentrations of midazolam during continuous subcutaneous administration in palliative care. Palliat Med. 1994;8:231–6. https://doi.org/10.1177/026921639400800307. PMID: 7952373
203. Breitbart W, Rosenfeld B, Gibson C, Pessin H, et al. Meaning centered group psychotherapy for patients with advanced cancer: a pilot randomized controlled trial. Psyhco-Oncology. 2010;19:21–8. https://doi.org/10.1002/pon.1556. PMID: 19274623 PMCID: PMC3648880
204. Breitbart W, Popito S, Rosenfeld B, Vickers AJ, et al. Pilot randomized controlled trial of individual meaning-centered psychotherapy for patients with advanced cancer. J Clin Oncol. 2012;30(12):1304–9. https://doi.org/10.1200/JCO.2011.36.2517. PMID: 22370330 PMCID: PMC3646315
205. Spiegel D, Bloom JR, Yalom I. Group support for patients with metastic cancer: a randomized outcome study. Arch Gen Psychiatry. 1981;38:527. PMID: 7235853
206. Spiegel D, Bloom JR. Group therapy and hypnosis to reduce breast cancer carcinoma pain. Psyhcosom Med. 1983;45:333. PMID: 6622622
207. Massie MJ, Holland JC, Straker N. Psychotherapuetic interventions. In: Holland JC, Rowland JH, editors. Handbook of psycho-oncology: psychological Care of the Patient with Cancer. New York: Oxford University Press; 1989. p. 455.
208. Chuckinov HM. Dignity-conserving care-a new model for palliative care: helping the patient feel valued. JAMA. 2002;287(17):2253–60. PMID: 11980525
209. Bausewein C, Booth S, Gyseis M, Higginson I. Non-pharmacological interventions for breathlessness in advanced stages of malignant and non-malignant diseases. Conchrane Database Syst Rev. 2008;2:CD005623. https://doi.org/10.1002/14651858.CD005623.pub2. PMID: 18425927
210. Block SD. Assessing and managing depression in the terminally ill patient. ACP-ASIM end-of-life consensus panel. American College of Physicians - American Society of Internal Medicine. Ann Intern Med. 2000:132–209. PMID: 10651602
211. Solomon BK, Wilson KG, Henderson PR, Poulin PA, et al. Loss of dignity in severe chronic obstructive pulmonary disease. J Pain Symptom Manag. 2016;51(3):529–37. https://doi.org/10.1016/j.jpainsymman.2015.11.007. Epub 2015 Nov 24. PMID: 26620235
212. Chochinov HM. Dignity-conserving care: a new model for palliative care. JAMA. 2002;287:22253–60. PMID: 11980525
213. Chuckinov HM, Hack T, Hassard T, et al. Dignity therapy: a novel psychotherapeutic intervention for patients nearing death. J Clin Oncol. 2005;23:5520–5. https://doi.org/10.1016/j.jpainsymman.2007.12.018. PMID: 18579340
214. Montross L, Winters KD, Irwin SA. Dignity therapy implementation in a community-based hospice setting. J Palliat Med. 2011;14:729. https://doi.org/10.1089/jpm.2010.0449. PMID: 21548823 PMCID: PMC3120093
215. Chochinov HM, Kristainson LJ, Breitbart W, McClements S, et al. Effect of dignity therapy on distress and end-of-life experience in terminally ill patients: a randomized controlled trial. Lancet Oncol. 2011;12:753. https://

doi.org/10.1016/S1470-2045(11)70153-X. PMID: 21741309 PMCID: PMC3185066
216. Vuksanovic D, Green HJ, Duck M, Morrissey SA. Dignity therapy and life review for palliative care patients: a randomized controlled trial. J Pain Symptom Manag. 2017;53:162. https://doi.org/10.1016/j.jpainsymman.2016.09.005. PMID: 27810568
217. Martinez M, Arantzamedi M, Belar A, et al. 'Dignity therapy,' a promising intervention in palliative care: a comprehensive literature review. Palliat Med. 2017;31:492. https://doi.org/10.1177/0269216316665562. PMID: 27566756 PMCID: PMC5405836
218. Greenstein M, Breitbart W. Cancer and the experience of meaning: a group psychotherapy program for people with cancer. Am J Psychother. 2000;54: 486. PMID: 11109133
219. Keall RM, Clayton JM, Butlow PN. Therapeutic life review in palliative care: a systematic review of qualitative evaluations. J Pain Symptom Manag. 2015; 49:747. https://doi.org/10.1016/j.jpainsymman.2014.08.015. PMID: 25261637
220. Breitbart W, Gibson C, Poppito S, Berg A. Psychotherapeutic interventions at the end of life: a focus on meaning and spirituality. Can J Psychiatr. 2004;49: 366–72. https://doi.org/10.1177/070674370404900605. PMID: 15283531
221. Fonzo-Christie C, Vukasovic C, Wasilewski-Rsaca AF, Bonnabry P. Subcutaneous administration of drugs in the elderly: survey of practice and systematic literature review. Palliat Med. 2005;19:208–19. https://doi.org/10.1191/0269216304pm1006oa. PMID: 15920935
222. Plaskota M, Lucas C, Evans R, Cook K, Pizzoferro K, et al. A hypnotherapy intervention for the treatment of anxiety in patients with cancer receiving palliative care. Int J Palliat Nurs. 2012;18(2):69–75. https://doi.org/10.12968/ijpn.2012.18.2.69. PMID: 22399044
223. Galfin JM, Watkins ER, Harlow T. A brief guided self-help intervention for psychological distress in palliative care patients: a randomized controlled trial. Palliat Med. 2012;26(3):197–205. https://doi.org/10.1177/0269216311414757. PMID: 21807750
224. Sharpe M, Strong V, Allen K, Rush R, et al. Management of major depression in outpatients attending a cancer center: a preliminary evaluation. Br J Cancer. 2004;90(2):310–3.
225. Greer S, Moorery S, Baruch JD, Watson M, et al. Adjuvant psychological therapy for patients with cancer: a prospective randomized trial. BMJ. 1992; 304:675–80. PMID: 1472184 PMCID: PMC1881503
226. McQuellon RP, Wells M, Hoffman S, Craven B, et al. Reducing distress in cancer patients with an orientation program. Psycho-Oncology. 1998;7:207–17. https://doi.org/10.1002/(SICI)1099-1611(199805/06)7:3<207::AID-PON304>3.0.CO;2-T. PMID: 9638782
227. Chen J, Chen C, Zhi S. Retrospective comparison of cognitive behavioral therapy and symptom-specific medication to treat anxiety and depression in throat cancer patients after laryngectomy. Shanghai Arch Psychiatry. 2014;26(2):95–100. https://doi.org/10.3969/j.issn.1002-0829.2014.02.006.
228. Barseveck AM, Sweeney C, Haney E, Chung E. A systematic qualitative analysis of psychoeducational interventions for depression patients with cancer. Oncol Nurs Forum. 2002;29:73–84. https://doi.org/10.1188/02.ONF.73-87. PMID: 11817494
229. Devine EC, Westlake SK. The effects of psychoeducational care provided to adults with cancer: meta-analysis of 116 studies. Oncol Nursing Forum. 1995;22:1369–81. PMID: 8539178
230. Sheard T, McGuire P. The effect of psychological interventions on axiety and depression in cancer patients: results of two meta-analyses. Br J Cancer. 1999;80:1770–80. https://doi.org/10.1038/sj.bjc.6690596. PMID: 10468295 PMCID: PMC2363129
231. Ell K, Xie B, Quon B, Quinn DI, et al. Randomized controlled trial of collaborative care management of depression among low-income patients with cancer. J Clin Oncol. 2008;26(27):4488–96. https://doi.org/10.1200/JCO.2008.16.6371.
232. Osborn RI, Demoncada AC, Feurestein M. Psychosocial interventions for depression and quality of life in cancer survivors: meta-analysis. Int J Psychiatry Med. 2006;36:13–34. https://doi.org/10.2190/EUFN-RV1K-Y3TR-FK0L. PMID: 16927576
233. Krebber AM, Jansen F, Witte BI, Cuijpers P, et al. Stepped care targeting psychological distress in head and neck cancer and lung cancer patients: a randomized, controlled trial. Ann Oncol. 2016;27(9):1754–60. https://doi.org/10.1093/annonc/mdw230. Epub 2016 Jun 10. DOI: 10.1093/annonc/mdw230, PMID: 27287209
234. Kwiatkowski F, Bignon YJ. To test the impact of hypnotherapy upon immunity and circadian rhythms among palliative cancer patients: a promising goal? Pathol Biol. 2007;55(3–4):186–93. https://doi.org/10.1016/j.patbio.2006.12.006. Epub 2007 Mar 27 PMID: 17391864
235. Check DK, Samuel CA, Rosenstein DL, Dusetzina SB. Investigation of racial disparities in early supportive medication use and end-of-life care among Medicare beneficiaries with stage IV breast cancer. J Clin Oncol. 2016;34(19): 2265–70. https://doi.org/10.1200/JCO.2015.64.8162. Epub 2016 May 9. PMID: 27161968 PMCID: PMC4962709
236. Balyn RE, Rubin JE. Psychiatric treatment challenges at the end of life. Clinical View. 2003;1(2):3–5. http://www.aagponline.org/clientuploads/Clinical%20View/clinicalView_v2n1.pdf
237. de Souza BF, Pires FH, Dewulf Nde L, Inocenti A, et al. Patients on chemotherapy: depression and adherence to treatment. Rev Esc Enferm USP. 2013;47(1):61–8. PMID: 23515804
238. Wang CW, Chow AY, Chan CL. The effects of life review interventions on spiritual well-being, psychological distress, and quality of life in patients with terminal or advanced cancer: a systematic review and metaanalysis of randomized controlled trials. Palliat Med. 2017;31(10):883–94. https://doi.org/10.1177/0269216317705101. PMID: 28488923
239. Scheffold K, Schulz-Kinderman F, Rosenberger C, Wollbrueck D, et al. Pilot results of the German managing concern and living meaningfully (CALM) RCT: a brief individual psychotherapy for advanced cancer patients. Psycho-Oncology. 2014;23(28) Doi:10111/j.1099-1611.2014.3693
240. Miller DK, Chibnall JT, Videen SD, Duckro PN. Supportive-affective group experience for persons with life-threatening illness: reducing spirtual, psychological, and death-related distress in dying patients. J Palliat Med. 2005;2(8):333–43. https://doi.org/10.1089/jpm.2005.8.333. PMID: 15890044
241. Steinhauser KE, Alexander SC, Byock IR, George LK, et al. Do preparation and life completion discussions improve functioning and quality of life in seriously ill patients? Pilot randomized control trial. J Palliat Med. 2008;9(11): 1234–40. https://doi.org/10.1089/jpm.2008.0078. PMID: 19021487
242. Johnson RJ. Cost-effectiveness of mental health services for persons with a dual diagnosis: a literature review and the CCMHCP. The cost-effectiveness of community mental health Care for Single and Dually Diagnosed Project. J Subst Abus Treat. 2000;18(2):119–27. PMID: 10716095
243. Kvale E, Balentine A, Walker E. Depression and fatigue. New York: Oxford University Press; 2015.
244. NCCN. Clinical Practice Guidelines in Oncology. Distress management. Version 3. 2015. National Comprehensive Cancer Network. Htpp://https://www.nccn.org/professionals/physician_gls/pdf/distress.pdf.

Does Chinese calligraphy therapy reduce neuropsychiatric symptoms

Kuan-Yu Chu[1,2,3*], Chih-Yang Huang[2] and Wen-Chen Ouyang[4,5]

Abstract

Background: There are currently no systematic reviews or meta-analyses of Chinese calligraphy therapy (CCT) to reduce neuropsychiatric symptoms. The aim of this systematic review and meta-analysis was to explore the efficacy of CCT for people with neuropsychiatric symptoms.

Methods: We searched Chinese and English databases, including the Cochrane Central Register of Controlled Trials and Wanfang Data for relevant articles published between the earliest year available and December 2016. The search was limited to randomized controlled trials and controlled clinical studies and the associated keywords were "handwriting," "Chinese calligraphy," "Chinese calligraphy therapy," "Calligraphy exercise," and "Calligraphy training." The 21 articles that met these criteria were used in the analysis. The Joanna Briggs Institute critical appraisal checklist was used to assess methodological quality.

Results: CCT significantly reduced psychosis (10 studies, 965 subjects, standardized mean difference [SMD] = − 0.17, 95% confidence intervals [CI] [− 0.30, − 0.40], $Z = 2.60$, $p < 0.01$), anxiety symptoms (9 studies, 579 subjects, SMD = − 0.78, 95% CI [− 0.95, − 0.61], $Z = 8.98$, $p < 0.001$), and depressive symptoms (7 studies, 456 subjects, SMD = − 0.69, 95% CI [− 0.88, − 0.50], $Z = 7.11$, $p < 0.001$). CCT also significantly improved cognitive function (2 studies, 55 subjects, MD = 2.17, 95% CI [− 0.03, 4.38], $Z = 1.93$, $p = 0.05$) and neurofeedback (3 studies, 148 subjects, SMD = − 1.09, 95% CI [− 1.44, − 0.73], $Z = 6.01$, $p < 0.001$). The therapy also significantly reduced the positive psychopathological expression of schizophrenia symptoms (4 studies, 287 subjects, SMD = − 0.35, 95% CI [− 0.59, − 0.12], $Z = 2.96$, $p = 0.003$) and reduced the negative symptoms of schizophrenia (4 studies, 276 subjects, SMD = − 1.39, 95% CI [− 1.65, − 1.12], $Z = 10.23$, $p < 0.001$).

Conclusions: CCT exerts a curative effect on neuropsychiatric symptoms, but the evidence remains insufficient. A large number of RCTs are needed to facilitate additional systematic reviews of evidence for CCT.

Keywords: Chinese calligraphy, Art therapy, Psychiatric disorders

Background

The term psychosis refers to a serious psychological disorder characterized by obvious and long-lasting abnormalities in understanding, emotion, cognition, behavior, and other psychological activities. Psychoses such as schizophrenia often involve cognitive impairment and comorbid anxiety and depression [1]. Pharmacological therapy often has a limited effect or produces side effects [2, 3]. Non-pharmacological therapies (such as psychotherapy, occupational therapy, and art therapy) for patients with psychiatric disorders are useful, adaptable, and potentially cost-effective approaches to improve outcomes and quality of life [4].

Chinese calligraphy therapy (CCT) is a branch of art therapy that involves visual–spatial patterning of characters. This type of calligraphy is more than an art therapy; in essence, it involves culture, health, behaviour treatment and rehabilitation. The art nature is only one of its varied roles and functions. It necessitates exercising motor control of the brush to follow

* Correspondence: kyc032@gmail.com
[1]Taoyuan General Hospital, Taoyuan City, Taiwan
[2]Department of Fine Art & Culture Creative Design, Hua-Fan University, New Taipei City, Taiwan
Full list of author information is available at the end of the article

specific character configurations based on a projection of the cognitive images of the characters [5]. CCT requires the use of a soft-tipped brush to reproduce Chinese glyphs. It combines physical, mental, and personal processes and integrates visual performance, spatial abilities, and cognitive planning [6].

Recent empirical studies have shown that the practice of calligraphy may improve behavioral and psychosomatic disorders and may have a therapeutic effect on attention and emotional stability [7]. CCT has been scientifically investigated within the contexts of psychology, cognitive science, and cognitive neuroscience, and the findings suggest that it can reduce neuropsychiatric symptoms [8].

There have been many systematic reviews of other art therapies, such as painting therapy, music therapy, and gardening therapy. However, there are no systematic reviews or meta-analyses of CCT's effect in reducing neuropsychiatric symptoms. Thus, the aim of this systematic review and meta-analysis was to explore the efficacy of CCT for people with neuropsychiatric symptoms.

Methods

Search strategy

A systematic search for articles was made in December 2016 using the databases MEDLINE, EMBASE, PsycINFO, Cochrane Central Register of Controlled Trials, and Wanfang Data. We searched for keywords and/or controlled vocabulary, such as medical subject headings and Emtree terms. Keywords were "handwriting," "Chinese calligraphy," "Chinese calligraphy therapy," "Calligraphy exercise," and "Calligraphy training."

Study selection

We included in the analysis studies that met the following criteria: (1) randomized controlled trial (RCT), cohort study, or case-control study, (2) published in Chinese or English, (3) subjects were either healthy or psychiatric patients, (4) experimental group intervention measures for Chinese calligraphy; the control group intervention could be general care, health education, or no care, and (5) measurement of physiological or mental indicators. The exclusion criteria were as follows: (1) not relevant to Chinese calligraphy/calligraphy therapy, (2) commentary, case report, or a review article, (3) experimental interventions other than calligraphy treatment, (4) and lack of a control group and/or overlapping populations.

Quality assessment

We used the guideline suggested by Queen's Joanna Briggs Collaboration critical appraisal checklist, Version 4.0 [9]. This scale contains 10 appraisal criteria that assess whether the assignment to treatment groups was truly random, participants were blinded to treatment allocation, allocation to treatment groups was concealed from the allocator, the outcomes of people who withdrew were described and included in the analysis, those assessing the outcomes were blind to the treatment allocation, the control and treatment groups were comparable at entry, the groups were treated identically other than for the named interventions, the outcomes were

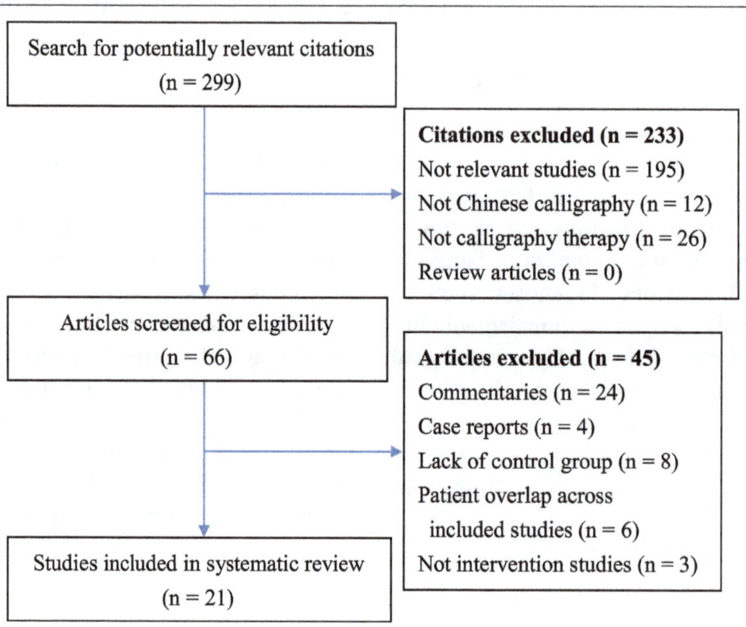

Fig. 1 Flow diagram of study selection

Table 1 Characteristics of studies that fulfilled inclusion criteria

Study	Inclusion criteria	No. of patients	Treatment duration	Ages (yrs) (mean ± SD)	Main measurement scale	Intervention
Luo 2000 [14]	Military college students	P: 31 C: 24	30 days	23.9	SCL-90	Calligraphy
Cui 2003 [11]	Senior college students	P: 60 C: 40	1 year	P: 65.4 ± 5.25 C: 64.8 ± 8.46	SCL-90	Calligraphy and painting
Zhou B 2005 [15]	Grade 3 elementary school students	P: 87 C: 37	2 years	–	CPQ	Calligraphy
Zhou GQ 2005 [16]	Patients with schizophrenia	P: 15 C: 21	20 weeks	P: 49.67 ± 6.9 C: 53.33 ± 6.64	PANSS TESS	Calligraphy
Dong 2006 [17]	Patients with anxiety	P: 28 C: 27	8 weeks	P: 32.4 ± 7.8 C: 30.5 ± 8.6	HAMA SAS, CGI	Calligraphy
Zhao 2006 [18]	Patients with chronic schizophrenia	P: 48 C: 50	8 weeks	P: 25 ± 8.6 C: 24 ± 7.8	SCL-90	Calligraphy
Guo 2007 [19]	Schizophrenic inpatients	P: 30 C: 30	2 months	P: 31.3 ± 11.6 C: 32.3 ± 11.7	SAS, SDS	Music, calligraphy, painting, and dancing
Zeng 2007 [20]	Patients with generalized anxiety	P: 34 C: 34	8 weeks	P: 32.49 ± 8.2 C: 33.2 ± 8.3	HAMA SAS	Calligraphy
Zheng 2008 [21]	Patients with depression	P: 31 C: 30	6 weeks	P: 37.5 ± 12.5 C: 36.6 ± 12.8	HAMA HAMD	Calligraphy
Li 2010 [22]	Schizophrenic inpatients	P: 30 C: 30	8 weeks	P: 32.6 ± 11.3 C: 32.1 ± 11.2	BPRS SANS	Calligraphy and painting
Yang 2010 [12]	NPC patients	P: 24 C: 29	4 weeks	49.63 ± 10.81	SDS POMS SF	Three groups: relaxation, calligraphy, and control
Zhou 2010 [23]	Schizophrenic inpatients	P: 30 C: 30	3 months	40.38 ± 11.20	BPRS SANS	Calligraphy and painting
Kwok 2011 [13]	Older people with MCI	P: 14 C: 17	8 weeks	P: 85.79 ± 4.93 C: 85.76 ± 6.93	CMMSE	Calligraphy
Tian 2012 [24]	Patients with chronic schizophrenia	P: 60 C: 60	6 months	36.21 ± 2.54	BPRS	Occupational therapy, fine art, and calligraphy
Zhang 2012 [25]	Schizophrenic inpatients	P: 30 C: 30	12 months	–	PANSS	Calligraphy and painting
Dong 2013 [26]	Patients with chronic schizophrenia	P: 35 C: 34	12 weeks	P: 32 ± 7 C: 31 ± 9	SCL-90 PANSS	Calligraphy or drawing
Xu 2013 [27]	Undergraduate students	P: 8 C: 8	10 days	–	EEG-theta waves	Calligraphy
Zhou 2013 [28]	Grade 3 to 4 elementary school students	P: 101 C: 69	2 school years	P: 8.60 ± 0.55 C: 8.59 ± 0.41	PANAC-c CERO-k	Calligraphy
Zhu 2014 [29]	Children with hyperarousal symptoms	P: 64 C: 38	30 days	P: 10.52 ± 1.16 C: 10.54 ± 1.15	Salivary cortisol level	Calligraphy
		P: 129		P: 10.51 ± 1.15	CRIES	

Table 1 Characteristics of studies that fulfilled inclusion criteria *(Continued)*

Study	Inclusion criteria	No. of patients	Treatment duration	Ages (yrs) (mean ± SD)	Main measurement scale	Intervention
		C: 81		C: 10.52 ± 1.13		
Tai 2016 [8]	Patients with AD	P: 14 C: 10	6 weeks	P: 70.21 ± 7.9 C: 76.3 ± 7.03	CDR-SB TC MMSE, GDS-S	Tai-chi, calligraphy, and drawing
Chan 2016 [30]	Individuals with MCI	P: 14 C: 16	8 weeks	P: 65.9 ± 5.0 C: 66.4 ± 3.65	Reaction time on the Chinese and digit 2-back and detection tasks	Calligraphy

Abbreviations: SCL-90 Symptom Checklist 90, *CPQ* Children's Personality Questionnaire, *PANSS* Positive and Negative Symptom Scale, *TESS* Treatment Emergent Symptom Scale, *HAMA* Hamilton Anxiety Scale, *SAS* Self-Rating Anxiety Scale, *CGI* Clinical Global Impression Scale, *SDS* Symptom Distress Scale, *HAMD* Hamilton Depression Rating Scale, *POMS SF* Profile of Mood State - Short Form, *BPRS* The Brief Psychiatric Rating Scale, *SANS* Scale for the Assessment of Negative Symptoms, *CMMSE* Chinese version of the Mini-Mental State Examination, *EEG* electroencephalogram, *PANAC-c* Positive and Negative Affect Scale for Children, *CERO-k* Child version of the Cognitive Emotion Regulation Questionnaire, *CRIES* Children's Revised Impact of Event Scale, *CDR-SB* Clinical Dementia Rating Sum of Boxes, *TC MMSE* Traditional Chinese version of the Mini-Mental State Examination, *GDS-S* Geriatric Depression Scale, *SD* standard deviation, *NPC* nasopharyngeal carcinoma, *AD* Alzheimer's disease, *MCI* mild cognitive impairment, *P* patient or experiment, *C* control, $^{*}p < 0.05$, $^{**}p < 0.01$

Study or Subgroup	Experimental Mean	Experimental SD	Experimental Total	Control Mean	Control SD	Control Total	Weight	Std. Mean Difference IV, Fixed, 95% CI	Year
Luo 2000	-0.25	0.29	31	-0.18	18	24	5.9%	-0.01 [-0.54, 0.53]	2000
Cui 2003	1.15	0.64	60	1.21	0.57	40	10.5%	-0.10 [-0.50, 0.30]	2003
Zhou B 2005	5.83	1.89	87	6.35	2.02	37	11.3%	-0.27 [-0.65, 0.12]	2005
Zhao 2006	1.39	0.61	48	1.4	0.72	50	10.7%	-0.01 [-0.41, 0.38]	2006
Dong 2006	2.51	0.63	28	2.95	0.98	27	5.8%	-0.53 [-1.07, 0.01]	2006
Zhang 2012	22.92	2.77	30	24.84	3.13	30	6.2%	-0.64 [-1.16, -0.12]	2012
Zhou 2013	29.86	10.6	101	30.41	11.9	69	17.9%	-0.05 [-0.36, 0.26]	2013
Dong 2013	1.38	0.49	35	1.4	0.53	34	7.5%	-0.04 [-0.51, 0.43]	2013
Zhu 2014	5.24	4.93	129	6.1	5.17	81	21.7%	-0.17 [-0.45, 0.11]	2014
Tai 2016	4.75	2.44	14	5.7	1.87	10	2.5%	-0.41 [-1.23, 0.41]	2016
Total (95% CI)			**563**			**402**	**100.0%**	**-0.17 [-0.30, -0.04]**	

Heterogeneity: $Chi^2 = 7.42$, df = 9 (P = 0.59); $I^2 = 0\%$
Test for overall effect: Z = 2.60 (P = 0.009)

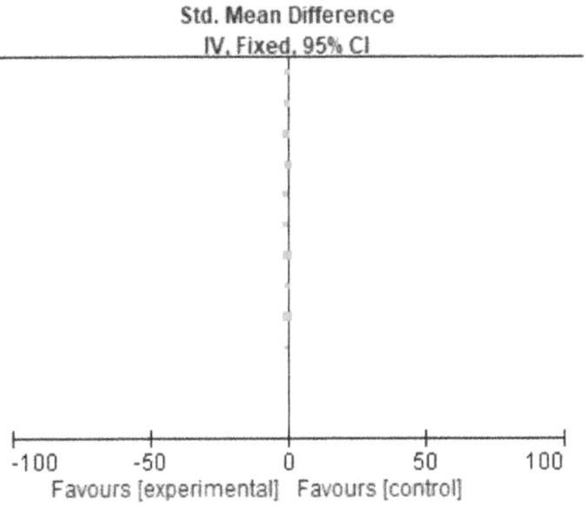

Fig. 2 Forest plot of comparison: Experimental (Chinese calligraphy therapy, etc.) versus Control. Outcome: index of psychosis

measured in the same way for all groups, the outcomes were measured in a reliable way, and the statistical analysis was appropriate. Two researchers extracted information and screened the quality of the articles independently. A third researcher was used to determine the quality of the studies in cases where it was difficult to reach a consensus.

Data analysis

Meta-analysis was performed using RevMan 5.3 software (Review Manager (RevMan) [Computer program]. Version 5.3. Copenhagen: The Nordic Cochrane Centre, The Cochrane Collaboration, 2014.). The mean and standard deviation of each group was calculated to determine the overall effect of the intervention. Chi-square was used to determine heterogeneity. In addition, I2 values were calculated to test the heterogeneity among the studies. When I2 was < 50%, a fixed-effects model was used to determine the homogeneity among studies [10]. However, if there were differences between the studies (such as study location, population, and intervention program), a random-effects model analysis was used to avoid underestimation of treatment variability. Odds ratios and mean differences were used to compare different measurement indexes, to obtain standardized mean differences (SMD), and to estimate the combined effect level. Based on the different psychiatric symptoms and diseases included in the studies, we divided the meta-analysis into six groups: group 1: psychosis, group 2: anxiety, group 3: depression, group 4: cognition, group 5: neurofeedback, and group 6: schizophrenia.

Results

Characteristics of the studies

Figure 1 shows the process of study selection. Our initial search strategy yielded 299 citations, 233 of which were ineligible based on our screening of titles and abstracts. Thus, we retrieved the full text of 66 studies. Of these, 24 were excluded because they were commentaries; 4 were case reports; 8 lacked a control group; 6 had study populations that overlapped with other included studies; and 3 did not meet the eligibility criteria because they were not intervention studies. Consequently, 21 eligible studies were analyzed.

Table 1 shows study characteristics and patient demographic data from each of the 21 studies included in the review. These studies were published between 2000 and 2016, and had sample sizes ranging from 16 to 224. Ten studies measured psychosis or general psychosis (the meta-analysis results and forest

Study or Subgroup	Experimental Mean	Experimental SD	Experimental Total	Control Mean	Control SD	Control Total	Weight	Std. Mean Difference IV, Fixed, 95% CI	Year
Luo 2000	-0.12	0.41	31	0.1	0.32	24	9.8%	-0.58 [-1.13, -0.04]	2000
Zhao 2006	1.23	0.66	48	1.82	0.56	50	16.5%	-0.96 [-1.38, -0.54]	2006
Dong 2006	10.86	6.98	28	14.58	8.65	27	10.1%	-0.47 [-1.00, 0.07]	2006
Guo 2007	41.61	9.12	30	49.31	9.28	30	10.4%	-0.83 [-1.35, -0.30]	2007
Zeng 2007	8.46	5.93	34	13.62	7.48	34	11.9%	-0.76 [-1.25, -0.26]	2007
Zheng 2008	8.45	2.81	31	12.45	3.92	30	9.7%	-1.16 [-1.71, -0.62]	2008
Yang 2009	3.5	1.69	24	4.04	1.54	29	9.8%	-0.33 [-0.88, 0.21]	2009
Li 2010	5.61	1.23	30	6.72	1.35	30	10.3%	-0.85 [-1.38, -0.32]	2010
Dong 2013	1.24	0.65	35	1.83	0.58	34	11.6%	-0.95 [-1.45, -0.45]	2013
Total (95% CI)			**291**			**288**	**100.0%**	**-0.78 [-0.95, -0.61]**	

Heterogeneity: $Chi^2 = 7.53$, df = 8 (P = 0.48); $I^2 = 0\%$
Test for overall effect: Z = 8.98 (P < 0.00001)

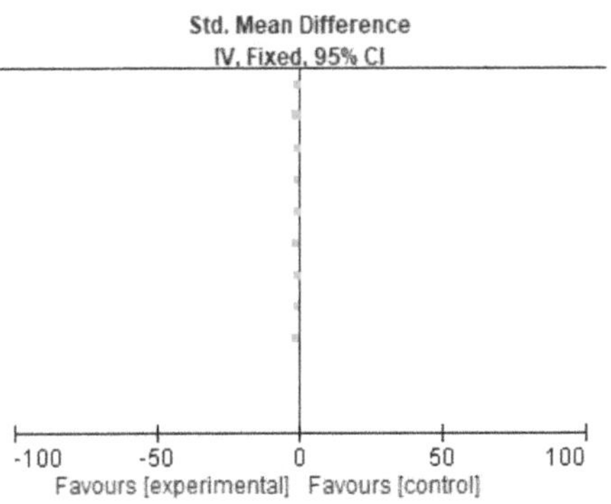

Fig. 3 Forest plot of comparison: Experimental (Chinese calligraphy therapy, etc.) versus Control. Outcome: index of anxiety

Study or Subgroup	Experimental Mean	Experimental SD	Experimental Total	Control Mean	Control SD	Control Total	Weight	Std. Mean Difference IV, Fixed, 95% CI	Year
Luo 2000	-0.31	0.39	31	-0.09	0.26	24	12.1%	-0.64 [-1.19, -0.09]	2000
Zhao 2006	1.49	0.71	48	1.83	0.65	50	22.3%	-0.50 [-0.90, -0.09]	2006
Guo 2007	42.32	9.21	30	50.58	8.84	30	12.7%	-0.90 [-1.44, -0.37]	2007
Zheng 2008	7.2	4.32	31	11.4	5.42	30	13.1%	-0.85 [-1.37, -0.32]	2008
Yang 2009	3.79	1.91	24	5.76	2.78	29	11.4%	-0.80 [-1.36, -0.24]	2009
Li 2010	5.61	1.23	30	6.72	1.35	30	12.8%	-0.85 [-1.38, -0.32]	2010
Dong 2013	1.5	0.72	35	1.84	0.67	34	15.7%	-0.48 [-0.96, -0.00]	2013
Total (95% CI)			**229**			**227**	**100.0%**	**-0.69 [-0.88, -0.50]**	

Heterogeneity: $Chi^2 = 3.09$, df = 6 (P = 0.80); $I^2 = 0\%$
Test for overall effect: Z = 7.11 (P < 0.00001)

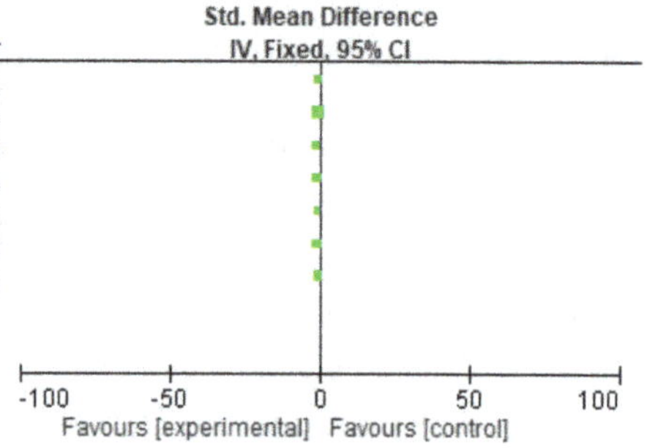

Fig. 4 Forest plot of comparison: Experimental (Chinese calligraphy therapy, etc.) versus Control. Outcome: index of depression

map are shown in Fig. 2). Nine studies on anxiety were analyzed; one study was removed [11] because the sensitivity analysis indicated large heterogeneity (Fig. 3). Seven studies on depression were analyzed (Fig. 4). Two studies on cognitive impairment were analyzed (Fig. 5) and three studies on neurofeedback were analyzed (Fig. 6).

Eight studies evaluated patients with schizophrenia, of which four measured positive psychopathology of schizophrenia and four measured negative syndromes of schizophrenia (see Figs. 7 and 8).

Table 2 shows the methodological quality of the 21 included studies. Two studies clearly documented the use of random allocation [12, 13]. The remaining quality criteria were scored based on the narrative of the studies. The scores for risk of bias ranged from 6 to 9 points. Agreement between the two reviewers was assessed using Cohen's kappa coefficient and was 0.891 ($p < 0.001$), indicating a high degree of consistency.

Figure 2 shows the meta-analysis results for group 1. Using a fixed-effects model, the heterogeneity test (I2) result for the seven studies was 0%, indicating homogeneity among the studies. The SMD was used to estimate the combined effect of measurements using different scales. The results showed that CCT can significantly reduce psychosis (10 studies, 965 subjects, SMD = – 0.17, 95% CI [– 0.30, – 0.04], Z = 2.60, $p = 0.009$).

Figure 3 shows the meta-analysis results for group 2. Using a fixed-effects model, the heterogeneity test (I2) was 0%, indicating that the nine studies were homogeneous. The SMD indicated that calligraphy treatment significantly reduced anxiety symptoms (9 studies, 579 subjects, SMD = – 0.78, 95% CI [– 0.95, – 0.61], Z = 8.98, $p < 0.001$).

Figure 4 shows the meta-analysis results for group 3. Using a fixed-effects model, the heterogeneity test (I2) was 0%, indicating that the seven studies were homogeneous. The SMD indicated that calligraphy treatment significantly reduced depressive symptoms (7 studies, 456 subjects, SMD = – 0.69, 95% CI [– 0.88, – 0.50], Z = 7.11, $p < 0.001$). Figure 5 shows the meta-analysis results for group 4. Using a fixed-effects model, the heterogeneity test (I2) was 0%, indicating that the two studies were homogeneous. The estimated combined effect showed that CCT significantly improved cognitive function (2 studies, 55 subjects, MD = 2.17, 95% CI [– 0.03, 4.38], Z = 1.93, $p = 0.05$). Figure 6 shows the meta-analysis results for group 5. Using a fixed-effects model, the heterogeneity test (I2) was 0%, indicating that the three studies were homogeneous. The estimated combined effect showed that CCT significantly improved neurofeedback (3 studies, 148 subjects, SMD = – 1.09, 95% CI [– 1.44, – 0.73], Z = 6.01, $p < 0.001$). Figure 7 shows the meta-analysis results for group 6–1 (schizophrenia-psychopathy). Using a fixed-effects model, the heterogeneity test (I2) was 0%, indicating that the four studies were homogeneous. The estimated combined effect showed that CCT significantly reduced positive psychopathological expression of schizophrenia symptoms (4 studies, 287 subjects, SMD = – 0.35, 95% CI [– 0.59, – 0.12], Z = 2.96, $p = 0.003$). Figure 8 shows the meta-analysis results for group 6–2 (schizophrenia-negative

Study or Subgroup	Experimental Mean	Experimental SD	Experimental Total	Control Mean	Control SD	Control Total	Weight	Mean Difference IV, Fixed, 95% CI	Year
Kwok 2011	25.07	3.1	14	22.47	3.99	17	78.1%	2.60 [0.10, 5.10]	2011
Tai 2016	19.86	6.7	14	19.2	5.07	10	21.9%	0.66 [-4.05, 5.37]	2016
Total (95% CI)			**28**			**27**	**100.0%**	**2.17 [-0.03, 4.38]**	

Heterogeneity: $Chi^2 = 0.51$, df = 1 (P = 0.48); $I^2 = 0\%$
Test for overall effect: Z = 1.93 (P = 0.05)

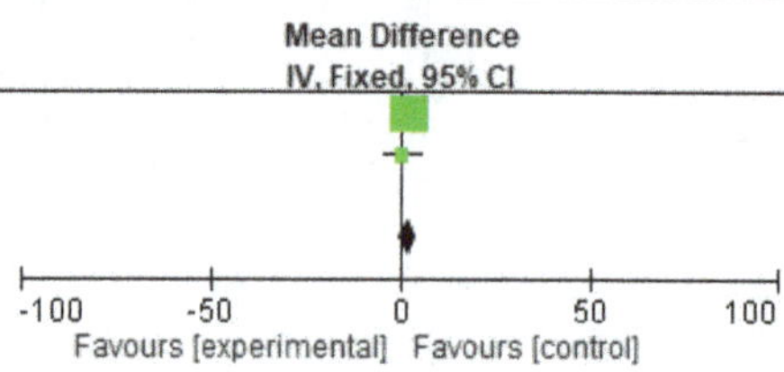

Fig. 5 Forest plot of comparison: Experimental (Chinese calligraphy therapy, etc.) versus Control. Outcome: index of cognitive function

Study or Subgroup	Experimental Mean	Experimental SD	Experimental Total	Control Mean	Control SD	Control Total	Weight	Std. Mean Difference IV, Fixed, 95% CI	Year
Xu 2013	9.6	2.16	8	10.96	2.16	8	12.4%	-0.60 [-1.60, 0.41]	2013
Zhu 2014	9.99	1.81	64	12.67	2.7	38	66.1%	-1.22 [-1.66, -0.78]	2014
Chan 2016	792.9	187.8	14	1,033.3	281.1	16	21.6%	-0.97 [-1.73, -0.20]	2016
Total (95% CI)			**86**			**62**	**100.0%**	**-1.09 [-1.44, -0.73]**	

Heterogeneity: Chi² = 1.36, df = 2 (P = 0.51); I² = 0%
Test for overall effect: Z = 6.01 (P < 0.00001)

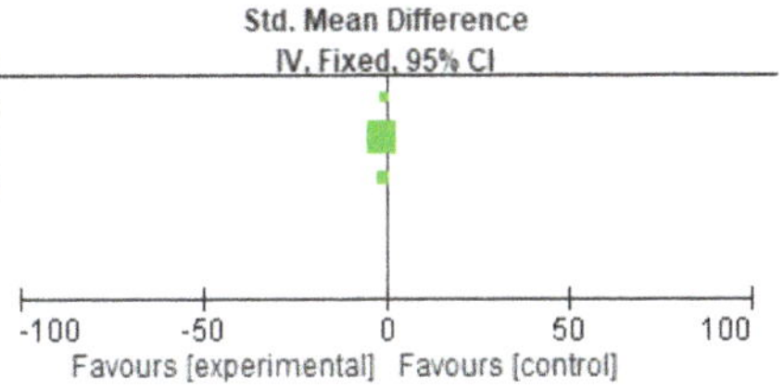

Fig. 6 Forest plot of comparison: Experimental (Chinese calligraphy therapy, etc.) versus Control. Outcome: index of neurofeedback

syndrome). Using a fixed-effects model, the heterogeneity test (I2) was 15%, indicating that the four studies were homogeneous. The estimated combined effect showed that CCT significantly reduced negative symptoms of schizophrenia (4 studies, 276 subjects, SMD = – 1.39, 95% CI [– 1.65, – 1.12], Z = 10.23, $p < 0.001$).

Discussion

The purpose of this study was to explore the effectiveness of calligraphy therapy in improving symptoms of psychiatric disorders by reviewing and analyzing relevant literature. Twenty-one studies met the inclusion criteria and were reviewed. Most of the evidence suggests that CCT can change targeted behaviors in individuals with neuropsychiatric symptoms and that CCT is associated with improvements in objective measurements of psychiatric performance.

Evidence from these kinds of studies is needed before CCT can be considered effective for neuropsychiatric symptoms. The study findings reviewed here suggest that, used as psychiatric therapy, CCT can significantly improve selected neuropsychiatric symptoms. The use of CCT in compensation-focused interventions and selected psychotherapeutic interventions may lead to neuropsychiatric changes and thus improve daily life.

RCTs provide the best evidence of the efficacy of CCT. In RCTs with large samples, there is more balance between the characteristics of participants in the treatment and control groups. In small-sample RCTs, some characteristics may not be balanced between groups. Table 1 shows that most of the sample sizes in each group were between 15 and 30. Only about half of the included studies had quality scores greater than 8 (Table 2). Therefore, more high-quality RCTs are needed to strengthen the evidence for CCT's effect in reducing neuropsychiatric symptoms. If more systematic reviews are produced to establish clinical guidelines, this could increase the clinical use of CCT.

A funnel plot of the CCT literature was symmetrical (i.e., showed no positive or negative relations between effect size and standard error). This indicates that there was no publication error. The best way to avoid publication bias is to begin with a rigorous examination of the literature.

As this is the first review of the efficacy of CCT for neuropsychiatric symptoms, we are unable to compare the findings with other similar studies. Compared with other non-pharmacological therapies like music therapy, painting therapy, or gardening therapy, CCT is perhaps a more culture-specific therapy, as it requires participants to learn Chinese writing and use a special soft calligraphy brush.

Our findings show that calligraphy therapy can significantly enhance cognitive function and relieve neuropsychiatric and depressive symptoms. However, there were some study limitations. First, studies varied markedly in their intervention approaches and selected outcome measures, and were frequently hampered by design limitations. Second, the pattern of effects on specific neuropsychiatric domains was inconsistent across studies. Additionally, some important outcomes, such as daily functioning, quality of life, and neuropsychiatric symptom severity, were assessed infrequently in the reviewed studies. Moreover, handwritten communication has largely been replaced by typed communications

Study or Subgroup	Experimental Mean	Experimental SD	Experimental Total	Control Mean	Control SD	Control Total	Weight	Std. Mean Difference IV, Fixed, 95% CI	Year
Zhao 2006	1.42	0.63	48	1.69	0.78	50	34.2%	-0.38 [-0.78, 0.02]	2006
Guo 2007	2.76	0.72	30	3.22	0.79	30	20.3%	-0.60 [-1.12, -0.08]	2007
Zhang 2012	10.75	1.23	30	11.17	1.18	30	21.0%	-0.34 [-0.85, 0.17]	2012
Dong 2013	17.8	5.91	35	18.64	7.56	34	24.5%	-0.12 [-0.60, 0.35]	2013
Total (95% CI)			**143**			**144**	**100.0%**	**-0.35 [-0.59, -0.12]**	

Heterogeneity: Chi² = 1.81, df = 3 (P = 0.61); I² = 0%
Test for overall effect: Z = 2.96 (P = 0.003)

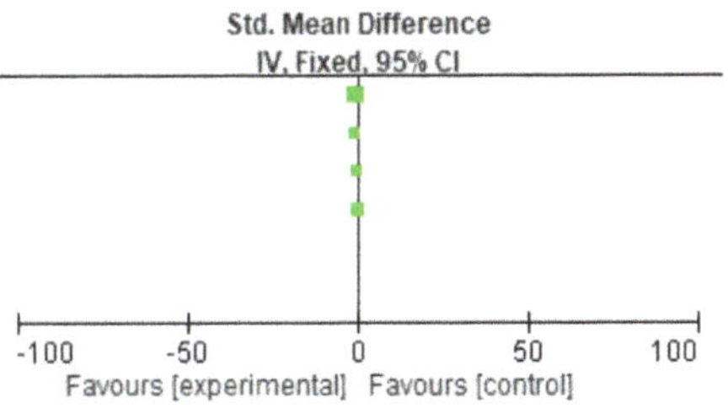

Fig. 7 Forest plot of comparison: Experimental (Chinese calligraphy therapy, etc.) versus Control. Outcome: index of schizophrenia-psychopathy

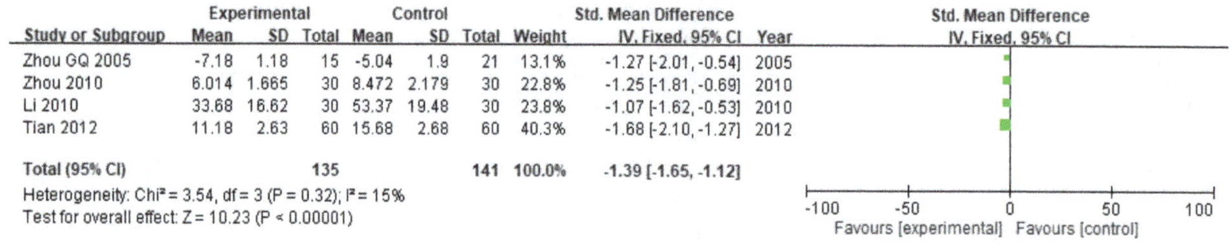

Fig. 8 Forest plot of comparison: Experimental (Chinese calligraphy therapy, etc.) versus Control. Outcome: index of schizophrenia-negative syndrome

(and, in more recent years, by mobile phone calls and texts). This may have affected the results.

Overall, the results from trials are promising but inconclusive. Additional well-designed and adequately powered trials are warranted. However, this evidence must be treated with caution because of methodological limitations. To better assess the value of non-pharmacological interventions for this population, we recommend the following: (1) RCTs should have a large size of over 30 subjects; (2) standards for cognitive/neuropsychiatric rehabilitation must be established for treatment of diseases, such as stroke, Alzheimer's disease and MCI; (3) general character templates for adaptation and modification in diverse fields of clinical trials must be standardized; (4) character form design must be set; (5) authority for standards of template designs, protocols for CCT and a large database for cases and trial follow ups must be established.

Table 2 Methodological quality assessment of the included studies (JBI)

Study	Study design	Score criteria										
		1	2	3	4	5	6	7	8	9	10	Total
Luo 2000	CCS	0	0	0	1	1	1	1	1	1	1	7
Cui 2003	CCS	0	0	0	1	1	1	1	1	1	1	7
Zhou B 2005	CS	0	0	0	1	0	1	1	1	1	1	6
Zhou GQ 2005	CCS	0	0	0	1	1	1	1	1	1	1	7
Dong 2006	RCT	1	1	1	0	1	1	1	1	1	1	9
Zhao 2006	RCT	1	1	0	1	1	1	1	1	1	1	9
Guo 2007	RCT	1	1	0	0	1	1	1	1	1	1	8
Zeng 2007	RCT	1	1	0	0	1	1	1	1	1	1	8
Zheng 2008	RCT	1	1	0	0	1	1	1	1	1	1	8
Li 2010	RCT	1	1	0	0	1	1	1	1	1	1	8
Yang 2010	RCT	1	1	0	1	1	1	1	1	1	1	9
Zhou 2010	RCT	1	1	0	0	1	1	1	1	1	1	8
Kwok 2011	RCT	1	0	0	0	1	1	1	1	1	1	6
Tian 2012	RCT	1	1	0	1	1	1	1	1	1	1	9
Zhang 2012	CCS	1	0	0	0	1	1	1	1	1	1	7
Dong 2013	RCT	1	1	1	0	1	1	1	1	1	1	9
Xu 2013	CCS	0	0	0	0	1	1	1	1	1	1	6
Zhou 2013	CS	0	0	0	1	0	1	1	1	1	1	6
Zhu 2014	RCT	1	1	0	0	1	1	1	1	1	1	8
Tai 2016	CCS	0	0	0	0	1	1	1	1	1	1	6
Chan 2016	RCT	1	1	0	0	1	1	1	1	1	1	8

Abbreviations: *JBI* Joanna Briggs Institute, *RCT* randomized controlled trial, *CCS* controlled clinical study, *CS* cohort study

Score criteria: 1. Was the assignment to treatment groups truly random? 2. Were participants blinded to treatment allocation? 3. Was allocation to treatment groups concealed from the allocator? 4. Were the outcomes of people who withdrew described and included in the analysis? 5. Were those assessing the outcomes blind to the treatment allocation? 6. Were control and treatment groups comparable at entry? 7. Were groups treated identically other than for the named interventions? 8. Were outcomes measured in the same way for all groups? 9. Were outcomes measured in a reliable way? 10. Was appropriate statistical analysis used?

Score descriptions: yes = 1, no = 0, unclear = 0, not applicable = 0

Conclusion

This study shows that CCT exerts a curative effect on neuropsychiatric symptoms, but the evidence remains insufficient. A large number of RCTs are needed to facilitate additional systematic reviews of evidence for CCT. In general, we hope that this paper offers a method for a systematic CCT review and meta-analysis, which may provide a basis for establishing standards for CCT in clinical trials and applications in the future.

Acknowledgments

We thank Diane Williams, PhD, from Edanz Group (www.edanzediting.com) for editing a draft of this manuscript.

Funding

This project received funding from Taoyuan General Hospital under agreement no. PTH10534. The corresponding author had full access to all data in the study and had final responsibility for the decision to submit for publication. The sponsor of the study had no role in the study design, data collection, analysis, interpretation, or writing of the paper.

Authors' contributions

KYC and CYH designed the study and contributed substantially to the design of the search strategy. KYC and CYH searched the literature and extracted data. WCO performed the analysis and interpreted the data. KYC wrote the first draft of the manuscript and CYH and WCO critically reviewed the manuscript. All authors read and approved the final manuscript.

Consent for publication

Not applicable.

Competing interests

The authors declare that they have no competing interests.

Author details
[1]Taoyuan General Hospital, Taoyuan City, Taiwan. [2]Department of Fine Art & Culture Creative Design, Hua-Fan University, New Taipei City, Taiwan. [3]College of General studies, Yuan-Ze University, Taoyuan City, Taiwan. [4]Jianan Psychiatric Center, Tainan City, Taiwan. [5]Department of Psychiatry, College of Medicine, Kaohsiung Medical University, Kaohsiung, Taiwan.

References

1. American Psychiatric Association. Diagnostic and statistical manual of mental disorders. 5th (DSM-5®). Arlington, VA: American Psychiatric Association; 2013.
2. Bet PM, Hugtenburg JG, Penninx BW, Hoogendijk WJ. Side effects of antidepressants during long-term use in a naturalistic setting. Eur Neuropsychopharmacol. 2013;23:1443–51.
3. Samaras K, Correll CU, Mitchell AJ, De Hert M. Diabetes risk potentially underestimated in youth and children receiving antipsychotics. JAMA Psychiat. 2014;71:209–10.
4. Rodakowski J, Saghafi E, Butters MA, Skidmore ER. Non-pharmacological interventions for adults with mild cognitive impairment and early stage dementia: an updated scoping review. Mol Asp Med. 2015;43-44:38–53.
5. HSR K. Shufa: Chinese calligraphic handwriting (CCH) for health and behavioural therapy. Int J Psychol. 2006;41:282–6.
6. HSR K, Zhu L, Chao AA, Chen HY, ICY L, Zhang M. Calligraphy and meditation for stress reduction: an experimental comparison. Psychol Res Behav Manag. 2014;7:47–52.
7. Zhou B. An experimental study on the influence of calligraphy exercises on children's behavior habits. Chinese calligraphy. Studies. 2007;4:72–80.
8. Tai SY, Hsu CL, Huang SW, Ma TC, Hsieh WC, Yang YH. Effects of multiple training modalities in patients with Alzheimer's disease: a pilot study. Neuropsychiatr Dis Treat. 2016;12:2843–9.
9. Aromataris, E., Fernandez, R. S., Godfrey, C., Holly, C., Khalil, H., & Tungpunkom, P. Methodology for JBI umbrella reviews. 2014.
10. Higgins J, Thompson SG, Deeks JJ, Altman DG. Measuring inconsistency in meta-analyses. Br Med J. 2003;327:557–60.
11. Cui M, Ao X. The effect of calligraphy and painting exercise on mental health of senile college students. Sichuan. Ment Health. 2003;16:85–6.
12. Yang XL, Li HH, Hong MH, HSR K. The effects of Chinese calligraphy handwriting and relaxation training in Chinese nasopharyngeal carcinoma patients: a randomized controlled trial. Int J Nurs Stud. 2010;47:550–9.
13. TCY K, Bai X, HSR K, JCY L, FKY H. Cognitive effects of calligraphy therapy for older people: a randomized controlled trial in Hong Kong. Clin Interv Aging. 2011;6:269–73.
14. Luo Z, Miao DM, Gao D. The emotion regulation of calligraphy training to military college students. Psychol Sci. 2000;23:564–7.
15. Zhou B, Liu J, Sang B. The effect of calligraphy on the development of children's personality. Psychol Sci. 2005;28:1266–8.
16. Zhou GQ, Wang J, Zheng H. Effect of painting and drawing therapy in the mental functional rehabilitation of patients with schizophrenia. Chin J Clin Rehab. 2005;9:50–1.
17. Dong XP, Jia JM, Wang J, Zhang R. A control study of calligraphy training plus venlafaxine in the treatment of anxiety disorder. Chin J Behav Med Sci. 2006;5:027.
18. Zhao J, Deng W, Wen J. Intervention of calligraphy therapy on rehabilitation of chronic schizophrenia. Modern. Nursing. 2006;12:357–8.
19. Guo QF, Tian D, Zhao F. Effect of psychological rehabilitation on comprehensive art intervention for patient with schizophrenia. J Nurs Sci. 2007;22:13–5.
20. Zeng Z. The effect of calligraphy training in the treatment of patient with generalized anxiety disorder. Chin J Health Psychol. 2007;15:483–4.
21. Zheng G, Wang P, Liu XB. The effects of handwriting artist therapy to depression. Med J Chin People's Health. 2008;5:061.
22. Li YM, Li ZQ, Zhang Y. The effect of painting and calligraphy behavior therapy among the clinical rehabilitation of schizophrenia inpatients. Int J Nurs. 2010;29:189–92.
23. Zhou Q. The application of chess painting and calligraphy in the treatment of inpatients with schizophrenia. Straint. Pharm J. 2010;22:173–5.
24. Tian JH. Chronic schizophrenia individualized therapy clinical research. Psychiatrist. 2012;105:13–4.
25. Zhang Z, Bei CL, Wang YL. Effectiveness of handwriting and drawing practice for chronic phase schizophrenia. Med J Chin People's Health. 2012;24:2115–7.
26. Dong ZQ, Shi LY. Art behaviorial therapy for chronic schizophrenia intervention study. Gansu medical. Journal. 2013;32:38–40.
27. Xu M, Kao HSR, Zhang M, Lam SPW, Wang W. Cognitive-neural effects of brush writing of Chinese characters: cortical excitation of theta rhythm. Evid Based Complement Alternat Med. 2013;2013::11. https://doi.org/10.1155/2013/975190.
28. Zhou B, Tang J, Li C, Tang H, Li J. Positive effect of practicing Chinese calligraphic handwriting on emotional regulation strategies in children. J Psychol Sci. 2013;36:98–102.
29. Zhu Z, Wang R, HSR K, Zong Y, Liu Z, Tang S, et al. Effect of calligraphy training on hyperarousal symptoms for childhood survivors of the 2008 China earthquakes. Neuropsychiatr Dis Treat. 2014;10:977–85.
30. Chan SC, Lam TL, Fong KN, Pang MY, Chan CC. Generalization of context-specific training in individuals with mild cognitive impairment: an event-related potential study. Dement Geriatr Cogn Disord Extra. 2016;6:568–79.

18

Behavioral activation versus treatment as usual in naturalistic sample of psychiatric patients with depressive symptoms

Kaisa E. Luoto[1,3*], Lars H. Lindholm[3], Vesa Paavonen[1], Antti Koivukangas[3], Antero Lassila[3], Esa Leinonen[1,2] and Olli Kampman[1,3]

Abstract

Background: More systematic use of evidence-based brief therapies is needed in the treatment of depression within psychiatric care. The aim of this study was to explore the impact of behavioral activation therapy (BA) for patients with depressive symptoms in a routine clinical setting of secondary psychiatric care.

Methods: The BA-treated intervention group ($n = 242$) comprised patients with depressive symptoms (Beck Depression Inventory (BDI) score ≥ 17 at baseline). The control group ($n = 205$) patients received treatment as usual in the same catchment area. The groups were matched at baseline using BDI and Alcohol Use Disorders Identification Test scores and inpatient/outpatient status. The groups were compared at 6-, 12- and 24-month follow-up points on functional outcome (Global Assessment of Functioning scale), service use, dropout and deaths. The Montgomery–Åsberg Depression Rating Scale was used to assess depressive symptoms in the intervention group.

Results: The estimated difference in GAF score between intervention and control group patients was significant at 12- and 24-months follow-up points in favor of intervention group (GAF score difference 4.85 points, $p = 0.006$ and 5.71 points, $p = 0.005$, respectively; estimate for patient group 2.26, $p = 0.036$). The rates of dropout, mortality and service use were similar between the groups. Among the intervention group patients, the estimated improvement in MADRS score compared to baseline was statistically significant throughout the follow-up ($p < 0.001$ at all follow-up points).

Conclusions: The systematic use of BA among secondary psychiatric care depressive patients provides encouraging results despite the patients had various comorbid non-psychotic disorders.

Keywords: Behavioral activation, Depressive disorder, Functional outcome, Naturalistic sample

Background

Depression is a leading cause of burden and often reduces the level of functioning [1]. Recurrent episodes and co-morbidity with other psychiatric symptoms make treatment challenging. Comorbidities of depression are very common in secondary psychiatric care [2] According to the guidelines of American Psychiatric Association and National Institute for Health and Care Excellence [3, 4], non-pharmacological therapeutic intervention should be included in the treatment of depression. Often, chosen therapeutic methods are not standardized or evidence based, although there are well-documented therapeutic options available [5, 6]. Evidence-based brief protocols should be used more widely; these are easy to implement among the usual psychiatric services [7].

It is not possible or necessary to offer every patient long-term therapies. Previous research indicates that some brief therapies are effective [8, 9]. One example of an

* Correspondence: kaisa.luoto@fimnet.fi
[1]Faculty of Medicine and Life Sciences, University of Tampere, PB 100, FI-33014 Tampere, Finland
[3]Department of Psychiatry, Seinäjoki Hospital District, Huhtalantie 53, 60220 Seinäjoki, Finland
Full list of author information is available at the end of the article

evidence-based brief intervention for treatment of depression is behavioral activation (BA) [10, 11]. BA is an application of cognitive-behavioral therapy and includes a maximum of 24 appointments. The aim is to explore the patient's actions in relation to his or her environment. The avoidance of certain actions, and the simultaneous avoidance of negative or otherwise uncomfortable feelings, can result in negative consequences and exacerbate depressive symptoms. BA focuses on helping the patient change this negative circle by changing his or her behavior. To our knowledge, there are no studies exploring the effectiveness of BA in a psychiatric naturalistic patient population. Patients with common comorbidities, such as problematic alcohol use and suicidal behavior, are often excluded from study samples.

The Ostrobothnia Depression Study (ODS) was a benchmark controlled trial (BCT) [12] which in practice means an observational intervention study. BCT can be used to assess the impact of clinical intervention in routine settings (in contrast to RCTs which usually assess the specific intervention in ideal settings). ODS aimed at developing a systematic model for assessment and treatment of patients with depression and comorbid non-psychotic disorders [13]. The purpose was to increase the effectiveness of psychiatric services by implementing a systematic use of brief therapy and improving the process of recognizing patients who could benefit from this type of therapy. The aim of the present study is to explore the benefits of BA in a heterogeneous group of depressed patients in a naturalistic setting and to compare BA with treatment as usual (TAU) in terms of functional recovery, service use, dropout and mortality.

Methods

Study setting and participants

According to the idea of BCTs, the aim of ODS was to study the impact of the selected intervention in real life setting of psychiatric secondary services. The comparisons were made with a control group representing as similar patient population as possible treated with TAU methods in the psychiatric services of the same area. This setting allowed the assessment of differences in outcomes between health care units treating similar patients with different methods (more structured brief intervention vs. treatment as usual).

ODS patients were recruited in five psychiatric outpatient clinics and one psychiatric hospital ward in the South Ostrobothnia hospital district of Finland (population 200,000) during October 2009–October 2013. Consecutive patients who were referred to adult psychiatric services because of depressive symptoms, anxiety, self-destructiveness, insomnia or substance-related problems were screened using the Beck Depression Inventory (BDI, version 1A) [14] . Those with a BDI score ≥ 17 (corresponding to at least moderate-level depression) at the screening phase were included in the intervention group (n = 242). In addition to having depressive symptoms, these patients had various other psychiatric diagnoses which is typical in psychiatric secondary services. Patients with a likely or verified psychotic disorder (other than psychotic depression, International Classification of Diseases [ICD]-10, F2*.**) [15] or organic brain disease were excluded.

The control group (n = 205) was recruited from the South Ostrobothnia hospital district database of psychiatric outpatient clinics not participating in the ODS study (time period: October 2009–December 2012) and from the same psychiatric hospital ward before the start of the ODS (i.e., before 30 September 2009). Patients with a new referral to adult psychiatric services were selected in chronological order if their BDI score was ≥17 at admission and the Alcohol Use Disorders Identification Test (AUDIT) [16] score at admission was available. Patients who had participated in the ODS study or had a likely or verified psychotic disorder (other than psychotic depression, ICD-10, F2*.**) or organic brain disease were excluded. The control group patients were matched with the intervention group patients by clustering according to the current psychiatric hospital contact (inpatient/outpatient), AUDIT score in four categories (0–7, 8–10, 11–19 and 20–40 points) and BDI score in two categories (17–29 or 30–60 points). Roughly 1650 patients' files were screened before the amount of patients in the control group was considered to be close enough to the intervention group. The main characteristics of intervention and control group patients at the baseline are presented in Table 1. The characteristics were mainly similar between the groups, only the baseline GAF score (p = 0.035) and the frequencies of personality disorders as a secondary psychiatric diagnosis (p = 0.037) were statistically significantly different between the groups. The psychiatric diagnoses were register based and determined by the responsible doctor in previous treatment contacts.

Antidepressive medication was used for 239 (98.8%) patients in the intervention group and for 203 (99.5%) patients in the control group (cumulative doses: 28.0 mg, standard deviation [SD] 20.6 mg vs. 26.7 mg, SD 21.2 mg fluoxetine equivalents [17, 18] , respectively). Sixty-six (27.3%) patients in the intervention group and 72 (35.1%) patients in the control group were using antipsychotic medication (cumulative doses: median 62.5 mg, interquartile range [IQR] 93.75 vs. 125 mg, IQR 187.5 chlorpromazine equivalents [19], respectively).

Information on somatic comorbidities was collected during the baseline assessment of the intervention group patients and from the psychiatric patient files of the control group patients. Thirteen patients in the intervention group and one patient in the control group had hypertension

Table 1 The main characteristics of patients at baseline

	Intervention group	Control group	
	n (%)	n (%)	p[e]
Number of patients	242	205	
Female / Male	148 (61.2) / 94 (38.8)	111 (54.1) / 94 (45.9)	0.135
Outpatient / Inpatient	189 (78.1) / 53 (21.9)	156 (76.1) / 49 (23.9)	0.615
Register based[f] clinical diagnosis (ICD-10):			
Primary psychiatric diagnosis			0.103
Depressive disorder (F32.x)	98 (40.5)	89 (50.0)	
Recurrent depressive disorder (F33.x)	92 (38.0)	48 (27.0)	
Bipolar disorder (F31.x)	19 (7.9)	17 (9.6)	
Anxiety disorders (F40–43.x)	9 (3.7)	20 (9.6)	
Other disorders	18 (7.4)	–	
Secondary psychiatric diagnosis			
Panic disorder (F41.x)	26 (10.7)	16 (7.8)	0.296
Phobic and other anxiety disorders (F40,42,43.x)	22 (9.1)	22 (10.8)	0.550
Personality disorder (F6x.x)	9 (3.7)	17 (8.4)	0.037
Tertiary psychiatric diagnosis			
Anxiety disorder (F4x.x)	12 (5.0)	5 (2.5)	0.168
Personality disorder (F6x.x)	8 (3.3)	10 (4.9)	0.393
Alcohol dependence (current)	47 (19.4)	n/a	
Use of other substance (last 12 months)	22 (9.1)	n/a	
	mean (SD)	mean (SD)	p
Age (years)	38.8 (12.2)	39.5 (12.7)	0.567
Baseline MADRS[a]	23.2 (6.7)	n/a	
Baseline BDI[b]	27.9 (7.3)	28.8 (7.9)	0.214
Baseline AUDIT[c]	10.7 (9.9)	9.8 (9.0)	0.319
Baseline GAF[d]	45.9 (10.7)	43.6 (11.7)	0.035

[a]Montgomery–Åsberg Depression Rating Scale
[b]Beck Depression Inventory
[c]Alcohol Use Disorders Identification Test
[d]Global Assessment of Functioning scale
[e]between groups (chi-square test)
[f]Register based diagnoses determined by the responsible doctor in previous treatment contacts

(I10). Four patients in the intervention group had diabetes mellitus type 1 (ICD-10, E10). Eight patients in the intervention group and one patient in the control group had diabetes mellitus type 2 (E11). In the intervention group, five patients had metabolic syndrome (E66), three patients had coronary heart disease (I25) and two patients had sequelae of cerebrovascular disease (I69). The patients in either group didn't have any current infections.

Baseline assessment

For the ODS intervention group, the baseline assessment was based on the Cube Method which is an integrated assessment method for comorbid psychiatric and substance use disorders in clinical settings; the method was developed by Kampman and Lassila in the South Ostrobothnia hospital district [20, 21]. Systematic assessment helps to target suitable treatment for each patient. The Cube Method was used to decide which patients would be additionally treated with motivational interviews. The baseline psychiatric diagnostic evaluation was performed using the Mini International Neuropsychiatric Interview (MINI) [22]. Depressive symptoms were rated using the Montgomery–Åsberg Depression Rating Scale (MADRS) [23] and level of functioning was assessed using the Global Assessment of Functioning scale (GAF) [24]. All evaluations were conducted by experienced psychiatrists or trained research nurses. The use of psychotropic medications was recorded using a paper-and-pencil diary. The study protocol is described in more detail in the Clinical Trials registry [13].

For the control group, all data were collected retrospectively from the hospital district patient registers. The diagnoses had been determined by the responsible doctor and were not confirmed using structured diagnostic interviews. GAF scores were estimated according to case notes by a trained research nurse supervised by a research doctor. In cases of insufficient information, scoring was omitted.

The GAF estimates were calibrated by prior rating of five test patients and comparing the possible differences between the raters (one research doctor and two research nurses). After the calibration process, the inter-rater correlations were strong ($r > 0.9$).

Procedures and follow-up

In the intervention group, BA and antidepressive medication were used for 239 patients. Additionally, motivational interviews (MIs) [25] were used during the first appointments with patients having alcohol use problems (baseline AUDIT ≥11) to be able to better ensure the patients engagement to the treatment. BA and MIs were implemented by the regional staff (registered psychiatric nurses, psychiatric practical nurses and psychologists) responsible for the patient. The regional staff was systematically trained to use the selected interventions [7]. The minimum duration of BA was set at four appointments. On request, we received information about the completed BA sessions from the therapists of 54 patients. The median number of sessions was 6.5 (IQR 8.25). The decision to start the medication and the type of medication used was based on clinical evaluation (at baseline and at 6 weeks) by the responsible doctor. If the baseline MADRS score was 20 or more the medication was started and the dose was elevated if necessary, or the type of antidepressive medication was changed (from selective serotonin reuptake inhibitors to serotonin–norepinephrine reuptake inhibitors). The follow-up included appointments with a clinical research nurse at 6, 12 and 24 months and depressive symptoms (MADRS) and the level of functioning (GAF) were checked (among other things, please see ClinicalTrials.gov Identifier NCT02520271).

All patients in the control group were treated in public psychiatric secondary care in the same organization and catchment area as the intervention group over the same time period. Control patients received TAU according to the protocols of the respective treatment unit and were followed-up according to the case notes at 6, 12 and 24 months by estimating GAF scores and obtaining information about possible alcohol use. In the area, psychiatric secondary care is always supervised by a specialized psychiatrist. The psychiatric TAU usually consists of regular individual visits to the outpatient clinic with varying frequency depending on each patient's situation. Most often, a nurse, psychologist or social worker is responsible for the individual visits; patients meet a doctor only at the beginning and end of the treatment and whenever the treatment plan is evaluated. The TAU methods varied according to the educational background and therapeutic training of the responsible staff.

For both groups, information about the frequency of outpatient visits, number of hospital days and dropouts was collected from patient registers at 6, 12 and 24 months follow-up points and information on mortality was collected from baseline (October 1, 2009) until March 30, 2016. The register data covered all cases during the whole follow up in both intervention and control groups (n = 242 and n = 205, respectively).

Statistical methods

The power calculations resulted in the following detectable limits for primary outcomes MADRS and GAF. Within intervention group including the current sample size, the paired analyses were able to detect a 1.7 point mean response difference in MADRS with a power of 0.8 and type I error probability of 0.05. Between intervention and control groups including the current number of pairs, the independent analyses were able to detect a 3.6 point mean response difference in GAF with a power of 0.8 and type I error probability of 0.05.

The independent samples t-test was used to compare the age distributions, GAF and AUDIT scores between the intervention and the control group at baseline. Chi-square tests were used to compare the frequencies of gender, inpatients and outpatients, psychiatric diagnoses and the patients hospitalized during the follow-up between the groups. A linear mixed model for repeated measures was used to analyze the changes in MADRS score from baseline to the three follow-up points in the intervention group patients and the changes in GAF score between the intervention and control groups. In the latter model, parameters time, patient group and an interaction term time*patient group were used in analyses. The Mann–Whitney U test was used to analyze antipsychotic medication doses and the number of days spent in hospital. The level of statistical significance was set at < 0.05. All calculations were performed using the software SPSS for Apple Macintosh version 24 (IBM SPSS Statistics, Armonk, NY) and PS: Power and Sample Size Calculation (version 3.1.2, Vanderbilt University, Nashville TN) [26].

Results

Depressive symptoms in the intervention group

Improvement of depressive symptoms in intervention group patients was analyzed using MADRS scores. The mean MADRS score for the intervention patients at baseline was 23.2 points (n = 228, SD 6.69), at 6 months 13.1 points (n = 156, SD 8.69), at 12 months 9.93 points (n = 135, SD 7.83) and at 24 months 8.31 points (n = 95, SD 7.58). The estimated change in MADRS score compared to baseline was statistically significant in every follow-up period. The results are presented in the Table 2.

Table 2 The results of linear mixed model for repeated measures of MADRS[a] score in the intervention group

Follow-up period	N	Estimate[b]	95% CI	SE	p
0–6 months	156	−10.06	−11.58 - -8.54	0.77	< 0.001
0–12 months	135	−13.15	−14.64 - -11.65	0.76	< 0.001
0–24 months	95	−14.82	−16.35 - -13.29	0.77	< 0.001

[a]Montgomery-Åsberg Depression Rating Scale
[b]Estimated change in MADRS scores from baseline

Level of functioning

At 12 months and 24 months follow-up points the estimated improvement in GAF score was significantly better in the intervention group patients (estimate for patient group 2.26, $p = 0.036$). At six months a similar difference was not found. For more detailed results please see Table 3. A sensitivity analysis was performed by excluding the patients with personality disorder as secondary clinical diagnoses ($n = 44$). The results were similar with the total sample analysis, with GAF estimates between intervention and control groups 0–6 months 2.84 ($p = 0.057$), 0–12 months 5.13 ($p = 0.006$), and 0–24 months 6.58 ($p = 0.002$).

Use of services

There were no between-group differences in number of outpatient visits (comparisons: no visits, one visit/month, two visits/month, more than two visits/month) during any of the follow-up periods (intervention group: $n = 242$, control group: $n = 205$; 0–6 months, $p = 0.74$; 6–12 months, $p = 0.56$; 12–24 months, $p = 0.52$). The need for hospitalization was measured in every follow-up period as "yes, patient was hospitalized" or "no, patient was not hospitalized." The number of hospitalized patients was similar in the intervention and control groups (intervention group: n = 242, control group: n = 205) during all periods: 0–6 months, 59 (24.4%) in the intervention group vs. 60 (29.6%) in the control group, $p = 0.22$; 6–12 months, 14 (5.8%) vs. 12 (5.9%), $p = 0.96$; 12–24 months, 16 (6.6%) vs. 15 (7.4%), $p = 0.75$). Among the patients who were hospitalized at baseline, the number of patients hospitalized during the follow-up periods was also similar between the groups ($p = 0.17$, $p = 0.95$, $p = 0.35$, respectively). The median number of days spent in hospital was analyzed for patients hospitalized during the respective follow-up periods. At 0–6 months, the median number of days hospitalized was 16 (IQR 17) in the study group ($n = 59$) and 18.5 (IQR 16.75) in the control group ($n = 60$), at 6–12 months it was 17 (IQR 12.75) ($n = 14$) and 19 (IQR 29.75) ($n = 12$), and at 12–24 months it was 10 (IQR 12.25) ($n = 16$) and 21 (IQR 31) ($n = 15$).

Dropout and deaths

There were no between-group differences in the number of patients who dropped out in any period ($p = 0.79$, $p = 0.86$, $p = 0.51$, respectively). There were four deaths in the intervention group and seven deaths in the control group (mortality rate: 1.7% vs. 3.4%, $p = 0.23$). Among these, the median time of death from baseline was 16 months (IQR 16) in the intervention group and 5 months (IQR 13) in the control group. We have no data on specific causes of death.

Discussion

The study setting, a benchmark controlled trial, allowed the evaluation of BA treatment among ordinary patients in a routine clinical setting of secondary psychiatric care. The findings provide essential information for the planning and development of a better treatment protocol for depressed patients. Since only patients with psychotic or organic pathologies were excluded, our study group was heterogeneous with various comorbidities and therefore representative of the usual patient population in everyday practice. The depressive symptoms among the intervention group patients seem to alleviate compared to baseline during the 2-years follow-up. Our results suggest that BA is a useful tool for this patient group although strong conclusions can't be drawn about the benefits compared to TAU. The intervention patients showed a greater improvement in functional ability than the control patients. This is an important finding, because functional recovery has a considerable effect on daily life and is particularly relevant from the patients' point of view. The ODS intervention did not change the need for outpatient visits or hospitalizations compared with TAU. This finding is surprising, since one could assume that the positive change in functional ability would reflect in a reduced need for inpatient treatment in the intervention group. The dropout rates indicated that adherence to treatment was similar in both groups.

In a review of studies of the impact of homework in cognitive-behavioral therapy, Thase and Callan concluded that homework adherence increases the possibility of

Table 3 The results of linear mixed model for repeated measures of GAF[a] score between the intervention and control groups

Follow-up period	Intervention (n)	Control (n)	Estimate[b]	95% CI	SE	p
0–6 months	167	159	2.65	−0.14 - 5.44	1.42	0.063
0–12 months	128	134	4.85	1.43–8.28	1.74	0.006
0–24 months	94	98	5.71	1.76–9.67	2.01	0.005

[a]Global Assessment of Functioning Scale
[b]Estimated difference in GAF score between intervention and control groups at the respective follow-up points

successful outcomes when treating depression [27]. This is one reason why BA was selected as an ODS treatment method instead of other evidence-based brief therapies. As BA aims to activate the patient (e.g., by homework and skills training) this may positively influence the overall functional ability of patients, resulting in functional recovery. The cost-effectiveness and outcomes of BA have been compared with those of more comprehensive cognitive-behavioral therapies in depressed adult patients and evidence indicates that BA is equally effective [28]. This suggests that brief interventions should be used at least in the public services, where the challenge is to provide effective treatment for a large number of patients despite limited resources. BA can be delivered successfully by mental health workers with no long-term training in psychological therapies [29] In the ODS, mental health workers with various backgrounds received short-term training in BA and delivered the intervention successfully. This indicates that this therapy could enhance the treatment of depression in the existing psychiatric health care system.

There are some limitations that should be considered when interpreting our results. BCTs are novel experimental designs which have yet to prove their methodological validity. Therefore, when considering the recommendations deriving from our paper it should be noted that this is a method that still needs to be validated against RCT (in this case BA vs treatment as usual groups). Data on intervention group patients was collected prospectively and data on control group patients was collected retrospectively. Data on intervention group patients was more comprehensive compared to the control patients. This is due to the inferior quality and the content of clinical information in the patient registers of the control group and it was not possible to complete the data afterwards. For example, it is possible that part of the information on somatic diagnoses of control patients is missing. We were unable to compare alleviation of depressive symptoms between the groups because of lack of information on BDI or MADRS scores for the control patients. Therefore, we could explore the effect of BA on the depression only in the intervention group. This is clearly a limitation when assessing our results in terms of the treatment of depressive symptoms. There was a slight between-group difference in baseline GAF scores. Thus, it was not possible to match the patients according to GAF levels at baseline. It could be argued that there is much inter-rater variation in GAF scores [30, 31] and that our results concerning GAF are therefore less reliable. We attempted to avoid this variation in scores using the calibration process described in section "Baseline assessment". Intervention group patients with comorbid alcohol use problems also received MIs (a maximum of five appointments), which was mainly targeted at engaging patients with the treatment and increasing the success of BA. This practice was chosen according to the strong evidence of MI for substance use disorders [25]. As the use of MI may have had an additional positive impact on the treatment of depressive symptoms among the patients with alcohol use problems, the trial can be regarded to evaluate not only BA, but also the combination of BA and MI in this group. We did not screen for possible personality disorders at baseline. Although 13.6% of the cohort patients had other diagnosis from mood disorders as primary research diagnoses, they all had depressive symptoms with at least moderate severity and only few of these patients were clinically diagnosed in the personality disorders category. When further exploring the register based clinical diagnoses of personality disorders, approximately 10% of the total sample were diagnosed in this category. As it is known, personality disorders have a close effect on treatment response. Therefore, it should be noted that personality disorder as a secondary psychiatric diagnosis was more common in the control group relative to the intervention group (9 patients (3.7%) vs. 17 patients (8.4%). Also, the antipsychotic exposure was higher in the control patients, suggesting the control group may have more complex depressive illness than the intervention group. It was anticipated that patients with serious complicating factors, such as personality problems, would not benefit sufficiently from BA and could then be assessed more thoroughly and offered more comprehensive intervention.

Conclusions

The systematic use of BA among secondary psychiatric care depressive patients provides encouraging results despite the patients had various comorbid non-psychotic disorders. Depressive symptoms alleviated and there was a trend towards better functional recovery among patients treated with BA compared to those treated with TAU in this study.

Abbreviations

AUDIT: Alcohol Use Disorders Identification Test; BA: behavioral activation; BDI: Beck Depression Inventory; GAF: Global Assessment of Functioning scale; IQR: interquartile range; MADRS: Montgåmery-Åsberg Depression Rating Scale; MINI: Mini International Neuropsychiatric Interview; ODS: The Ostrobothnia Depression Study; SD: standard deviation; TAU: treatment as usual

Acknowledgements

We thank the research nurses Susanna Hotakainen, Marja Koivumäki and Kati Huhtala for their important work on the ODS project. We thank our colleagues in the PhD seminars at the Department of Psychiatry, School of Medicine, University of Tampere for their valuable comments and help in preparing this manuscript. We thank Diane Williams, PhD, from Edanz Group (www.edanzediting.com/ac) for editing a draft of this manuscript.

Funding

The ODS was supported by the South Ostrobothnia Hospital District research fund, grant number EVO1114. The preparation of the manuscript was supported by a grant from the Finnish Research Foundation of Psychiatry.

Authors' contributions

OK, AL and EL conceived the study and participated in its design. AK participated in coordinating the study and the data collection. OK, VP and KL performed the statistical analysis. OK, LL and KL drafted the manuscript. All authors read and approved the final manuscript.

Consent for publication

Not applicable.

Competing interests

The authors declare that they have no competing interests.

Author details

[1]Faculty of Medicine and Life Sciences, University of Tampere, PB 100, FI-33014 Tampere, Finland. [2]Department of Psychiatry, Tampere University Hospital, PB 2000, FI-33521 Tampere, Finland. [3]Department of Psychiatry, Seinäjoki Hospital District, Huhtalantie 53, 60220 Seinäjoki, Finland.

References

1. Ferrari AJ, Charlson FJ, Norman RE, Patten SB, Freedman G, Murray CJ, Vos T, Whiteford HA. Burden of depressive disorders by country, sex, age, and year: findings from the global burden of disease study 2010. PLoS Med. 2013; 10(11):e1001547.
2. Melartin TK, Rytsälä HJ, Leskelä US, Lestelä-Mielonen PS, Sokero PT, Isometsä ET. Current comorbidity of psychiatric disorders among DSM-IV major depressive disorder patients in psychiatric care in the Vantaa depression study. J clinical psychiatry. 2002;63(2):126–34.
3. American Psychiatric Association Practice Guidelines
. http://psychiatryonline.org/guidelines. Accessed 2017.
4. National Institute for Health and Care Excellence Guidance. https://www.nice.org.uk/guidance. Accessed 2017.
5. Cuijpers P, van Straten A, Andersson G, van Oppen P. Psychotherapy for depression in adults: a meta-analysis of comparative outcome studies. J Consult Clin Psychol. 2008;76(6):909–22.
6. Barth J, Munder T, Gerger H, Nüesch E, Trelle S, Znoj H, Jüni P, Cuijpers P. Comparative Efficacy of Seven Psychotherapeutic Interventions for Patients with Depression: A Network Meta-Analysis. PLoS Med. 2013;10(5):e1001454.
7. Lindholm LH, Koivukangas A, Lassila A, Kampman O. Early assessment of implementing evidence-based brief therapy interventions among secondary service psychiatric therapists. Evaluation and Program Planning. 2015;52: 182–8.
8. Knekt P, Lindfors O, Laaksonen MA, Renlund C, Haaramo P, Härkänen T, Virtala E. Quasi-experimental study on the effectiveness of psychoanalysis, long-term and short-term psychotherapy on psychiatric symptoms, work ability and functional capacity during a 5-year follow-up. J Affect Disord. 2011;132(1):37–47.
9. Nieuwsma JA, Trivedi RB, McDuffie J, Kronish I, Benjamin D, Williams JW. Brief psychotherapy for depression: a systematic review and meta-analysis. Int J Psychiatry Med. 2012;43(2):129–51.
10. Kanter JW, Manos RC, Bowe WM, Baruch DE, Busch AM, Rusch LC. What is behavioral activation? A review of the empirical literature. Clin Psychol Rev. 2010;30(6):608–20.
11. Cuijpers P, van Straten A, Warmerdam L. Behavioral activation treatments of depression: a meta-analysis. Clin Psychol Rev. 2007;27(3):318–26.
12. Malmivaara A. Benchmarking controlled trial-a novel concept covering all observational effectiveness studies. Ann Med. 2015;47(4):332–40.
13. ClinicalTrials.gov, Identifier NCT02520271. Ostrobothnia Depression Study (ODS). https://clinicaltrials.gov/ct2/show/NCT02520271. Accessed 2015.
14. Beck AT, Ward CH, Mendelson M, Mock J, Erbaugh J. An inventory for measuring depression. Arch Gen Psychiatry. 1961;4:561–71.
15. WHO | International Classification of Diseases. http://www.who.int/classifications/icd/en/. Accessed 2017.
16. Saunders JB, Aasland OG. Babor TF, de la Fuente, J R, grant M: development of the alcohol use disorders identification test (AUDIT): WHO collaborative project on early detection of persons with harmful alcohol consumption--II. Addiction. 1993;88(6):791–804.
17. David Taylor D, Paton C, Kapur S, editors. The Maudsley Prescribing Guidelines in Psychiatry. 11th ed. UK: Wiley-Blackwell; 2012.
18. Hansen RA, Moore CG, Dusetzina SB, Leinwand BI, Gartlehner G, Gaynes BN. Controlling for drug dose in systematic review and meta-analysis: a case study of the effect of antidepressant dose. Med Decis Mak. 2009;29(1):91–103.
19. Aronson JK, editor. Meyler's Side Effects of Psychiatric Drugs. 1st ed. UK: Elsevier Science; 2009.
20. Kampman O, Lassila A. Samanaikaisen mielenterveys- ja päihdeongelman hoitoon on kehitetty integroitu arviointimalli. Suom Lääkäril. 2007;47:4447–51.
21. Luoto KE, Koivukangas A, Lassila A, Kampman O. Outcome of patients with dual diagnosis in secondary psychiatric care. Nord J Psychiatry. 2016;70(6): 470–6.
22. Sheehan DV, Lecrubier Y, Sheehan KH, Amorim P, Janavs J, Weiller E, Hergueta T, Baker R, Dunbar GC. The Mini-International Neuropsychiatric Interview (M.I.N.I.): the development and validation of a structured diagnostic psychiatric interview for DSM-IV and ICD-10. J Clin Psychiatry. 1998;59(Suppl 20):57.
23. Montgomery SA, Asberg M. A new depression scale designed to be sensitive to change. Br J Psychiatry. 1979;134:382–9.
24. Aas IHM. Guidelines for rating global assessment of functioning (GAF). Ann General Psychiatry. 2011;10(1):2.
25. Lundahl B, Burke BL. The effectiveness and applicability of motivational interviewing: a practice-friendly review of four meta-analyses. J Clin Psychol. 2009;65(11):1232–45.
26. Dupont WD, Plummer WD. Power and Sample Size Calculations for Studies Involving Linear Regression. Control Clin Trials. 1998;19:589–601.
27. Thase ME, Callan JA. The role of homework in cognitive behavior therapy of depression. J Psychother Integr. 2006;16(2):162–77.
28. Richards DA, Ekers D, McMillan D, Taylor RS, Byford S, Warren FC, Barrett B, Farrand PA, Gilbody S, Kuyken W, O'Mahen H, Watkins ER, Wright KA, Hollon SD, Reed N, Rhodes S, Fletcher E, Finning K. Cost and outcome of Behavioural activation versus cognitive Behavioural therapy for depression (COBRA): a randomised, controlled, non-inferiority trial. Lancet. 2016; 388(10047):871–80.
29. Ekers D, Richards D, McMillan D, Bland JM, Gilbody S. Behavioural activation delivered by the non-specialist: phase II randomised controlled trial. Br J Psychiatry. 2011;198(1):66–72.
30. Grootenboer EM. Giltay EJ, van der Lem R, van Veen T, van der wee, N J, Zitman FG: reliability and validity of the global assessment of functioning scale in clinical outpatients with depressive disorders. J Eval Clin Pract. 2012; 18(2):502–7.
31. Söderberg P, Tungström S, Armelius BA. Reliability of global assessment of functioning ratings made by clinical psychiatric staff. Psychiatr Serv. 2005; 56(4):434–8.

19

Problematic internet use and psychiatric co-morbidity in a population of Japanese adult psychiatric patients

Hille T. de Vries[1], Takashi Nakamae[2*], Kenji Fukui[3], Damiaan Denys[4,5] and Jin Narumoto[2]

Abstract

Background: Many studies reported the high prevalence of problematic internet use (PIU) among adolescents (13–50%), and PIU was associated with various psychiatric symptoms. In contrast, only a few studies investigated the prevalence among the adult population (6%). This study aimed to investigate the prevalence of PIU and psychiatric co-morbidity among adult psychiatric patients.

Methods: Three hundred thirty-three adult psychiatric patients were recruited over a 3-month period. Two hundred thirty-one of them completed the survey (response rate: 69.4%, 231/333; Male/Female/Transgender: 90/139/2; mean age = 42.2). We divided participants into "normal internet users" and "problematic internet users" using a combination of Young's Internet Addiction Test (IAT) and the Compulsive Internet Use Scale (CIUS). Demographic data and comorbid psychiatric symptoms were compared between the two groups using self-rating scales measuring insomnia (Athens Insomnia Scale, AIS), depression (Beck Depression Inventory, BDI), anxiety (State-trait Anxiety Inventory, STAI), attention deficit hyperactivity disorder (ADHD) (Adult ADHD Self-report Scale, ASRS), autism (Autism Spectrum Quotient, AQ), obsessive-compulsive disorder (OCD) (Obsessive-Compulsive Inventory, OCI), social anxiety disorder (SAD) (Liebowitz Social Anxiety Scale, LSAS), alcohol abuse, and impulsivity (Barratt Impulsive Scale, BIS).

Results: Among 231 respondents, 58 (25.1%) were defined as problematic internet users, as they scored high on the IAT (40 or more) or CIUS (21 or more). The age of problematic internet users was significantly lower than that of normal internet users ($p < 0.001$, Mann–Whitney U test). The problematic internet users scored significantly higher on scales measuring sleep problems (AIS, 8.8 for problematic internet users vs 6.3 for normal internet users, $p < 0.001$), depression (BDI, 27.4 vs 18.3, $p < 0.001$), trait anxiety (STAI, 61.8 vs 53.9, p < 0.001), ADHD (ASRS, part A 3.1 vs 1.8 and part B 3.5 vs 1.8, $p < 0.001$), autism (AQ, 25.9 vs 21.6, $p < 0.001$), OCD (OCI, 63.2 vs 36.3, $p < 0.001$), SAD (LSAS, 71.4 vs 54.0, $p < 0.001$), and impulsivity (BIS, 67.4 vs 63.5, $p = 0.004$).

Conclusions: The prevalence of PIU among adult psychiatric patients is relatively high. As previous studies reported in the general population, lower age and psychiatric comorbidity were associated with PIU among adult psychiatric patients. More research is needed to determine any causal relations between PIU and psychopathological illnesses.

Keywords: Internet addiction, Problematic internet use, Prevalence, Japan

* Correspondence: nakamae@koto.kpu-m.ac.jp
[2]Department of Psychiatry, Graduate School of Medical Science, Kyoto Prefectural University of Medicine, 465 Kajii-cho, Kawaramachi-Hirokoji, Kamigyo-ku, Kyoto 602-8566, Japan
Full list of author information is available at the end of the article

Background

With internet access and use pervading society worldwide, concerns have been raised about the potential damage of excessive internet use [1]. 'Internet Addiction (Disorder)', 'Problematic Internet Use', 'Pathological Internet Use', 'Internet Addictive Behaviour' and other terms have been used to describe the combination of addiction-like symptoms and social problems seen in individuals spending huge amounts of time using the internet [2, 3]. However, this proposed disorder is still under discussion concerning its definition, validity as a construct, proposed diagnostic criteria, preferred measuring instruments, and treatment [4, 5]. Proponents of the disorder have made considerable efforts to see it included in the American Psychiatric Association (APA)'s Diagnostic and Statistical Manual of Mental Disorders (DSM), resulting in the inclusion of Internet Gaming Disorder in section III under the heading "Conditions for Further Study" [6].

Previous epidemiological studies used some measurements including the Young Diagnostic Questionnaire (YDQ), the Internet Addiction Test (IAT), and the Compulsive Internet Use Scale (CIUS) to assess excessive internet use. High prevalence of internet addiction among adolescents and students has been reported by many authors. Cheng et al. [7] conducted a meta-analysis including 89.281 participants from 31 nations and estimated prevalence of internet addiction defined as a YDQ score from 5 to 8 or an IAT score from 70 to 100 to be 6.0% among adolescents and youth. Tsitsika et al. [8] reported that prevalence of dysfunctional internet behavior defined as an IAT score from 40 to 100 among 14–17-year old students to be 13.9% in European countries (N = 13.284) while Mak et al. [9] reported its prevalence to range from 13.7 to 50.9% among 12–18-year-old students in Asian countries (N = 5.366).

In contrast, only a few studies investigated the prevalence among the adult population. Bakken et al. [10] reported the prevalence of internet addiction (YDQ score 5–8) and at-risk internet users (YDQ score 3–4) to be 1.0 and 5.2% respectively in 3.399 Norwegian subjects. Zadra et al. [11] reported that 685 out of 15.023 subjects (4.5%) showed 21 points and more on the CIUS. Thus, the problem of excessive internet use in adults should not be underestimated, even though its prevalence may be lower in adults than among students.

A number of studies have identified the correlation between problematic internet use (PIU) and psychiatric disorders [12–16], including a systematic review by Carli et al. [3] and most notably a meta-analysis by Ho et al. [2]. PIU was shown to be associated with alcohol abuse, attention deficit hyperactivity disorder (ADHD), depression, and anxiety. The correlation with depression has also been found in longitudinal studies [17–19], with individuals overly exposed to the internet having a higher risk of developing depression. Furthermore, PIU has also been found to correlate with sleep problems and these also have their effects on patients' well-being [20–23]. Therefore, we deemed it necessary to assess the correlation between PIU and comorbid psychiatric symptoms among patients with psychiatric disorders as their psychiatric symptoms could affect PIU or vice versa.

As far as we know, however, there have been no studies as of yet investigating the prevalence and comorbidity of PIU in a psychiatric population. Psychiatric symptoms might either induce PIU in patients with psychiatric illnesses, or PIU might induce or aggravate psychiatric symptoms. Therefore, this study aims to investigate the prevalence of PIU among adult psychiatric patients, and to reveal the degree of co-morbidity between PIU and psychiatric symptoms.

We hypothesize that the prevalence of PIU among psychiatric patients to be higher than among the general population. PIU might be associated with sleep problems, depression, anxiety, ADHD, autism, obsessive-compulsive disorder (OCD), social anxiety disorder (SAD), alcohol abuse, and impulsivity as previous studies reported in adolescents and students.

Methods

Study design and population

A cross-sectional study was performed using online questionnaires. Participants were recruited through their treating physicians at the outpatient clinic of psychiatry, University Hospital, Kyoto Prefectural University of Medicine from January 2016 to April 2016, for which Kyoto Prefectural University of Medicine Research Ethics Committee approved all procedures (ERB-C-485). After obtaining both oral and written consent, participants were asked to fill in an electronic questionnaire either at home or on tablets provided by the researchers.

In- and exclusion criteria

Participants were included if they had been diagnosed with a psychiatric diagnosis from the tenth revision of the International Classification of Diseases and Related Health Problems (ICD-10) [24] categories F1 (Mental and behavioural disorders due to psychoactive substance use), F2 (Schizophrenia, schizotypal and delusional disorders), F3 (Mood [affective] disorders), F4 (Neurotic, stress-related and somatoform disorders), or F5 (Behavioural syndromes associated with physiological disturbances and physical factors).

Participants were excluded if they were below 20 years of age, did not have access to the internet, or were in such a clinically bad shape that their treating physician preferred not to ask them to fill out the questionnaire.

In order to prevent and assess possible selection bias, whether or not the patient met the inclusion criterion for diagnosis or had to be excluded due to age was judged beforehand by the researchers by accessing the medical files for each patient scheduled for an appointment at the psychiatry outpatient department. If any of the treating physicians were unable to recruit a patient due to the patient's clinical condition being too severe (i.e. the patient was not able to fill out the questionnaire), the patient not agreeing to participate in the research, or not turning up for their appointment, physicians were asked to note this on a form provided to them by the researchers.

Measurements

To assess internet addiction, we administered both IAT developed by Young [25] and the CIUS developed by Meerkerk et al. [26], both translated into and validated in Japanese [27]. There seem to be different versions of the IAT in use. The validated Japanese version used in this research has 20 questions that can be answered on a Likert-scale of 1 to 5, with proposed cut-off points of 40 (problematic internet use), as also used in the large studies by Tsitsika et al. [8] and Mak et al. [9]. The cut-off for PIU on the CIUS was defined as 21 points, as suggested by Guertler et al. [28]. To measure sleep problems, we administered the validated Japanese version of the Athens Insomnia Scale [29, 30]. To measure the severity of other symptoms of mental disorders, we administered the validated Japanese versions of the Beck Depression Inventory II (BDI-II) [31, 32], the State-Trait Anxiety Inventory (STAI) [33, 34], the Adult ADHD Self-report Scale (ASRS) [35], the Autism Spectrum Quotient (AQ) [36, 37], the Obsessive-Compulsive Inventory (OCI) [38, 39], the Liebowitz Social Anxiety Scale (LSAS) [40, 41], the Alcohol Use Disorders Identification Test (AUDIT) [42, 43], the Barratt Impulsive Scale (BIS) [44, 45], and questions regarding the amount and nature of internet use and the patients' background (Appendix).

The physicians diagnosed their patients based on ICD-10 criteria, and then assessed the severity using the Clinical Global Impression Severity (CGI-S) [46].

Data was only sent when participants completely finished the questionnaire. Any participants who might have completed only part of the questionnaire were thus counted as non-respondent, as we did not receive any of their data.

Statistical analysis

Continuous variables were shown as mean (± standard deviation) or median (interquartile range), and categorical variables were presented as numbers and percentages. To study statistically significant differences between problematic internet users and normal internet users, we divided our sample in two groups. Respondents who scored 40 or higher on the IAT [8, 9] or 21 or higher on the CIUS [28] were defined as problematic internet users, while those who scored below those values on both were defined as normal internet users. Categorical variables were compared between two groups using chi-square test while Fisher's exact test was performed in tables larger than 2 × 2 using R version 3.3.1 (http://www.r-project.org/). As results apparently didn't follow a Gaussian distribution, differences in ordinal and interval variables between the two groups were assessed using the Mann–Whitney U test. The software used was SPSS for Windows version 23. Bonferroni correction was applied for multiple comparisons.

Results

Demographics and internet use

As shown in Figs. 1, 1.220 patients visited the hospital during the 3 months of our recruitment period and 333 of them were included in this study. Two hundred thirty-one patients completed the survey, making the response rate at 69.4% (231/333). Fifty patients (21.6%, 50/231) scored above the 40 points thresholds on the IAT. Furthermore, 43 patients (18.6%, 43/231) scored 21 or higher on the CIUS. This brought the total number of patients we defined as "problematic internet users", those who scored either 40 or higher on the IAT or 21 or higher on the CIUS, to 58 (25.1%, 58/231).

The proportion of problematic internet users is remarkably higher in the younger age groups and unemployed group (Table 1). Sex, education level, living alone or with others, and marital status do not seem to significantly affect internet addiction scores. Furthermore, PIU did not seem to differ greatly between the ICD-10 categories of the respondent's main diagnosis (as reported by their treating physicians). CGI-S scores of patients with PIU assessed by their treating physicians were significantly higher than those of normal internet users.

Psychiatry scale scores

Problematic internet users scored higher on all scales measuring co-morbid psychiatry showing a significantly uneven distribution of scores between the problematic and normal internet users, with the exception of the state subscale of STAI and AUDIT (Table 2).

Sleep habits

Some of the questions regarding to internet use (Appendix) revolved around the amount of internet use before sleep. The question "After you've gone to bed but before you sleep, how much on average per day do you use the smartphone or tablet?" (median < 10 min vs 30 min-1 h, Mann–Whitney U test, $p < 0.001$) and "When you wake up during your sleep, how much do you use your smartphone or tabled in bed?" (median "I don't use it at all" vs "I hardly

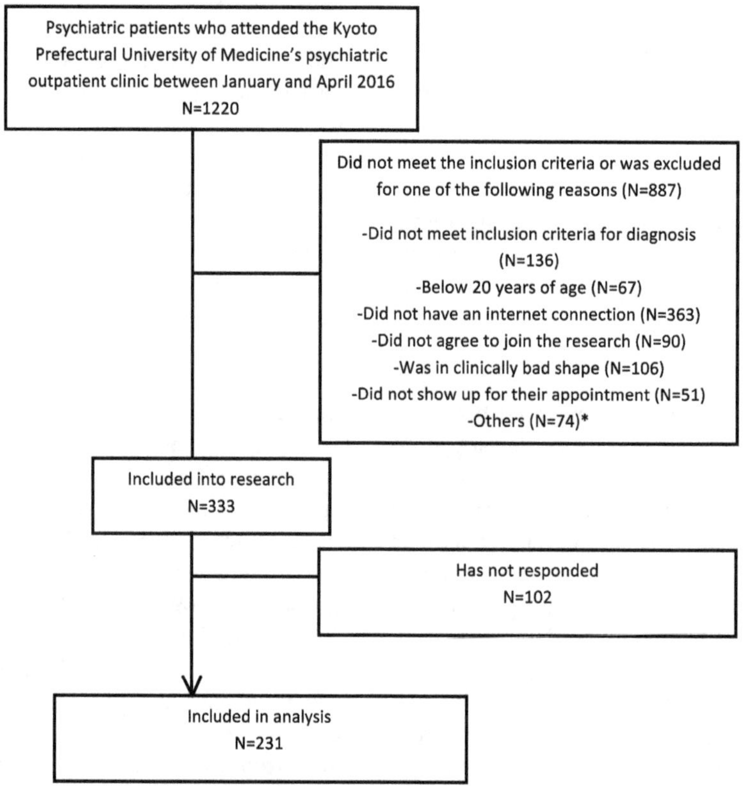

Fig. 1 Flowchart of the inclusion of patients

use it", Fisher's exact test, $p < 0.001$) got significantly higher answers from problematic internet users than from normal internet users (Additional file 1: Tables S1 and S2).

Internet activities

While problematic internet users do not use the internet for work significantly more than normal internet users, they do use it more for private purposes (median 1 h–3 h vs >3 h, Mann–Whitney U test, $p < 0.001$) (Table 3). Several private activities on the internet seemed more closely associated with PIU (Additional file 1: Table S3). Problematic internet users seem to spend more private time on the internet for the purposes of communicating, looking up information, reading blogs/forums or making blog/forum posts, surfing social networking sites, and watching videos or listening to music.

Other results

We also asked about the different devices participants used to access the internet (Appendix). Of these devices, only smartphone use was reported significantly more often by problematic internet users than normal internet users in all samples (median "I often use it" vs "I use it really often", Fisher's exact test, $p < 0.001$) (Additional file 1: Table S4). When the data was analyzed by age, only the twenties showed the significant difference in smartphone use frequency between the two groups (Table 4). However, this finding was not significant after Bonferroni correction.

Discussion

To our knowledge, this is the first study that investigated the prevalence of PIU, and degree of co-morbidity between PIU and psychiatric symptoms among adult psychiatric patients.

We identified 58 problematic internet users who scored either high IAT (40 and more) or CIUS (21 and more) out of 231 patients (25.1%). Although their demographic background was different, Osaki et al. [47] reported only 4.0% of people scored 40 and more on the IAT in the Japanese general population ($N = 4.153$). Bakken et al. [10] in Norway found percentages for at-risk internet users (YDQ score 3–4) and internet addiction (YDQ score 5–8) of 5.2% (177/3.393) and 1.0% (35/3.393) respectively. Zadra et al. [11] reported that 685 out of 15.023 German general population (4.5%) showed 21 points and more on the CIUS. Thus, the prevalence of problematic internet users among the general population might be estimated to be 4.0 to 6.2%. Bakken et al. [10] reported that 13.0% of their respondents did not use the internet at all, which means 6.0% of their internet using population displayed at-risk internet users, and

Table 1 Demographics of the respondents

		Normal internet users (N = 173)	Problematic internet users (N = 58)	p
Sex	Male	69 (39.9%)	21 (36.2%)	0.10[a]
	Female	104 (60.1%)	35 (60.3%)	
	Transgender	0	2 (3.4)	
Age	Mean, years (standard deviation)	43.6 (12.7)	35.9 (11.9)	<0.001[b]**
	20–29	26 (15.0%)	23 (39.7%)	
	30–39	37 (21.4%)	14 (24.1%)	
	40–49	60 (34.7%)	12 (20.7%)	
	50–59	29 (16.8%)	6 (10.3%)	
	60–69	16 (9.2%)	3 (5.2%)	
	70–79	5 (2.9%)	0	
Education (highest level)	Junior high school	8 (4.6%)	5 (8.6%)	0.59[a]
	High school	57 (32.9%)	23 (39.7%)	
	Junior college	25 (14.5%)	6 (10.3%)	
	University	76 (43.9%)	22 (37.9%)	
	Graduate school	7 (4.0%)	2 (3.4%)	
Employment status	Employed/homemaker/studying	113 (65.3%)	29 (50.0%)	0.04[c]*
	Unemployed	60 (34.7%)	29 (50.0%)	
Living situation	With others	138 (79.8%)	47 (81.0%)	0.84[c]
	Alone	35 (20.2%)	11 (19.0%)	
Marital status	Married/living together	67 (38.7%)	17 (29.3%)	0.20[c]
	Unmarried/divorced/separated/widowed	106 (61.3%)	41 (70.7%)	
Diagnosis	ICD-10 F1	4 (2.3%)	1 (1.7%)	0.79[c]
	ICD-10 F2	20 (11.6%)	6 (10.3%)	0.80[c]
	ICD-10 F3	56 (32.4%)	17 (29.3%)	0.66[c]
	ICD-10 F4	94 (54.3%)	37 (63.8%)	0.21[c]
	ICD-10 F5	13 (7.5%)	3 (5.2%)	0.54[c]
Clinical Global Impression-Severity	Median (interquartile range)	3 (3–4)	4 (3–4)	0.009[b]*

Number of persons in each sex, age, education, employment, living situation, marital status, and diagnosis category
[a]Fisher's exact test
[b]Mann-Whitney U test
[c]Chi-square test
*: $p < 0.05$, **: $p < 0.001$

1.2% internet addiction. Considering these results, the prevalence of PIU among psychiatric patients could be much higher compared to that of general population.

There may be several reasons explaining the high prevalence of PIU among psychiatric patients. First, our study found that problematic internet users scored higher on scales measuring sleep problems, depression, trait anxiety, ADHD, autism, OCD, SAD, and impulsivity. This is in line with previous research in non-psychiatric students and adolescents [2, 3, 12]. The severity of these psychiatric symptoms in our samples may very well be higher than that of previous studies' subjects because all of our subjects were diagnosed with at least one of primary psychiatric disorders. Therefore, it is reasonable to assume that the more severe the psychiatric illness of the studied population, the higher the prevalence of PIU. Then, some measurements used in our study such as STAI, AQ, and BIS assess the inherent characteristics of each subject, and these measurements also showed a significant difference between the two groups. Due to its cross-sectional nature, this study is unable to identify any causal relationships between PIU and psychiatric disorders [3], but intrinsic characteristics that predispose towards anxiety, autism, and impulsiveness may be the same characteristics that cause people to develop PIU. Further study to reveal the causal relationship between psychiatric symptoms and PIU is needed. In contrast to previous research [2], we did not find PIU to be associated with alcohol abuse. This is likely due to the small number of patients with alcohol abuse attending our psychiatric outpatient clinic, as these

Table 2 Average scores (and standard deviation) for the different scales measuring psychopathological co-morbidity of normal internet users compared with problematic internet users

	Normal internet users ($N = 173$)	Problematic internet users ($N = 58$)	p (Mann–Whitney U test)
Athens Insomnia Scale	6.3 (4.5)	8.8 (4.8)	<0.001*
Beck Depression Inventory	18.3 (12.7)	27.4 (11.9)	<0.001*
State-trait Anxiety Inventory (State)	49.3 (12.1)	54.0 (12.0)	0.013
State-trait Anxiety Inventory (Trait)	53.9 (11.0)	61.8 (8.5)	<0.001*
Adult ADHD Self-report Scale part A	1.8 (1.5)	3.1 (1.6)	<0.001*
Adult ADHD Self-report Scale part B	1.8 (2.3)	3.5 (2.5)	<0.001*
Autism Spectrum Quotient	21.6 (7.1)	25.9 (7.1)	<0.001*
Obsessive-compulsive Inventory	36.3 (31.7)	63.2 (34.1)	<0.001*
Liebowitz Social Anxiety Scale	54.0 (33.9)	71.4 (32.2)	<0.001*
Alcohol Use Disorders Identification Test	3.2 (4.4)	4.3 (5.5)	0.357
Barratt Impulsiveness Scale	63.5 (8.2)	67.4 (8.2)	0.004*

P-values represent the significance of uneven distribution between normal and problematic internet users on each of the scale scores, according to the Mann–Whitney U test
*Significant after Bonferroni correction

patients are often referred to other hospitals where specialized treatment is available for alcohol addicts and abusers. Further studies that include a larger number of alcohol addiction patients are necessary.

The study also showed a strong inverse association of PIU and age, which might be caused by the high amount of smartphone use among the younger population. There is also a number of studies done in student and adolescent populations which also show an inverse association between PIU and age [12]. An investigation done by the Japanese Ministry of Internal Affairs and Communications among Japanese high schoolers showed figures of 4.6% of high school students scoring 70 or higher on the IAT, and 55.2% scoring between 40 and 70 ($N = 14.071$) [48]. The group closest in age to these studies was our group of respondents between the ages of 20 and 29, which showed a percentage of 46.0 of problematic internet users. Due to the strong apparent inverse correlation between age and PIU, it is very well possible that psychiatric patients of high school age would score higher than older psychiatric patients or healthy high school students. Further studies should clarify the prevalence of PIU among adolescent patients with psychiatric illnesses.

There was no significant difference in time spent for work-related activities on the internet between the two groups, while problematic internet users spent significantly longer private time compared to normal internet users. Regarding time spent for various private activities on the internet, amount spent for activities such as blogging, social networking, and watching movies would be associated with PIU. These findings offer an important suggestion in clinical settings, as it shows that psychiatric patients need not avoid using the internet for work. Furthermore, physicians could suggest their patients to restrict their internet use to specific activities in order to prevent PIU. Lastly, patients with PIU seem to use their smartphone a lot after they have gone to bed, or when they wake up during sleep. Physicians could help their patients by discouraging this bad sleep hygiene.

This investigation is limited by the relatively small sample size. Only patients who were examined at the University Hospital, Kyoto Prefectural University of Medicine's Psychiatry outpatient clinic were recruited. Due to the small population size, we were unable to divide our population into groups with a specific psychiatric diagnosis and analyse correlations with scores on the questionnaires. Another limitation is the cross-sectional nature of the study. Because we did not measure our population repeatedly over time, there can be no conclusions drawn regarding causality. Furthermore, this study using an online questionnaire is likely to have greatly improved response rates (69.4%) among people with familiarity to the internet, but prevented us from collecting data on patients who were not used to

Table 3 Reported time spent for work and private related activities on the internet among problematic internet users compared with normal internet users

Activities	Normal internet users, n (%) ($N = 173$)						Problematic internet users, n (%) ($N = 58$)						p (Mann–Whitney U test)
	None	<30 m	30 m-1 h	1 h–3 h	3 h–5 h	>5 h	None	<30 m	30 m-1 h	1 h–3 h	3 h–5 h	>5 h	
Work	51(29.5)	40(23.1)	31(17.9)	26(15.0)	11(6.4)	14(8.1)	25(43.1)	10(17.2)	6(10.3)	6(10.3)	4(6.9)	7(12.1)	0.300
Private	10(5.8)	23(13.3)	27(15.6)	69(39.9)	26(15.0)	18(10.4)	6(10.3)	1(1.7)	3(5.2)	12(20.7)	7(12.1)	29(50.0)	<0.001*

*: $p < 0.001$

Table 4 Comparison of smartphone use frequency between normal internet users and problematic internet users

Age	Smartphone use frequency	Normal internet users, n (%) ($N = 173$)	Problematic internet users, n (%) ($N = 58$)	p (Fisher's exact test)
Total ($N = 231$)	I don't use it at all	48 (27.7)	13 (22.4)	<0.001**
	I hardly use it	8 (4.6)	1 (1.7)	
	I sometimes use it	21 (12.1)	0	
	I often use it	40 (23.1)	2 (3.4)	
	I use it really often	56 (32.4)	42 (72.4)	
20–29 ($N = 49$)	I don't use it at all	2 (7.7)	2 (8.7)	0.016*
	I hardly use it	1 (3.8)	0	
	I sometimes use it	2 (7.7)	0	
	I often use it	8 (30.8)	1 (4.3)	
	I use it really often	13 (50.0)	20 (87.0)	
30–39 ($N = 51$)	I don't use it at all	5 (13.5)	3 (21.4)	0.12
	I hardly use it	3 (8.1)	0	
	I sometimes use it	2 (5.4)	0	
	I often use it	9 (24.3)	0	
	I use it really often	18 (48.6)	11 (78.6)	
40–49 ($N = 72$)	I don't use it at all	20 (33.3)	4 (33.3)	0.14
	I hardly use it	3 (5.0)	0	
	I sometimes use it	11 (18.3)	0	
	I often use it	12 (20.0)	1 (8.3)	
	I use it really often	14 (23.3)	7 (58.3)	
50–59 ($N = 35$)	I don't use it at all	7 (24.1)	2 (33.3)	0.29
	I hardly use it	1 (3.4)	1 (16.7)	
	I sometimes use it	3 (10.3)	0	
	I often use it	9 (31.0)	0	
	I use it really often	9 (31.0)	3 (50.0)	
60–69 ($N = 19$)	I don't use it at all	9 (56.3)	2 (66.7)	1.00
	I hardly use it	0	0	
	I sometimes use it	3 (18.8)	0	
	I often use it	2 (12.5)	0	
	I use it really often	2 (12.5)	1 (33.3)	
70 < (N = 5)	I don't use it at all	5 (100.0)	0	1.00
	I hardly use it	0	0	
	I sometimes use it	0	0	
	I often use it	0	0	
	I use it really often	0	0	

*: $p < 0.05$, **: $p < 0.001$

answering questionnaires online and who did not have internet connection. In our study, we also didn't employ more advanced statistical methods such as bootstrapping to address the deviations from normality in our data. Finally, the questionnaire relied on self-report. One of the strengths of this study is that many different scales were filled in by each respondent, providing a clear and broad overview of any overlapping or co-morbid illness in every patient.

Future research could aim at finding causal relationships between PIU and various co-morbidities. Future research could also investigate the effectiveness of specialized treatment for psychiatric patients with PIU, due to the high degree of co-morbidity.

Conclusion

This study in adult psychiatric patients suggest that the prevalence of PIU is higher (25%) than that of general population

(6%). In addition, PIU in psychiatric patients is associated with higher scores on questionnaires investigating sleep problems, depression, trait anxiety, ADHD, autism, OCD, SAD, and impulsivity. More research is needed to determine the causal relation between PIU and psychiatric symptoms.

Abbreviations

ADHD: attention deficit hyperactivity disorder; APA: American Psychiatric Association; AQ: The Autism Spectrum Quotient; ASRS: The Adult ADHD Self-report Scale; AUDIT: The Alcohol Use Disorders Identification Test; BDI-II: The Beck Depression Inventory II; BIS: The Barratt Impulsive Scale; CGI-S: The Clinical Global Impression Severity; CIUS: The Compulsive Internet Use Scale; DSM: Diagnostic and Statistical Manual of Mental Disorders; IAT: Young's Internet Addiction Test; ICD-10: The tenth revision of the International Classification of Diseases and Related Health Problems; LSAS: The Liebowitz Social Anxiety Scale; OCD: Obsessive-compulsive disorder; OCI: The Obsessive-Compulsive Inventory; PIU: Problematic internet use; SAD: Social anxiety disorder; STAI: The State-Trait Anxiety Inventory; YDQ: The Young Diagnostic Questionnaire

Acknowledgements

We thank Y. Abe, N. Ayani, H. Fujimoto, Y. Hatano, N. Iida, T. Matsuoka, A. Minamisawa, Y. Mizuhara, I. Nishimura, J. Ono, Y. Sakai, T. Tominaga, Y. Wada, A. Watanabe and T. Yoshii for their assistance in collecting data.

Funding

This work was supported by MEXT KAKENHI Grant Number 26461753.

Authors' contributions

All authors contributed in study design. HdV TN contributed in data collection, statistical analysis, and article writing. HdV TN JN contributed in interpretation of the results. KF DD JN supervised the study and contributed in critical revision of the article. All authors read and approved the final article.

Consent for publication

Not applicable.

Competing interests

The authors declare that they have no competing interests.

Author details

[1]Academic Medical Center, University of Amsterdam, Meibergdreef 9, 1105, AZ, Amsterdam, the Netherlands. [2]Department of Psychiatry, Graduate School of Medical Science, Kyoto Prefectural University of Medicine, 465 Kajii-cho, Kawaramachi-Hirokoji, Kamigyo-ku, Kyoto 602-8566, Japan. [3]Health Care Center, Kyoto Prefectural University of Medicine, 465 Kajii-cho, Kawaramachi-Hirokoji, Kamigyo-ku, Kyoto 602-8566, Japan. [4]Department of Neuropsychiatry, Academic Medical Center, University of Amsterdam, Meibergdreef 9, 1105, AZ, Amsterdam, the Netherlands. [5]The Netherlands Institute for Neuroscience, an institute of the Royal Netherlands Academy of Arts and Sciences, Meibergdreef 47, 1105, BA, Amsterdam, the Netherlands.

References

1. Young KS. Psychology of computer use: XL. Addictive use of the internet: a case that breaks the stereotype. Psychol Rep. 1996;79(3 Pt 1):899–902.
2. Ho RC, Zhang MW, Tsang TY, Toh AH, Pan F, Lu Y, Cheng C, Yip PS, Lam LT, Lai CM, et al. The association between internet addiction and psychiatric co-morbidity: a meta-analysis. BMC Psychiatry. 2014;14:183.
3. Carli V, Durkee T, Wasserman D, Hadlaczky G, Despalins R, Kramarz E, Wasserman C, Sarchiapone M, Hoven CW, Brunner R, et al. The association between pathological internet use and comorbid psychopathology: a systematic review. Psychopathology. 2013;46(1):1–13.
4. Shaffer HJ, Hall MN, Vander Bilt J. "Computer addiction": a critical consideration. Am J Orthop. 2000;70(2):162–8.
5. Subramaniam M. Re-thinking internet gaming: from recreation to addiction. Addiction. 2014;109(9):1407–8.
6. American Psychiatric A, American Psychiatric Association DSMTF. Diagnostic and statistical manual of mental disorders : DSM-5. 5th ed: American Psychiatric Pub; 2013.
7. Cheng C, Li AY. Internet addiction prevalence and quality of (real) life: a meta-analysis of 31 nations across seven world regions. Cyberpsychol Behav Soc Netw. 2014;17(12):755–60.
8. Tsitsika A, Janikian M, Schoenmakers TM, Tzavela EC, Olafsson K, Wojcik S, Macarie GF, Tzavara C, Richardson C. Internet addictive behavior in adolescence: a cross-sectional study in seven European countries. Cyberpsychol Behav Soc Netw. 2014;17(8):528–35.
9. Mak KK, Lai CM, Watanabe H, Kim DI, Bahar N, Ramos M, Young KS, Ho RC, Aum NR, Cheng C. Epidemiology of internet behaviors and addiction among adolescents in six Asian countries. Cyberpsychol Behav Soc Netw. 2014;17(11):720–8.
10. Bakken IJ, Wenzel HG, Gotestam KG, Johansson A, Oren A. Internet addiction among Norwegian adults: a stratified probability sample study. Scand J Psychol. 2009;50(2):121–7.
11. Zadra S, Bischof G, Besser B, Bischof A, Meyer C, John U, Rumpf HJ. The association between internet addiction and personality disorders in a general population-based sample. J Behav Addict. 2016;5(4):691–9.
12. Ko CH, Yen JY, Yen CF, Chen CS, Chen CC. The association between internet addiction and psychiatric disorder: a review of the literature. Eur Psychiatry. 2012;27(1):1–8.
13. Wei HT, Chen MH, Huang PC, Bai YM. The association between online gaming, social phobia, and depression: an internet survey. BMC Psychiatry. 2012;12:92.
14. Goel D, Subramanyam A, Kamath R. A study on the prevalence of internet addiction and its association with psychopathology in Indian adolescents. Indian J Psychiatry. 2013;55(2):140–3.
15. Huang AC, Chen HE, Wang YC, Wang LM. Internet abusers associate with a depressive state but not a depressive trait. Psychiatry Clin Neurosci. 2014; 68(3):197–205.
16. Park S, Hong KE, Park EJ, Ha KS, Yoo HJ. The association between problematic internet use and depression, suicidal ideation and bipolar disorder symptoms in Korean adolescents. Aust N Z J Psychiatry. 2013;47(2):153–9.
17. Lam LT, Peng ZW. Effect of pathological use of the internet on adolescent mental health: a prospective study. Arch Pediatr Adolesc Med. 2010;164(10):901–6.
18. Dong G, Lu Q, Zhou H, Zhao X. Precursor or sequela: pathological disorders in people with internet addiction disorder. PLoS One. 2011;6(2):e14703.
19. Gentile DA, Choo H, Liau A, Sim T, Li D, Fung D, Khoo A. Pathological video game use among youths: a two-year longitudinal study. Pediatrics. 2011; 127(2):e319–29.
20. Van den Bulck J. Television viewing, computer game playing, and internet use and self-reported time to bed and time out of bed in secondary-school children. Sleep. 2004;27(1):101–4.
21. Dworak M, Schierl T, Bruns T, Struder HK. Impact of singular excessive computer game and television exposure on sleep patterns and memory performance of school-aged children. Pediatrics. 2007;120(5):978–85.
22. Shochat T, Flint-Bretler O, Tzischinsky O. Sleep patterns, electronic media exposure and daytime sleep-related behaviours among Israeli adolescents. Acta Paediatr. 2010;99(9):1396–400.
23. Brunborg GS, Mentzoni RA, Molde H, Myrseth H, Skouveroe KJ, Bjorvatn B, Pallesen S. The relationship between media use in the bedroom, sleep habits and symptoms of insomnia. J Sleep Res. 2011;20(4):569–75.
24. World Health Organization. The ICD-10 classification of mental and behavioural disorders : clinical descriptions and diagnostic guidelines. Geneva: World Health Organization; 1992.
25. Young KS. Caught in the net : how to recognize the signs of internet addiction, and a winning strategy for recovery: Wiley; 1998.

26. Meerkerk GJ, Van Den Eijnden RJ, Vermulst AA, Garretsen HF. The compulsive internet use scale (CIUS): some psychometric properties. Cyberpsychol Behav. 2009;12(1):1–6.
27. Yong KFR: The reliability and validity of three internet addiction instruments in the Japanese population. http://hdl.handle.net/2261/55608. 2012.
28. Guertler D, Rumpf HJ, Bischof A, Kastirke N, Petersen KU, John U, Meyer C. Assessment of problematic internet use by the compulsive internet use scale and the internet addiction test: a sample of problematic and pathological gamblers. Eur Addict Res. 2014;20(2):75–81.
29. Okajima I, Nakajima S, Kobayashi M, Inoue Y. Development and validation of the Japanese version of the Athens insomnia scale. Psychiatry Clin Neurosci. 2013;67(6):420–5.
30. Soldatos CR, Dikeos DG, Paparrigopoulos TJ. Athens insomnia scale: validation of an instrument based on ICD-10 criteria. J Psychosom Res. 2000; 48(6):555–60.
31. Beck AT, Steer RA, Brown G. Manual for the Beck depression inventory-II. San Antonio: Psychological Corporation; 1996.
32. Kojima M, Furukawa TA, Takahashi H, Kawai M, Nagaya T, Tokudome S. Cross-cultural validation of the Beck depression inventory-II in Japan. Psychiatry Res. 2002;110(3):291–9.
33. Spielberger CD, Reheiser EC. Assessment of emotions: anxiety, anger, depression, and curiosity. Applied Psychology: Health and Well-Being. 2009; 1(3):271–302.
34. Nakazato K, Mizuguchi T. Development and validation of Japanese version of state-trait anxiety inventory: a study with female subjects. hinshin Igaku [in Japanese]. 1982;22(s):107–12.
35. Kessler RC, Adler LA, Gruber MJ, Sarawate CA, Spencer T, Van Brunt DL. Validity of the World Health Organization adult ADHD self-report scale (ASRS) screener in a representative sample of health plan members. Int J Methods Psychiatr Res. 2007;16(2):52–65.
36. Woodbury-Smith MR, Robinson J, Wheelwright S, Baron-Cohen S. Screening adults for Asperger syndrome using the AQ: a preliminary study of its diagnostic validity in clinical practice. J Autism Dev Disord. 2005;35(3):331–5.
37. Wakabayashi A, Tojo Y, Baron-Cohen S, Wheelwright S. The autism-Spectrum quotient (AQ) Japanese version: evidence from high-functioning clinical group and normal adults. Shinrigaku Kenkyu. 2004;75(1):78–84.
38. Foa EB, Kozak MJ, Salkovskis PM, Coles ME, Amir N. The validation of a new obsessive-compulsive disorder scale: the obsessive-compulsive inventory. Psychol Assess. 1998;10:206–2014.
39. Ishikawa R, Kobori O, Shimizu E. Development and validation of the Japanese version of the obsessive-compulsive inventory. BMC Res Notes. 2014;7:306.
40. Heimberg RG, Horner KJ, Juster HR, Safren SA, Brown EJ, Schneier FR, Liebowitz MR. Psychometric properties of the Liebowitz social anxiety scale. Psychol Med. 1999;29(1):199–212.
41. Asakura S, Inoue S, Sasaki F, Sasaki Y, Kitagawa N, Inoue T, Denda K, Koyama T. Reliability and validity of the Japanese version of the Liebowitz social anxiety scale. Seishin Igaku [in Japanese]. 2002;44(10):1077–84.
42. Daeppen JB, Yersin B, Landry U, Pecoud A, Decrey H. Reliability and validity of the alcohol use disorders identification test (AUDIT) imbedded within a general health risk screening questionnaire: results of a survey in 332 primary care patients. Alcohol Clin Exp Res. 2000;24(5):659–65.
43. Kawada T, Inagaki H, Kuratomi Y. The alcohol use disorders identification test: reliability study of the Japanese version. Alcohol. 2011;45(3):205–7.
44. Patton JH, Stanford MS, Barratt ES. Factor structure of the Barratt impulsiveness scale. J Clin Psychol. 1995;51(6):768–74.
45. Someya T, Sakado K, Seki T, Kojima M, Reist C, Tang SW, Takahashi S. The Japanese version of the Barratt impulsiveness scale, 11th version (BIS-11): its reliability and validity. Psychiatry Clin Neurosci. 2001;55(2):111–4.
46. Busner J, Targum SD. The clinical global impressions scale: applying a research tool in clinical practice. Psychiatry (Edgmont). 2007;4(7):28–37.
47. Osaki Y, Kinjo A. Epidemiology on addictive disorders and behaviors in Japan. Nippon Rinsho [in Japanese]. 2015;73(9):1459–64.
48. Ministry of Internal Affairs and Communications: The survey report of smartphone-app usage and tendency of internet addiction among Japanese high school students. [in Japanese] http://www.soumu.go.jp/main_content/000302914.pdf. 2014.

20

Risk of dementia in patients with primary insomnia: a nationwide population-based case-control study

Chao-Ming Hung[1], Ying-Chun Li[2], Han-Jung Chen[2,3], Kang Lu[2,3], Cheng-Loong Liang[3], Po-Chou Liliang[4], Yu-Duan Tsai[3] and Kuo-Wei Wang[4*]

Abstract

Background: To investigate the association between primary insomnia and dementia using a Taiwanese population-based database.

Methods: This case-control study involved a subset of Taiwan's National Health Insurance Research Database of reimbursement claims. We included 51,734 patients who were diagnosed with primary insomnia from 2002 to 2004 as the test group and 258,715 nonprimary insomnia participants aged 20 years or older as the reference group. We excluded patients under 20 and those with depression, post-traumatic stress disorder, and/or sleep disorders caused by organic lesion(s), drugs, or alcohol. We used a Cox proportional hazards model to assess the primary insomnia on the risk of developing dementia after adjusting for sociodemographic characteristics and comorbidities.

Results: The primary insomnia cohort had a higher prevalence of diabetes, dyslipidemia, hypertension, coronary heart disease, chronic liver disease, and chronic kidney disease at baseline. After adjusting for select comorbidities, primary insomnia remained a significant predisposing factor for developing dementia, and was associated with a 2.14-fold (95% confidence interval, 2.01–2.29) increase in dementia risk. We also found a higher risk of dementia in younger patients.

Conclusions: Taiwanese patients with primary insomnia, especially those under 40, had a higher risk of developing dementia than those without primary insomnia.

Keywords: Insomnia, Sleep disorder, Dementia, Neurodegeneration, Epidemiology

Background

Insomnia is defined as difficulty in initiating sleep, maintaining sleep, and/or struggling with frequent early morning awakenings. Difficulty in sleeping significantly interfering with daily functioning is an important factor considered before diagnosing a patient with insomnia [1]. Primary insomnia is sleeplessness that is not attributable to a medical, psychiatric, or environmental cause. The predominant symptom is difficulty initiating or maintaining sleep, or suffering from nonrestorative sleep, for at least 1 month. The sleep disturbance causes clinically significant distress or impairment in social, occupational, or other important areas of functioning [2]. Primary insomnia is also associated with hypertension, diabetes, myocardial infarction, stroke, and transient ischemic attack [3, 4]. Although an association between sleep and neurological disorders is widely acknowledged [5, 6], most studies of this association have focused on sleep apnea [7, 8]. Few studies have investigated the relationship between primary insomnia and the prevalence of neurological diseases.

Dementia is a condition involving a significant decrease in cognitive abilities, including memory deficits, mood changes, and problems in communication and reasoning. Approximately 1% of the 35 million people worldwide aged 65 to 69 years are affected by this condition [9], and its prevalence increases with age of the population. The percentage of the Taiwanese population aged 65 and above has increased over the past 27 years

* Correspondence: wang11290713@hotmail.com.tw
[4]Department of Neurosurgery, E-Da Cancer Hospital, I-Shou University, Kaohsiung, Taiwan
Full list of author information is available at the end of the article

from 4.1% in 1980 to 10.2% in 2007 [10]. In 2007, the estimated average life expectancy was 81 and 75 years for women and men, respectively. Therefore, dementia is one of the biggest threats to the health of the Taiwanese population.

In this study, we investigated whether primary insomnia was associated with an increased risk of dementia using the Taiwan Longitudinal Health Insurance Database (LHID 2000). In addition, we investigated whether this association was moderated by age.

Methods

Database

This study consisted of a nationwide population-based case-control design. The data were retrieved from the Longitudinal Health Insurance Database (LHID 2000) of Taiwan's National Health Institute Research Database (NHIRD) [11, 12]. This program is a universal health insurance program that was launched in March 1995 in Taiwan. LHID 2000, which is made available to scientists in Taiwan for research purposes, contains comprehensive healthcare data for 1 million people who were randomly selected from original insurance claim data and the registration files of all beneficiaries, representing more than 99% of the 23.37 million people living in Taiwan from 1996 to 2010. The study was approved by the National Health Research Institutes, Taiwan. The database information was anonymized.

Study sample

For the study cohort, we were interested in determining the effects of primary insomnia on the development of dementia. The diagnoses were based on the International Classification of Diseases, Ninth Revision, Clinical Modification (ICD-9-CM). Initially, we included patients who had visited ambulatory care centers for the treatment of primary insomnia from 2002 to 2004 (n = 51,743) [307.4 (specific disorders of sleep of nonorganic origin), 780.5 (sleep disturbance), 780.50 (sleep disturbance, unspecified), 780.52 (insomnia, unspecified), 780.54 (hypersomnia, unspecified), 780.55 (disruptions of the 24-h sleep-wake cycle, unspecified), 780.56 (dysfunctions associated with sleep stages or arousal from sleep), 780.58 (sleep-related movement disorder, unspecified), and 780.59 (sleep disturbance, other)] [13]. Patients were diagnosed with a sleep disorder when at least two ambulatory care claims were recorded [14, 15]. We excluded patients younger than 20 years of age and those with depression, post-traumatic stress disorder, and sleep disorders caused by organic lesion(s), drugs or alcohol [291.82 (alcohol-induced sleep disorders), 292.85 (drug-induced sleep disorders], 309.1 (prolonged depressive reaction), 309.81 (post-traumatic stress disorder), 327.0 (organic disorders of initiating and maintaining sleep), 327.4 (organic parasomnia), 327.5 (organic sleep-related movement disorders), and 327.8 (other organic sleep disorders)]. Dementia is not a specific disease. It is a descriptive term for a collection of symptoms that can be caused by several disorders that affect the brain. People with dementia have significantly impaired intellectual functioning that interferes with normal activities and relationships. They also lose their ability to solve problems and maintain emotional control, and they may experience personality changes and behavioral problems, such as agitation, delusions, and hallucinations [16]. In addition, patients who were diagnosed with dementia [290.0 (senile dementia, uncomplicated), 290.1 (presenile dementia), 290.2 (senile dementia with delusional or depressive features), 290.3 (senile dementia with delirium), 290.4 (arteriosclerotic dementia), 294.1 (dementia in conditions classified elsewhere), 331.0 (Alzheimer's disease), 331.1 (Pick disease), and 331.2 (senile degeneration of the brain)] prior to the index use of health care facilities were identified and excluded from the study. A total of 51,743 primary insomnia patients were included in this study. The study flow chart is shown in Fig. 1.

The comparison cohort (5 comparison subjects for every patient with sleep disorders) was randomly selected from the remaining age- and sex-matched insured controls that used the health service during the same period. A total of 258,715 controls were enrolled in this study, none of whom had been diagnosed with dementia before their initial clinic visits.

Main outcome measures

The primary endpoint of this study was the diagnosis of dementia during hospitalization. Dementia diagnosis in the follow-up years was based on the presence of ICD-9-CM codes 290.0, 290.1, 290.2, 290.3, 290.4, 294.1, 331.0, 331.1, and 331.2 [11, 12]. Each patient was followed for a 3-year period after their sleep disorder diagnosis to identify those patients who subsequently developed dementia. We also explored the relationship between primary insomnia and dementia in different age groups.

Statistical analysis

Our study used Pearson's χ^2 tests to examine the differences in sociodemographic characteristics among patients with and without primary insomnia and select comorbid medical disorders. Selected comorbidities that occurred either in the inpatient setting or in two or more ambulatory care claims and that were recorded 1 year before the index ambulatory care visit were considered in our study. We used the Kaplan–Meier method and log-rank test to estimate the 3-year dementia-free rate and compared the risk of dementia for these two cohorts. In addition, a stratified Cox proportional hazard regression (HR; stratified by age group:

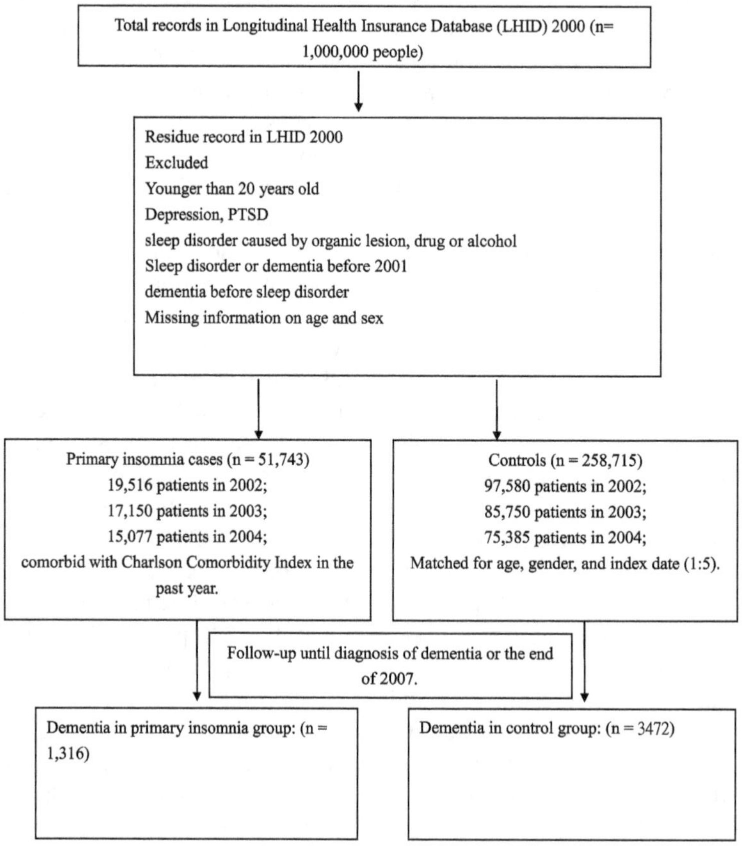

Fig. 1 Flow chart describing the study population

20–39, 40–59, 60–74, and ≥75) was conducted to calculate the 3-year dementia-free rate between patients with and without primary insomnia. The HR values and 95% confidence intervals were computed with a significance level of 0.05. All statistical analyses were conducted using SAS 9.2 statistical software (SAS Institute, Inc., Cary, NC, USA).

Results

Table 1 shows the sociodemographic characteristics and baseline comorbidity statuses of the patients in the primary insomnia and non-primary insomnia cohorts. A total of 51,743 patients who were diagnosed with primary insomnia matched the inclusion criteria; 258,715 patients were included in the comparison cohort. Patients with primary insomnia were more likely to have diabetes (8.25% vs. 6.47%, $p < 0.0001$), dyslipidemia (8.63% vs. 6.05%, $p < 0.0001$), hypertension (18.43% vs. 13.55%, $p < 0.0001$), coronary heart disease (7.35% vs. 4.57%, $p < 0.0001$), chronic liver disease (10.82% vs. 6.43%, $p < 0.0001$), and chronic kidney disease (3.16% vs. 1.96%, $p < 0.0001$).

Table 2 shows the prevalence of dementia in the study subjects. During the 3-year follow-up period, 1316 patients with primary insomnia (2.54% of the study cohort) and 3472 patients with non-primary insomnia (1.34% of the comparison cohort) developed dementia. Compared with patients without primary insomnia, patients with primary insomnia had a higher risk of developing dementia (HR = 2.17; 95% CI, 2.04–2.32; $p < 0.05$). After adjusting for geographic location, residential area, and select premorbid comorbidities, primary insomnia remained a significant predisposing factor for developing dementia, and was associated with a 2.14-fold (95% CI, 2.01–2.29) increase in dementia risk.

Table 3 shows the relative risk of dementia according to age. In the stratified Cox proportional HR, the dementia risk yielded the following results for the 3-year period: in those aged 20–39 years, the HR of patients with primary insomnia was 4.88 (95% CI, 2.98–7.99; $p < 0.05$) compared with patients with non-primary insomnia; in subjects aged 40–59, the HR was 3.56 (95% CI, 2.91–4.36; $p < 0.05$); and, in the 60–74 age group, the HR was 2.21 (95% CI, 2.00–2.44; $p < 0.05$). The HR for those older than 75 years was 1.96 (95% CI, 1.79–2.15; $p < 0.05$). Furthermore, we found that the adjusted HR for dementia within the 3-year period in patients with primary insomnia aged 20–39 years was 4.77 (95% CI, 2.92–7.84; $p < 0.05$), aged

Table 1 Comparison of the Demographic Characteristics and Comorbidities between Patients with and without Primary insomnia

	Patients With primary insomnia		Comparison Patients		
	(*N* = 51,743)		(*N* = 258,715)		
Characteristic	*N*	%	*N*	%	*P*
Sex					1.0000a
Male	20,878	40.35	104,390	40.35	
Female	30,865	59.65	154,325	59.65	
Age, mean ± SD	47.39 ± 15.69		47.39 ± 15.69		1.0000b
Year					1.0000a
≦39	17,637	34.09	88,185	34.09	
40–59	22,081	42.67	110,405	42.67	
60–74	8890	17.18	44,450	17.18	
≥ 75	3135	6.06	15,675	6.06	
Geographic region					<.0001a
Northern	22,354	43.20	123,645	47.79	
Central	14,241	27.52	53,729	20.77	
Southern	12,622	24.39	68,637	26.53	
Eastern	1194	2.31	6362	2.46	
Missing	1332	2.57	6342	2.45	
Comorbidities					
diabetes	4267	8.25	16,750	6.47	<.0001a
dyslipidemia	4465	8.63	15,656	6.05	<.0001a
hypertension	9538	18.43	35,067	13.55	<.0001a
coronary heart disease	3803	7.35	11,824	4.57	<.0001a
chronic liver disease	5597	10.82	16,630	6.43	<.0001a
chronic kidney disease	1636	3.16	5069	1.96	<.0001a

SD standard deviation; *a* chi-square test; *b* t-test

40–59 years was 3.24 (95% CI, 2.91–4.36; $p < 0.05$), the corresponding value in patients aged 60–74 years was 2.12 (95% CI, 1.92–2.34; $p < 0.05$), and in patients older than 75 years, the adjusted HR value was 1.95 (95% CI, 1.77–2.14; $p < 0.05$).

Discussion

In the present study, patients with primary insomnia showed an increased prevalence of dementia risk factors, such as hypertension, diabetes, hyperlipidemia, and coronary heart disease. Our findings were concurrent with meta-analyses and community-based reports showing that primary insomnia is associated with an increased prevalence of hypertension, diabetes, myocardial infarction, stroke, and transient ischemic attack [17]. Patients with primary insomnia have a greater risk of being diagnosed with dementia. During the 3-year follow up, 2.54% of patients with primary insomnia (1316 patients) compared with 1.34% of patients without primary insomnia (3472 patients) were diagnosed with dementia. After adjusting for age, sex, region of residence, and selected comorbidities, a primary insomnia diagnosis was independently associated with a 2.17-fold higher risk of subsequent development of dementia. When the results were further stratified according to sex and other covariates were controlled, the adjusted HR was 2.14-fold (95% CI, 2.01–2.29). Younger patients with primary insomnia had a higher risk of developing dementia.

The mechanism underlying the association between primary insomnia and dementia is unclear. Sleep disturbances are common in the general population. A recent study conducted in older adults reported that insomnia was associated with a significantly increased risk of all-cause dementia [18]. Another recent study also demonstrated that sleep disturbances can enhance the risk of developing dementia, and insomnia may increase the risk of Alzheimer's disease. These findings elucidate the influence of sleep disturbances on the incidence of dementia, especially in older adults [19]. In the US, 35–40% of the adult population is reported to suffer from sleep disorders. There is increasing evidence from large screening surveys showing that primary insomnia is associated with hypertension, diabetes, myocardial infarction, stroke, and transient ischemic attack [20–24],

Table 2 Dementia risk among sampled patients during the 3-year follow-up period after index healthcare utilization

Type of sleep disorder	n	Persons-years	dementia case	Unadjusted		Adjusted	
				HR	95% CI	HR	95% CI
No insomnia	258,715	1,303,464.02	3472	1.00	(reference)	1.00	(reference)
Primary insomnia	51,745	233,853.23	1316	2.17*	(2.04-2.32)	2.14*	(2.01-2.29)

CI confidence interval
*$p < 0.05$ The Hazard Ratio (HR) was calculated by using the stratified Cox proportional regression method (stratified by sex, age group, and year of index healthcare use) during the 3-year follow-up period. Adjustments were made for the following selected comorbidities in the patients: diabetes, hyperlipidemia, hypertension, coronary heart disease, chronic liver disease, and chronic kidney disease

which suggests that sleep disorders should be considered a new cardiovascular risk factor. Because diabetes, hypertension, myocardial infarction, and stroke are known risk factors for dementia, these findings suggest that patients with primary insomnia have higher cognitive dysfunction [11, 12].

Several recently published studies support the results of the present study. A study by Monlar et al. showed that restless legs syndrome was associated with an 88% increase in mortality risk, and the risk of coronary heart disease and stroke increased almost four times [25]. Stroke and coronary heart disease are risk factors for dementia [3, 4]. However, the data collected in this study described the risk factors in patients with chronic kidney disease in US veterans and not in the general population. Another study by Sung et al. showed that non-apnea sleep disorders might be an early indicator of cognitive dysfunction, especially in the younger population [26], even though those without non-apnea sleep disorders were not included in this study. There was a small group of patients with subjective insomnia (ICD-9-CM codes 307.42, 307.49, and 780.52). This type of insomnia is also known as sleep state misperception. Personality traits, anxiety, rumination, and pre-sleep worry have been suggested to be associated with such cases of insomnia. The somatic preoccupations of these insomniacs are most likely not hypochondriacal in nature but rather reflect true physiological and physical changes that occur as a result of chronic activation of the stress system. The distinct psychological profiles between insomnia subtypes based on objective sleep duration have showed that patients with subjective insomnia have higher neuroticism, higher scores on the psychasthenia and schizophrenia scales, higher anxiety, lower mood, more dysfunctional sleep-related cognitions, and fewer somatic complaints compared to patients with objective insomnia [27]. This type of insomnia is related to stress.

Another mechanism that possibly links primary insomnia to dementia is amyloid β-related neurodegenerative pathophysiological processes [9]. Proteins, including amyloid β and tau, which are linked to neurodegenerative diseases, are present in the interstitial space surrounding brain cells [28]. Cerebrospinal fluid

Table 3 Crude and adjusted Hazard Ratios (HRs) for dementia among sampled patients of different age groups during the 3-year follow-up period after index healthcare utilization

	n	dementia case	Unadjusted		Adjusted	
			HR	95% CI	HR	95% CI
20–39						
No insomnia	88,185	34	1.00	(reference)	1.00	(reference)
Primary insomnia	17,637	30	4.88*	(2.98- 7.99)	4.77*	(2.90-7.84)
40–59						
No insomnia	110,405	253	1.00	(reference)	1.00	(reference)
Primary insomnia	22,081	155	3.56*	(2.91- 4.36)	3.24*	(2.64-3.97)
60–74						
No insomnia	44,450	1392	1.00	(reference)	1.00	(reference)
Primary insomnia	8890	533	2.21*	(2.00- 2.44)	2.12*	(1.92-2.34)
≥ 75						
No insomnia	15,675	1793	1.00	(reference)	1.00	(reference)
Primary insomnia	3135	598	1.96*	(1.79- 2.15)	1.95*	(1.77-2.14)

*$p < 0.05$ The HR was calculated by using the stratified Cox proportional regression method (stratified by sex, age group, and the year of index healthcare use) during the 3-year follow-up period. Adjustments were made for the following selected comorbidities in the patients: diabetes, hyperlipidemia, hypertension, coronary heart disease, chronic liver disease, and chronic kidney disease

recirculates throughout the brain, interchanges with interstitial fluid, and removes interstitial proteins, including amyloid β. Amyloid β clearance is increased during sleep, and the sleep-wake cycle regulates lymphatic clearance [29]. Primary insomnia therefore leads to an accumulation of amyloid β deposits, potentially triggering earlier cognitive decline [29]. Age-dependent amyloid β deposits are related to Alzheimer's disease and sleep abnormalities [30]. Other studies have reported that amyloid deposits in the preclinical stage of Alzheimer's disease are associated with worse sleep quality, but not quantity [31]. These studies support the hypothesis that primary insomnia is a potential risk factor for subsequent dementia.

There were several advantages to our study. Our study was based on a nationwide population-based case-control study. Secondly, sleep disorders can lead to stroke, Alzheimer's disease, multiple sclerosis, deep vein thrombosis, and poorer hospital outcomes [20–24]. However, most epidemiological studies have focused on obstructive sleep apnea [7, 8]. Sleep disorders can be divided into primary insomnia, insomnia associated with medical or mental diseases, and insomnia associated with the consumption or abuse of substances. It is difficult to establish the impact of primary insomnia on disease development. In our study, we excluded patients with insomnia due to medical disease, mental diseases, the consumption or abuse of substances, and organic lesions. Therefore, the main finding of our study was that primary insomnia was a potential risk factor for subsequent dementia. In addition, we found that the risk of developing dementia associated with sleep disorder was higher in younger patients. Several studies have shown that total sleep time, sleep efficiency, and percentage of slow-wave sleep all significantly decrease with age, thus showing that young adults are not able to obtain enough time for sleep. Changes in sleep patterns earlier in life have a greater impact on health. Most dementia studies have focused on older individuals. However, the age of onset is an important consideration for dementia patients [31]. Savva et al. have shown that the association between the pathological features of Alzheimer's disease and dementia is stronger in younger persons than in their older counterparts. Age will be an important factor to consider while considering the effects of dementia and developing effective strategies for dealing with this condition [32, 33].

Some important limitations in this study need to be addressed. First, detailed information regarding smoking, alcohol consumption, socioeconomic status, and family history of systemic diseases were not available from the NHIRD. Second, the follow-up period may not have been long enough for patients to develop dementia in our study. Third, the quality of evidence from a nationwide population-based case-control study is lower than that from randomized trials.

Conclusions

The results of our study supported the hypothesis that patients with primary insomnia have a higher longitudinal risk of developing dementia. Young patients with primary insomnia showed a greater incidence of dementia than older patients. However, very little is known about the type, frequency, or level of insomnia necessary to induce dementia; further research in this area is necessary to confirm our findings.

Abbreviations

LHID 2000: Longitudinal Health Insurance Database; NHIRD: National Health Institute Research Database

Acknowledgements

This study was based in part on data from the National Health Insurance Research Database provided by the Bureau of National Health Insurance, Department of Health, Taiwan, and managed by the National Health Research Institutes. The interpretations and conclusions contained herein do not represent those of the Bureau of National Health Insurance, Department of Health, or National Health Research Institutes.

Funding

The study was not supported by any source of funding.

Authors' contributions

CMH data collection. YCI and HJC data analysis. KL, CLL, PCL, YDT, and KWW analysis of conclusions and completion of paper. All authors read and approved the final manuscript.

Consent for publication

The manuscript did not contain any individual person's data in any form (including individual details, images or videos).

Competing interests

The authors declare that they have no competing interests.

Author details

Department of General Surgery, E-Da Cancer Hospital, I-Shou University, Kaohsiung, Taiwan. [2]Institute of Health Care Management, National Sun Yat-Sen University, Kaohsiung, Taiwan. [3]Department of Neurosurgery, E-Da Hospital, I-Shou University, Kaohsiung, Taiwan. [4]Department of Neurosurgery, E-Da Cancer Hospital, I-Shou University, Kaohsiung, Taiwan.

References

1. Corine H, Jaap L, Jan BR, et al. Adherence to technology-mediated insomnia treatment: a meta-analysis, interviews, and focus groups. J Med Internet Res. 2015;17(9):e214.
2. Diagnostic and Statistical Manual of Mental Disorders, Fourth Edition, Text Revision (DSM-IV-TR). Washington, DC: American Psychiatric Press; 2000. 553–557.
3. Altman NG, Izci-Balserak B, Schopfer E, Jackson N, Rattanaumpawan P, Gehrman PR, et al. Sleep duration versus sleep insufficiency as predictors of cardiometabolic health outcomes. Sleep Med. 2012;13(10):1261–70.
4. Valham F, Mooe T, Rabben T, Stenlund H, Wiklund U, Franklin KA. Increased risk of stroke in patients with coronary artery disease and sleep apnea: a 10-year follow-up. Circulation. 2008;118(9):955–60.

5. Watson NF, Viola-Saltzman M. Sleep and comorbid neurologic disorders. Continuum (Minneap Minn). 2013;19(1):148–69.
6. Benca RM, Obermeyer WH, Thisted RA, Gillin JC. Sleep and Psychiatric disorders. A meta-analysis. Arch Gen Psychiatry. 1992;49(8):651–68.
7. Chen PL, Lee WJ, Sun WZ, Oyang YJ, Fuh JL. Risk of dementia in patients with insomnia and long-term use of hypnotics: a population-based retrospective cohort study. PLoS One. 2012;7(11):e49113.
8. Chang WP, Liu ME, Chang WC, Yang AC, Ku YC, Pai JT, Huang HL, Tsai SJ. Sleep apnea and the risk of dementia: a population-based 5-year follow-up study in Taiwan. PLoS One. 2013;8(10):e78655.
9. Querfurth HW, LaFerla FM. Alzheimer's disease. N Engl J Med. 2010; 362(4):329–44.
10. Fuh JL, Wang SJ. Dementia in Taiwan: past, present, and future. Acta Neurol Taiwanica. 2008;17(3):153–61.
11. Wang HK, Lin SH, Sung PS, et al. Population based study on patients with traumatic brain injury suggests increased risk of dementia. J Neurol Neurosurg Psychiatry. 2012;83(11):1080–5.
12. Wang HK, Tsai KJ, Huang CY, Wang LC, Lu K, Chen HJ, et al. Newly diagnosed dementia and increased risk of hemorrhagic stroke: a Nationwide population-based study. Curr Alzheimer Res. 2014;11(3):291–8.
13. Roberts RE, Roberts CR, Chen IG. Impact of insomnia on future functioning of adolescents. J Psychosom Res. 2002;53(1):561–9.
14. Hsieh CY, Chen CH, Li CY, Lai ML. Validating the diagnosis of acute ischemic stroke in a National Health Insurance claims database. J Formos Med Assoc. 2015;114(3):254–9.
15. Lin CC, Lai MS, Syu CY, Chang SC, Tseng FY. Accuracy of diabetes diagnosis in health insurance claims data in Taiwan. J Formos Med Assoc. 2005;104(3): 157–63.
16. National Institute of Neurological Disorders and Stroke (https://www.ninds.nih.gov/).
17. Spiegelhalder K, Scholtes C, Riemann D. The association between insomnia and cardiovascular diseases. Nat Sci Sleep. 2010;2:71–8.
18. de Almondes KM, Costa MV, Malloy-Diniz LF, Diniz BS. Insomnia and risk of dementia in older adults: systematic review and meta-analysis. J Psychiatr Res. 2016;77:109–15.
19. Shi L, Chen SJ, Ma MY, Bao YP, Han Y, Wang YM, Shi J, Vitiello MV, Lu L. Sleep disturbances increase the risk of dementia: A systematic review and meta-analysis. Sleep Med Rev. 2017. https://doi.org/10.1016/j.smrv.2017.06.010.
20. Narang I, Manlhiot C, Davies-Shaw J, Gibson D, Chahal N, Stearne K, et al. Sleep disturbance and cardiovascular risk in adolescents. CMAJ. 2012; 184(17):E913–20.
21. Shankar A, Syamala S, Kalidindi S, "Insufficient rest or sleep and its relation to cardiovascular disease, diabetes and obesity in a national, multiethnic sample, " PLoS One, vol. 5, no. 11, pp. e14189, 2010.
22. Grandner MA, Jackson NJ, Pak VM, Gehrman PR. Sleep disturbance is associated with cardiovascular and metabolic disorders. J Sleep Res. 2012; 21(4):427–33.
23. Magee CA, Kritharides L, Attia J, McElduff P, Banks E. Short and long sleep duration are associated with prevalent cardiovascular disease in Australian adults. J Sleep Res. 2012;21(4):441–7.
24. Najafian J, Mohamadifard N, Siadat ZD, Sadri G, Rahmati MR. Association between sleep duration and diabetes mellitus: Isfahan healthy heart program. Niger J Clin Pract. 2013;16(1):59–62.
25. Molnar MZ, Lu JL, Kalantar-Zadeh K, Kovesdy CP. Association of incident restless legs syndrome with outcomes in a large cohort of US veterans. J Sleep Res. 2016;25(1):47–56.
26. Sung PS, Yeh CC, Wang LC, Hung PH, Muo CH, Sung FC, Chen CH, Tsai KJ. Increased risk of dementia in patients with non-apnea sleep disorder. Curr Alzheimer Res. 2016; [Epub ahead of print]
27. Fernandez-Mendoza J, Calhoun SL, Bixler EO, Karataraki M, Liao D, Vela-Bueno A, Ramos-Platon MJ, Sauder KA, Basta M, Vgontzas AN. Sleep misperception and chronic insomnia in the general population: the role of objective sleep duration and psychological profiles. Psychosom Med. 2011; 73(1):88–97.
28. Iliff JJ, Wang M, Liao Y, Plogg BA, Peng W, Gundersen GA, et al. A paravascular pathway facilitates CSF flow through the brain parenchyma and the clearance of interstitial solutes, including amyloid β. Sci Transl Med. 2012;4(147):147.
29. Mander BA, Winer JR, Jagust WJ, Walker MP. Sleep: a novel mechanistic pathway, biomarker, and treatment target in the pathology of Alzheimer's disease? Trends Neurosci. 2016;39(8):552–66.
30. Wisor JP, Edgar DM, Yesavage J, Ryan HS, McCormick CM, Lapustea N, Murphy GM Jr. Sleep and circadian abnormalities in a transgenic mouse model of Alzheimer's disease: a role for cholinergic transmission. Neuroscience. 2005;131(2):375–85.
31. Ju YE, McLeland JS, Toedebusch CD, Xiong C, Fagan AM, Duntley SP, Morris JC, Holtzman DM. Sleep quality and preclinical Alzheimer disease. JAMA Neurol. 2013;70(5):587–93.
32. Villa MP, Rizzoli A, Rabasco J, Vitelli O, Pietropaoli N, Cecili M, Marino A, Malagola C. Rapid maxillary expansion outcomes in treatment of obstructive sleep apnea in children. Sleep Med. 2015;16(6):709–16.
33. Savva GM, Wharton SB, Ince PG, Forster G, Matthews FE, Brayne C, et al. Age, neuropathology, and dementia. N Engl J Med. 2009;360:2302–9.

21

Mental health outcomes among Arab refugees, immigrants, and U.S. born Arab Americans in Southeast Michigan

Sanjana Pampati[1*], Zaineb Alattar[1], Evette Cordoba[2], Madiha Tariq[3] and Carlos Mendes de Leon[1]

Abstract

Background: Arab refugees and immigrants living in the United States may be exposed to political, economic, social, and environmental stressors that may affect their mental health. Yet, little is known regarding mental health outcomes among Arab Americans. The purpose of this study was to measure depression and anxiety levels among Arabs in Southeast Michigan and determine whether these levels differ by resident status: refugee, immigrant, or U.S. born.

Methods: We conducted a cross-sectional study in a convenience sample of 275 adults who self-identify as Arab living in Southeast Michigan. Participants were recruited from a non-profit health and social services organization between August–November 2015. Data were collected via self-administered questionnaires, using standardized instruments to assess depression and anxiety symptoms.

Results: All three resident groups exhibited high mean levels of depression and anxiety. Refugees reported higher levels of depression and anxiety than either immigrants or U.S. born Arab Americans. After adjustment for sociodemographics, differences between U.S. born Arab Americans and refugees were statistically significant for depression (b = 2.84; 95% CI: 0.21, 5.47), but not for anxiety. Refugees had significantly higher depression scores (b = 3.18, 95% CI: 1.52, 4.84) and anxiety scores (b = 1.31, 95% CI: 0.11, 2.50) than immigrants. Those reporting political violence and religious persecution as reasons for immigration had the highest levels of depression and anxiety.

Conclusions: This convenience sample of Arab Americans reported high levels of depression and anxiety symptoms. Refugees appear to have poorer mental health outcomes than either immigrants or U.S.-born Arab Americans.

Keywords: Refugee, Immigrant, Arab-American, Depression, Anxiety

Background

The overall purpose of this study is to provide an initial examination of mental health outcomes among Arab refugees, immigrants, and U.S. born Arab Americans in Southeast Michigan. Over the last few decades, the United States has become home to a growing population of refugees from Arab countries in the Middle East and North Africa (MENA) [1, 2]. The majority of those refugees in the past decade have fled war, political oppression, and persecution in Iraq and Syria [3, 4]. Given the many social, political, environmental, and economic stressors that refugees and immigrants may be exposed to before, during, and after their journey, this population may be at high risk of developing adverse mental health outcomes [5–11]. Pre-migration stressors can include war, political conflict, persecution based on religion, race, ethnicity, gender, sexual orientation, or other social group membership, and economic stress [5, 6, 12]. Post-migration stressors can include acculturative stress associated with resettlement, language barriers, social

* Correspondence: spampati@umich.edu
[1]University of Michigan School of Public Health, 1415 Washington Heights, Ann Arbor, MI 48109, USA
Full list of author information is available at the end of the article

isolation, xenophobia, Islamophobia, discrimination, and difficulty accessing secure employment, housing, and transportation [5, 6, 12–14].

Many Arab refugees and immigrants enter and settle in Southeast Michigan, which is one of the largest recipient regions in the U.S. for this population [3, 15]. In the past decade (FY2008-FY2018), Michigan has received 35,009 refugees, including 20,362 Iraqis and 2256 Syrians; that is 14% of all Iraqi/Syrian refugees arriving to the U.S. during this period, and more than any other state after California [16]. Historically, most Arab refugees and immigrants in Michigan have settled around the Detroit Metro Area, which has been drawing immigrants going back to the late nineteenth century with the booming automotive industry [2]. Today, the city of Dearborn is home to the largest proportion of Arabs in the U.S., with Arab Americans representing 49.8% of the population [17]. There is very little systematic information on the mental health needs of the Arab-origin population in the U.S. The small number of studies thus far suggest that Arab Americans experience greater mental health challenges relative to majority non-Hispanic Whites. For example, data from the National Health Interview Survey indicate that foreign-born adults from the Middle East report significantly more serious psychological distress compared with foreign-born adults from Europe, or U.S.-born non-Hispanic Whites [18]. Data from a 2004 internet-based non-probability convenience sample of Arab Americans revealed much higher depression and anxiety levels in this population relative to normative data from non-Hispanic Whites and other ethnic groups, with about 50% reporting depression scores that met clinical case criteria, and about one-fourth reporting moderate to severe anxiety [19].

In addition, there may also be important mental health differences within the Arab American population itself, especially as a function of immigrant status (refugee, immigrant, or U.S. born). According to data from the 2003 Detroit Arab American Study, Arab immigrants reported poorer self-rated health than U.S. born Arab Americans [20]. Similarly, a study on older Arab Americans living in the Detroit Metro Area, age 56 and older, also found that immigrants report more frequent feelings of depression and lower life satisfaction than their U.S. born counterparts [21]. Further, among Arab Americans age 60 and older, higher levels of depression have also been found among refugees as compared to citizens, permanent residents, and visa holders [22]. Previous research in other immigrant populations suggests that refugees tend to have more mental health issues compared with immigrants. For example, Tamil refugees and asylum seekers reported more symptoms of anxiety, depression, and post-traumatic stress than Tamil immigrants [23]. Similarly, female refugees in Sweden had a significantly higher likelihood of purchasing psychotropic drugs, a proxy measure for mental health problems, compared to non-refugee immigrants [24]. Recent conflicts in the MENA region may put immigrants and refugees from that region at particular risk for adverse mental health outcomes, even relative to those with the same heritage but born in the U.S. However, the degree to which differences in country of birth (U.S. versus MENA) and refugee status affect mental health in Arab Americans is currently unknown.

In this study, we examine (1) the degree to which resident status (refugee, immigrant, U.S. born) is associated with depression and anxiety in Arab Americans, (2) whether duration living in the U.S. moderates the relationship between resident status and these mental health outcomes, and (3) the association between specific reasons for migration and each of these mental health outcomes among Arab immigrants and refugees.

Methods

Study background

This is a cross-sectional study of a convenience sample of adults who self-identify as Arab. Between August 2015 to November 2015, participants ($n = 309$) were recruited from the health and social services waiting room of the Arab Community Center for Economic and Social Services (ACCESS) in Dearborn, Michigan. ACCESS is the largest Arab American community nonprofit organization in the U.S. Founded in Dearborn, Michigan in 1971 with the purpose of helping Arab immigrants adjust to their new life in the U.S., it has since expanded and now provides a variety of health, education, employment, and social services to different communities in Southeast Michigan [25]. Although ACCESS' services are open to a diverse population, clients tend to come from low-income backgrounds and are typically more recent immigrants and refugees. Eligibility for this study was restricted to those who were at least 18 years old and self-identified as being of Arab origin. Standardized English questionnaires covering basic demographic information, health conditions, mental health, and risk behaviors were translated into Modern Standard Arabic and back-translated into English independently by 2 bilingual study staff members. A consensus approach was used to resolve any differences. All participants completed either a self-administered English or Arabic-language paper questionnaire after providing written informed consent. IRB approval was received from the University of Michigan. Participants were compensated $10 for their time and effort.

Measures

Depression was measured using the Center for Epidemiologic Studies Depression Short Form (CES-D-SF), a shorter, 8 item version of the CES-D [26]. The CES-D-SF assesses the frequency of common depressive symptoms over the past 14 days, rated on a frequency scale as follows: not at all, several days, more than half the days, and nearly every day. The internal consistency of the CES-D-SF was found to be high (Cronbach coefficient alpha = 0.84). The CES-D has been successfully used to measure depression among Arab populations in the Middle East as well as Arab Americans [14, 27–29]. Summary scores of depressive symptomatology (referred to as depression scores) were calculated by summing the responses to the 8 items (range 0–24). We used mean imputation for participants with one missing item (n = 36). Depression scores for participants with ≥ 2 items missing were set to missing (n = 19). Anxiety was measured using 4 items from the Generalized Anxiety Disorder (GAD-4) scale [30]. The GAD-4 scale assesses the frequency of GAD symptoms over the past 14 days using the same 4-point scale as the CES-D-SF. The internal consistency of the GAD-4 instrument was high (Cronbach coefficient alpha = 0.90). Summary scores of anxiety symptomatology (referred to as anxiety scores) were calculated by summing the responses to the 4 items (range 0–12).

Resident status was ascertained based on 3 questions: "What country were you born in?", "Do you have legal refugee status?", and "If you were not born in the United States, in what year did you first enter the United States to live?" Participants who responded that they were born in the U.S. were categorized as U.S. born Arab Americans. Participants who responded that they had legal refugee status were categorized as refugees. Participants who listed another country besides the "United States" as their nation of birth or participants who reported a year of immigration to the U.S. and did not report legal refugee status were categorized as immigrants. We did not assess asylum status due to the very limited number of Arab-origin individuals granted asylum in the U.S. [3].

Duration living in the U.S. was modelled as a continuous variable, determined based on the reported year of immigration. For U.S. born Arab Americans, duration was set to their current age. Highest educational attainment was modelled as an ordinal variable and categorized as less than high school, high school/GED, college, or greater than college (graduate work). Marital status was categorized as married, divorced/separated, widowed, or never married, and modeled as married versus non-married in the regression analyses.

Reasons for immigrating to the U.S. were assessed by asking "If you immigrated to the United States, for what reason did you leave your home country?" Possible responses included political violence, religious persecution, seeking educational opportunity, seeking economic opportunity, and all of the above. These categories were not mutually exclusive and multiple responses could be selected. Participants were also permitted to write in a response. Write-in responses were either re-classified into one of the existing categories or were classified in the new response category "family reasons," as it mostly included family reunification. U.S. born Arab Americans who responded to this question were set to missing.

Analysis

The analysis for this study was restricted to those with complete self-reported age, sex, and resident status information (n = 275). The sample consisted of refugees (n = 67), immigrants (n = 153), and U.S. born Arab Americans (n = 55). To test the association between resident status and depression and anxiety outcomes, we fitted a linear regression model for each outcome with U.S. born Arab Americans serving as reference category for resident status. Each model also included control variables for age, sex, duration living in the U.S., education, and marital status. In both models, interaction between resident status and duration living in the U.S. were tested to see if mental health outcomes associated with resident status varied as a function of time since arriving in the U.S. In order to test differences between refugees and immigrants, we repeated the aforementioned models with immigrants as reference group. All models were fitted in SAS 9.4. An exploratory analysis examining mean depression and anxiety levels by reason for immigration was also conducted.

Results

Participant characteristics

Of the 275 participants with complete sociodemographic information, the majority resided in Dearborn (n = 156), Dearborn Heights (n = 58), or Detroit (n = 18). Most of them identified as Muslim (n = 255), while a small minority identified as Christian (n = 11; data not shown). Of the 275 participants, several were missing information on relevant covariates, including marital status (n = 6), duration in the U.S. (n = 21), depression (n = 19), and anxiety (n = 4). Thus, the depression analysis included a sample size of 233 and the anxiety analysis included a sample size of 245. Sociodemographic characteristics of the total analytic sample (n = 275) and by resident status are shown in Table 1. Mean age for the total sample was 38.7 years (SD = 1.7 years; range = 18–85 years) and the majority was female (61.8%). Although the mean age of refugees (42.8 ± 3.4 years) and immigrants (41.2 ± 2.2 years) were similar, U.S. born Arab Americans were considerably younger (26.5 ± 3.2 years). Educational attainment varied based on resident status, with one third (34.3%) of refugees, 55% (46.4% + 8.5%) of immigrants, and three-quarters (61.8% + 14.6%) of U.S. born Arab Americans reporting a college degree or more. Most participants were married (58.0%), with U.S. born participants less likely to be married (24.5%) than either

Table 1 Characteristics of the Study Sample by Resident Status

	Total (n = 275), No. (%), or Mean (95% CI)	Refugee (n = 67), No. (%), or Mean (95% CI)	Immigrant (n = 153), No. (%), or Mean (95% CI)	U.S. Born (n = 55), No. (%), or Mean (95% CI)
Age, years	38.7 (36.9, 40.4)	42.8 (39.4, 46.3)	41.2 (39.0, 43.3)	26.5 (23.3, 29.8)
Female	170 (61.8%)	33 (49.2%)	97 (63%)	40 (72.7%)
Education				
< High school	45 (16.4%)	15 (22.4%)	27 (17.6%)	3 (5.4%)
High school/GED	81 (29.4%)	29 (43.3%)	42 (27.4%)	10 (18.2%)
College	128 (46.5%)	23 (34.3%)	71 (46.4%)	34 (61.8%)
> College	21 (7.6%)	0 (0.0%)	13 (8.5%)	8 (14.6%)
Marital Status				
Married	156 (58.0%)	48 (73.8%)	95 (62.9%)	13 (24.5%)
Divorced or separated	32 (11.9%)	5 (7.7%)	25 (16.6%)	2 (3.8%)
Widowed	11 (4.1%)	3 (4.6%)	7 (4.6%)	1 (1.9%)
Never married	70 (26.0%)	9 (13.8%)	24 (15.9%)	37 (69.8%)
Duration in U.S.				
≤ 5 years	52 (20.5%)	25 (39.7%)	27 (19.8%)	0 (0.0%)
6–14 years	53 (20.9%)	19 (30.2%)	34 (25.0%)	0 (0.0%)
≥ 15 years	149 (58.7%)	19 (30.2%)	75 (55.2%)	55 (100%)
Depression score	8.85 (5.52)	11.93 (5.35)	8.04 (5.46)	7.39 (4.55)
Anxiety score	4.77 (3.77)	5.88 (3.68)	4.41 (3.79)	4.51 (3.65)
Reasons for immigration[a]				
Political violence	95 (45.5%)	46 (69.7%)	49 (34.3%)	–
Religious persecution	39 (18.7%)	13 (19.7%)	26 (18.2%)	–
Educational opportunity	70 (33.5%)	10 (15.2%)	60 (42.0%)	–
Economic opportunity	91 (43.5%)	17 (25.8%)	74 (51.8%)	–
Familial reasons	24 (11.5%)	4 (6.1%)	20 (14.0%)	–

[a]Categories not mutually exclusive; participants could select more than one reason

refugees (73.8%) or immigrants (62.9%). Refugees reported a shorter duration of being in the U.S. than immigrants; 39.7% of them had lived in the U.S. ≤ 5 years compared with 19.8% of immigrants. Mean depression scores were 8.85 (SD = 5.52) for the total sample, and 11.93 (SD = 5.35), 8.04 (SD = 5.46), and 7.39 (SD = 4.55) for refugees, immigrants, and U.S. born Arab Americans, respectively. Mean anxiety scores were 4.77 (SD = 3.77) for the total sample, and 5.88 (SD = 3.68), 4.41 (SD = 3.79), and 4.51 (SD = 3.65) for refugees, immigrants, and U.S. born Arab Americans, respectively.

Regression analyses

In regression analyses controlling for age, sex, marital status, education, and duration living in the U.S., refugee status was associated with significantly higher depression scores (b = 2.84; 95% CI: 0.21, 5.47) relative to U.S. born Arab Americans (Table 2, Model 1). Depression scores were not significantly different between immigrants and U.S. born Arab Americans. Using immigrants as the referent group in an additional model, we found that refugees had significantly higher depression scores than immigrants (b = 3.18, 95% CI: 1.52, 4.84; data not shown). Of the other covariates in the model, only educational attainment was significantly associated with depression scores, such that higher education was associated with

Table 2 Linear Regression Analyses Predicting Depression and Anxiety Scores

Variable	Model 1: Depression Score (n = 233) b (95% CI)	Model 2: Anxiety Score (n = 245) b (95% CI)
Resident status		
Refugee	2.84 (0.21, 5.47)	1.38 (−0.52, 3.27)
Immigrant	−0.34 (−2.43, 1.75)	0.07 (−1.44, 1.57)
U.S. Born (ref)	–	–
Age	0.05 (−0.02, 0.11)	0.01 (−0.04, 0.06)
Female	0.79 (−0.63, 2.22)	0.88 (−0.14, 1.89)
Married	−1.02 (−2.51, 0.47)	−0.47 (−1.54, 0.59)
Education	−0.99 (−1.39, −0.59)	−0.42 (−0.70, −0.14)
Duration in U.S.	−0.03 (−0.09, 0.04)	0.01 (−0.04, 0.05)

lower depressive scores (b = – 0.99; 95% CI: -1.39, – 0.59). Interaction effects between duration living in the U.S. and refugee and immigrant status were tested but did not yield significant results (data not shown).

In regression analyses for anxiety scores controlling for the same set of covariates, neither refugee status (b = 1.38; 95% CI: -0.52, 3.27) nor immigrant status (b = 0.07; 95% CI: -1.44, 1.57) were associated with significantly different anxiety scores relative to U.S. born Arab Americans (see Table 2, Model 2). Using immigrants as the referent group in an additional model, we found that refugees had significantly higher anxiety scores than immigrants (b = 1.31, 95% CI: 0.11, 2.50; data not shown). Of the other covariates, only educational attainment was significantly associated with anxiety scores, such that higher education was associated with lower anxiety scores (b = – 0.42; 95% CI: -0.70, – 0.14). Interaction effects between duration living in the U.S. and refugee and immigrant status were tested in both models but did not yield significant results (data not shown).

Reasons for immigration

The exploratory analysis of mental health outcomes by reasons for immigration revealed that those reporting political violence and religious persecution had the highest levels of depression and anxiety (see Table 3). This was particularly the case if these were the only reasons they listed for immigration to the U.S. In contrast, those reporting educational opportunity or economic opportunity, especially as the sole reason for immigration, had the lowest levels of depression and anxiety. Immigrants and refugees reporting family reasons for coming to the U.S. had average levels of depression and anxiety in this sample.

Discussion

Our findings suggest potentially important differences in mental health outcomes within the Arab American population. Overall, and not unexpectedly, Arab refugees appear to experience higher depression and anxiety symptom levels than U.S. born Arab Americans, even if these differences were statistically significant only for depression among refugees after adjustment for relevant correlates. Further, they also experienced higher depression and anxiety symptom levels than immigrants. Due to the stressors that Arab refugees may experience before and after resettlement, they may well be at particular risk of adverse mental health outcomes [5–11]. Other challenges that may contribute to higher depression among refugees compared to the U.S. born include difficulties in integrating into society and accessing opportunities in employment and other social domains [5, 6, 12, 13]. In addition, in an exploratory analysis, we found that those reporting political violence and religious persecution as reasons for immigration had the highest levels of depression and anxiety.

Table 3 Depression and Anxiety Scores by Reason for Immigration

Reason for Immigration	Depression		Anxiety	
	N	Mean (SD)	N	Mean (SD)
Political violence only	49	10.90 (5.90)	52	5.21 (3.85)
Political violence and other	38	9.48 (6.16)	40	4.72 (3.53)
Religious persecution only	5	14.60 (1.95)	5	10.80 (1.30)
Religious persecution and other	32	9.40 (6.46)	34	4.47 (3.26)
Educational opportunity only	26	6.49 (5.13)	27	4.18 (4.00)
Educational opportunity and other	38	9.16 (6.48)	42	5.05 (3.87)
Economic opportunity only	46	8.92 (5.41)	50	3.96 (3.23)
Economic opportunity and other	36	9.02 (6.70)	40	4.92 (3.93)
Familial reasons only	22	9.50 (4.42)	24	4.96 (3.62)

Our findings suggest that there is greater mental health suffering among Arab Americans not born in the U.S., especially those that came as refugees. The relatively lower depression scores found among U.S. born Arab Americans in this study are consistent with past findings of greater perceived well-being, including less frequent feelings of depression, among older U.S. born Arab Americans in the Detroit Metro Area, compared to immigrants [21]. According to their findings, access to human capital, such as language acquisition, may mediate the association between immigrant status and perceived well-being, with U.S. born Arab Americans' relatively greater English proficiency facilitating more integration opportunities, and therefore contributing to greater well-being [21]. Although that study only compared immigrants and U.S. born Arab Americans, the potential mediating effect of human capital may still be relevant when comparing refugees and U.S. born Arab Americans. Other possible mediating factors may be differential exposure to stressors or sense of control between refugees and U.S. born Arab Americans.

Differences in mental health were also apparent between refugees and immigrants. This pattern is consistent with the small number of previous studies directly comparing refugees and immigrants [20, 23, 24], and speaks to the particular mental health challenges refugees face as they enter the U.S., regardless of country of origin. While adverse mental health outcomes did not appear to vary as a function of duration since initial entry into the U.S., this may be due to the relatively small number of refugees in our sample. This is consistent with another study which found that length of time in the U.S. was not significantly associated with well-being, or frequency of feeling depressed, among older Arab American immigrants in the Detroit Metro Area [21]. More systematic studies of the mental health risks in refugee populations are needed, including a focus on the severity and course of these mental health conditions after longer periods of settlement.

In an exploratory analysis, we found that refugees and immigrants reporting political violence or religious persecution as reasons for immigration had the highest levels of depression and anxiety, especially those who listed these as the only reason for coming to the U.S. These findings are consistent with other studies that have found an association between pre-migration exposure to political violence and subsequent negative mental health outcomes such as depression and post-traumatic stress disorder among both Arab and non-Arab populations [31–33]. We also found that Arab American immigrants reporting educational opportunity or economic opportunity as reasons for coming to the U.S. had relatively lower depression and anxiety levels. Taken together, this suggests that escaping political violence or religious persecution in one's home country is more traumatizing and has more adverse mental health consequences than leaving one's home country in search of educational or economic opportunity. Given the small sample size and the lack of a more systematic sampling method, these findings are suggestive at best, and larger and more detailed studies are urgently needed to examine these important aspects of Arab refugee and immigrant mental health. Nevertheless, these findings may underscore the need for ensuring adequate mental health services for immigrants and refugees, especially for those who have been exposed to political violence and religious persecution.

Overall, the findings further suggest that Arab Americans in Southeast Michigan experience high levels of depressive and anxiety symptoms. The average depression score in our sample was 8.85. While this symptom level cannot be compared directly to those reported in previous studies, it is worth noting that this depressive symptom level is substantially higher than those reported for other major U.S population groups based on a nationally representative sample using the identical measure, which reported depression scores of 3.96 for African Americans, 4.38 for Hispanics, and 3.27 for non-Hispanic Whites [34]. Similarly, anxiety levels in our sample of Arab Americans also appeared substantially higher than those reported previously. For example, the Detroit Neighborhood Health Study (DNHS), a population-based study of adult (≥ 18 years old) residents of Detroit (the same geographic area as the present study) using the identical anxiety measure reported mean anxiety scores of 1.27, 2.56, and 1.10 for African Americans, Hispanic and non-Hispanic White residents, respectively (unpublished data). These levels compare to a mean anxiety score of 4.77 that we found in our sample of Arab Americans.

Overall, our findings are suggestive of considerable mental health needs in the Arab American population in Southeast Michigan, which could be due to a number of reasons. Since 9/11, there have been an increasing number of anti-Arab incidents of discrimination, such as ethnic-based harassment and hate crimes as well as discrimination in employment, housing, and other services [19]. Additionally, the majority of our sample is Muslim, putting them at added risk for Islamophobia-motivated forms of discrimination. The fear and social isolation that may result from this discrimination may well have contributed to the high levels of depression and anxiety across all Arab Americans in our sample. While these findings are limited to Arab Americans who reside in Southeast Michigan, this area is one of the largest population centers of Arab Americans in the country, including those who settled several generations ago as well as more recent immigrants and refugees. They are also consistent with previous research that have found higher levels of depression among Arab Americans relative to other ethnic groups in the Detroit Metro Area [31]. Our findings also corroborate those of Amer et al. (2011), who found higher levels of depression and anxiety in a large geographically and socio-demographically diverse sample of Arab Americans compared to other minority groups [19]. Taken together, these findings emphasize the importance of public health research to recognize the growing Arab population in the U.S. as a distinct entity and the unique mental health challenges they may face.

There are several limitations of this study. The measures to capture depression and anxiety have not been specifically validated for use in Arab Americans. The CESD-SF and GAD-4 focus primarily on mood, such as feelings of sadness or nervousness. However, it is possible that Arab Americans experience symptoms of depression and anxiety in slightly different ways; for example, Arab Americans may focus more on physical attributes such as chest tightness, body aches, and fatigue to convey experiences of depression and anxiety, as has been noted in other Asian populations as well [35–37]. Further, due to the stigma associated with mental illness, both generally and particularly in Arab communities, participants may have been reluctant to respond honestly to questions about depression and anxiety [38–40]. While the high levels of depression and anxiety symptoms we observed in our sample make under-estimation of these symptoms less of a concern, more research is needed with measures that are more sensitive to the cultural nuances with which mental disorders are expressed in Arab-origin populations, including Arab Americans. In addition, our measure of resident status did not assess asylum status. However, a comparatively low number of Arab-origin individuals are granted asylum status in the U.S. [4]. We were also unable to validate participants' self-reported refugee status. It may be possible that individuals did not want to share their refugee status due to stigma or were not certain about their own status. Further, many individuals likely meet the U.S. criteria for determining refugee status but never formally applied for it. It is also important to note that data for this study came from a convenience sample of Arab Americans recruited from ACCESS, which provides health and social services to predominantly low-income clients. As a result, our findings are not necessarily generalizable to the entire Arab American population in Southeast Michigan. However, ACCESS' client-base does include people with a range of sociodemographic backgrounds, which is reflected in our sample which similarly includes participants with a broad spectrum of background characteristics such as age, marital status, and educational attainment. In addition, the sample consisted of Arab Americans who differed in resident status, including refugees, immigrants, and U.S. born residents. Still, it is possible that this sample has greater health needs than the Arab American population more generally, and this may have contributed to the high levels of depression and anxiety symptoms found in this study. Additionally, nearly all of the sample identified as Muslim (93%), likely due to the large population of Muslim Arabs in Dearborn where ACCESS is located. However, this is not representative of the larger Arab American community in Southeast Michigan which also includes a substantial Christian population, further limiting the generalizability of our findings. It is important to note that recruiting a random sample is difficult, as the U.S. Census does not include an Arab or Middle East and North Africa (MENA) identifier. More systematic studies in this population are urgently needed, and would be greatly facilitated by the re-introduction of Arab-origin or MENA ethnicity identifiers on the U.S. Census. Nonetheless, our study serves as an initial investigation of the mental health needs in the Arab American population.

In addition, although the findings are based on cross-sectional data, reporting errors in resident status or other key variables due to mental health seem an unlikely source of bias. Although the survey was administered anonymously, participants may have been reluctant to share potentially stigmatizing (e.g., depressive thoughts) or criminalizing (e.g., unlawful resident status) information due to fear of government surveillance or disclosure of information to their community. Also, no information was available on pre-immigration experiences to specify or validate the circumstances that led to decisions to immigrate, which prevented a more in-depth analysis of the role of pre-immigration exposures in post-settlement mental health. Future studies should conduct a more in-depth evaluation of mental health needs of Arab Americans. Despite these limitations, this is one of a very limited number of studies to assess the mental health of the growing Arab refugee and immigrant population in the U.S.

Conclusions

In sum, this study provides important new information on mental health outcomes of Arab-origin adults in the U.S. The findings suggest that our sample of Arab Americans report very high levels of depression and anxiety symptoms. In particular, Arab-origin refugees and immigrants who have resettled in the U.S. to escape political violence or religious persecution experience higher levels of depression and anxiety compared to those immigrating for other reasons. While such pre-migration stressors are not the focus of this paper, mental health outcomes among immigrants and refugees may also be affected by stressors that occur after resettlement, such as discrimination, social isolation, and difficulty obtaining employment. In order to make mental health intervention and prevention efforts more effective in this population, future research should aim to identify the unique stressors that contribute to these adverse mental health outcomes in Arab Americans. With the growing population of Arab Americans more generally, including Arab-origin immigrants and refugees in the U.S., more systematic efforts are required to examine and address the scope and determinants of their mental health needs.

Abbreviation

MENA: Middle East and North Africa

Acknowledgements

We thank the clients and staff of ACCESS for their participation in this project.

Funding

This work was supported by a pilot project grant from the Robert Wood Johnson Foundation Health and Society Scholars Program (# 70278).

Authors' contributions

SP, ZA, and CML were major contributors in the writing of the manuscript. SP conducted the analysis under the guidance of CML In addition, EC conducted analyses using comparable data from the Detroit Neighborhood Health Study. SP, ZA, CML, EC, and MT provided substantial feedback, read, and approved the final manuscript.

Consent for publication

Not applicable.

Competing interests

The authors declare that they have no competing interests.

Author details

[1]University of Michigan School of Public Health, 1415 Washington Heights, Ann Arbor, MI 48109, USA. [2]University of North Carolina Gillings School of Global Public Health, 135 Dauer Dr., Chapel Hill, NC 27599, USA. [3]Arab Community Center for Economic and Social Services (ACCESS), 2651 Saulino Ct., Dearborn, MI 48120, USA.

References

1. Arab American Institute Foundation. Demographics. 2014. http://www.aaiusa.org/demographics. Accessed 10 Feb 2017.
2. Shryock A, Abraham N. On margins and mainstreams. In: Abraham N, Shryock A, (eds). Arab Detroit: From margin to mainstream. Detroit: Wayne State University Press; 2000. p. 15–35.
3. Mossaad N. Annual Flow Report: Refugees and Asylees: 2015. 2016. https://www.dhs.gov/sites/default/files/publications/Refugees_Asylees_2015.pdf. Accessed 10 Nov 2018.
4. U.S. Department of Homeland Security. Refugees & Asylees 2015 Data Tables. 2016. https://www.dhs.gov/immigration-statistics/refugees-asylees. Accessed 10 Nov 2018.
5. Mawani FN. Social determinants of refugee mental health. In: Simich, L., & Andermann, L. Refuge and resilience: Promoting resilience and mental health among resettled refugees and forced migrants. Dordrecht: Springer; 2014. p. 27–50.
6. Shannon PJ, Vinson GA, Cook TL, Lennon E. Characteristics of successful and unsuccessful mental health referrals of refugees. Adm Policy Ment Heal Ment Heal Serv Res. 2016;43:555–68.
7. Thomson MS, Chaze F, George U, Guruge S. Improving immigrant populations' access to mental health services in Canada: a review of barriers and recommendations. J Immigr Minor Health. 2015;17:1895–905.
8. Moradi B, Hasan NT. Arab American persons' reported experiences of discrimination and mental health: the mediating role of personal control. J Couns Psychol. 2004;51:418.
9. Padela AI, Heisler M. The association of perceived abuse and discrimination after September 11, 2001, with psychological distress, level of happiness, and health status among Arab Americans. Am J Public Health. 2010;100: 284–91.
10. Wright AM, Aldhalimi A, Lumley MA, Jamil H, Pole N, Arnetz JE, et al. Determinants of resource needs and utilization among refugees over time. Soc Psychiatry Psychiatr Epidemiol. 2016;51:539–49.
11. Centers for Disease Control and Prevention. Iraqi Refugee Health Profile. 2014. http://www.cdc.gov/immigrantrefugeehealth/pdf/iraqi-refugee-health-profile.pdf. Accessed 10 Nov 2018.
12. Porter M, Haslam N. Predisplacement and postdisplacement factors associated with mental health of refugees and internally displaced persons: a meta-analysis. JAMA. 2005;294:602–12.
13. Stewart MJ. Social support in refugee resettlement. In: Simich, L., & Andermann, L. Refuge and resilience: Promoting resilience and mental health among resettled refugees and forced migrants. Dordrecht: Springer; 2014. p. 91–107.
14. Amer MM, Hovey JD. Socio-demographic differences in acculturation and mental health for a sample of 2nd generation/early immigrant Arab Americans. J Immigr Minor Health. 2007;9:335.
15. Arab American Institute Foundation. Arab American Populations in 50 States - Michigan. 2015. https://d3n8a8pro7vhmx.cloudfront.net/aai/pages/7706/attachments/original/1461267434/Michigan_2015.pdf?1461267434. Accessed 13 Dec 2017.
16. U.S. Department of State. Refugee Arrivals From October 1, 2007 through September 30, 2018. 2018. http://ireports.wrapsnet.org/. Accessed 1 May 2018.
17. U.S. Census Bureau. American Community Survey 1-Year Estimates: DP02 - Selected Social Characteristics in the United States: Dearborn city, Michigan: Ancestry. 2016. https://factfinder.census.gov. Accessed 2 May 2018.
18. Dallo FJ, Kindratt TB, Snell T. Serious psychological distress among non-Hispanic whites in the United States: the importance of nativity status and region of birth. Soc Psychiatry Psychiatr Epidemiol. 2013;48:1923–30.
19. Amer MM, Hovey JD. Anxiety and depression in a post-September 11 sample of Arabs in the USA. Soc Psychiatry Psychiatr Epidemiol. 2012;47: 409–18.
20. Abdulrahim S, Baker W. Differences in self-rated health by immigrant status and language preference among Arab Americans in the Detroit metropolitan area. Soc Sci Med. 2009;68:2097–103.
21. Ajrouch KJ. Resources and well-being among Arab-American elders. J Cross Cult Gerontol. 2007;22:167–82.
22. Wrobel NH, Farrag MF, Hymes RW. Acculturative stress and depression in an elderly Arabic sample. J Cross Cult Gerontol. 2009;24:273–90.
23. Silove D, Steel Z, McGorry P, Mohan P. Trauma exposure, postmigration stressors, and symptoms of anxiety, depression and post-traumatic stress in Tamil asylum-seekers: comparison with refugees and immigrants. Acta Psychiatr Scand. 1998;97:175–81.
24. Hollander A-C, Bruce D, Burström B, Ekblad S. Gender-related mental health differences between refugees and non-refugee immigrants-a cross-sectional register-based study. BMC Public Health. 2011;11:180.
25. Our Roots. Arab Community Center for Economic and Social Services. https://www.accesscommunity.org/about. Accessed 10 Feb 2017.
26. Radloff LS. The CES-D scale: a self-report depression scale for research in the general population. Appl Psychol Meas. 1977;1:385–401.
27. Ghubash R, Daradkeh TK, Al Naseri KS, Al Bloushi NBA, Al Daheri AM. The performance of the Center for Epidemiologic Study Depression Scale (CES-D) in an Arab female community. Int J Soc Psychiatry. 2000;46:241–9.
28. Beshai S, Dobson KS, Adel A. Psychometric properties of the Center for Epidemiologic Studies Depression Scale in an Egyptian student sample: a preliminary report. Middle East Curr Psychiatry. 2013;20:223–8.
29. Kazarian SS, Taher D. Validation of the Arabic center for epidemiological studies depression (CES-D) scale in a Lebanese community sample. Eur J Psychol Assess. 2010;26:68–83.
30. Spitzer RL, Kroenke K, Williams JBW, Löwe B. A brief measure for assessing generalized anxiety disorder: the GAD-7. Arch Intern Med. 2006;166:1092–7.
31. Jamil H, Grzybowski M, Hakim-Larson J, Fakhouri M, Sahutoglu J, Khoury R, et al. Factors associated with self-reported depression in Arab, Chaldean, and African Americans. Ethn Dis. 2007;18:464–70.
32. Steel Z, Chey T, Silove D, Marnane C, Bryant RA, Van Ommeren M. Association of torture and other potentially traumatic events with mental health outcomes among populations exposed to mass conflict and displacement: a systematic review and meta-analysis. JAMA. 2009;302:537–49.
33. Rousseau C, Drapeau A. Premigration exposure to political violence among independent immigrants and its association with emotional distress. J Nerv Ment Dis. 2004;192:852–6.
34. Mulia N, Ye Y, Zemore SE, Greenfield TK. Social disadvantage, stress, and alcohol use among black, Hispanic, and white Americans: findings from the 2005 US National Alcohol Survey. J Stud Alcohol Drugs. 2008;69:824–33.
35. Al-Krenawi A, Graham JR. Culturally sensitive social work practice with Arab clients in mental health settings. Health Soc Work. 2000;25:9–22.
36. Al-Krenawi A. Mental health practice in Arab countries. Curr Opin Psychiatry. 2005;18:560–4.
37. Marsella AJ, Sartorius N, Jablensky A, Fenton FR. Cross-cultural studies of depressive disorders: An overview. Cult Depress Stud Anthropol Cross-Cultural Psychiatry Affect Disord. 1985;16:299.
38. Ciftci A, Jones N, Corrigan PW. Mental health stigma in the Muslim community. J Muslim Ment Health. 2013;7;17–32.
39. Youssef J, Deane FP. Factors influencing mental-health help-seeking in Arabic-speaking communities in Sydney, Australia. Ment Health Relig Cult. 2006;9:43–66.
40. Coker EM. Selfhood and social distance: toward a cultural understanding of psychiatric stigma in Egypt. Soc Sci Med. 2005;61:920–30.

Permissions

All chapters in this book were first published in PSYCHIATRY, by BioMed Central; hereby published with permission under the Creative Commons Attribution License or equivalent. Every chapter published in this book has been scrutinized by our experts. Their significance has been extensively debated. The topics covered herein carry significant findings which will fuel the growth of the discipline. They may even be implemented as practical applications or may be referred to as a beginning point for another development.

The contributors of this book come from diverse backgrounds, making this book a truly international effort. This book will bring forth new frontiers with its revolutionizing research information and detailed analysis of the nascent developments around the world.

We would like to thank all the contributing authors for lending their expertise to make the book truly unique. They have played a crucial role in the development of this book. Without their invaluable contributions this book wouldn't have been possible. They have made vital efforts to compile up to date information on the varied aspects of this subject to make this book a valuable addition to the collection of many professionals and students.

This book was conceptualized with the vision of imparting up-to-date information and advanced data in this field. To ensure the same, a matchless editorial board was set up. Every individual on the board went through rigorous rounds of assessment to prove their worth. After which they invested a large part of their time researching and compiling the most relevant data for our readers.

The editorial board has been involved in producing this book since its inception. They have spent rigorous hours researching and exploring the diverse topics which have resulted in the successful publishing of this book. They have passed on their knowledge of decades through this book. To expedite this challenging task, the publisher supported the team at every step. A small team of assistant editors was also appointed to further simplify the editing procedure and attain best results for the readers.

Apart from the editorial board, the designing team has also invested a significant amount of their time in understanding the subject and creating the most relevant covers. They scrutinized every image to scout for the most suitable representation of the subject and create an appropriate cover for the book.

The publishing team has been an ardent support to the editorial, designing and production team. Their endless efforts to recruit the best for this project, has resulted in the accomplishment of this book. They are a veteran in the field of academics and their pool of knowledge is as vast as their experience in printing. Their expertise and guidance has proved useful at every step. Their uncompromising quality standards have made this book an exceptional effort. Their encouragement from time to time has been an inspiration for everyone.

The publisher and the editorial board hope that this book will prove to be a valuable piece of knowledge for researchers, students, practitioners and scholars across the globe.

List of Contributors

Yuki Sakai
Faculty of Medicine and Health sciences, Institute for Mental Health, Norwegian University of Science and Technology, Trondheim, Norway

Valentina Iversen and Solveig Klæbo Reitan
Faculty of Medicine and Health sciences, Institute for Mental Health, Norwegian University of Science and Technology, Trondheim, Norway
Department of Mental health, St. Olav's University Hospital, Trondheim, Norway

Patrizia Zeppegno
Department of Translational Medicine, Azienda Ospedaliero Universitaria Maggiore della Carità, University of Piemonte Orientale, Via Solaroli 17, 28100 Novara, Italy
Institute of Psychiatry, Maggiore della Carità Hospital of Novara, C.so Mazzini 18, 28100 Novara, Italy

Miriam Iosue
Department of Health Sciences, University of Molise, Via Francesco De Sanctis, 1, 86100 Campobasso, Italy

Vladimir Carli
National Centre for Suicide Research and Prevention of Mental Ill-Health (NASP), Karolinska Institute, -171 77 Stockholm, SE, Sweden

Laura Mandelli
Department of Biomedical and Neuromotor Sciences, Institute of Psychiatry, University of Bologna, Via Altura 3, 40139 Bologna, Italy

Alessandro Serretti
Department of Biomedical and Neuromotor Sciences, Institute of Psychiatry, University of Bologna, Via Altura 3, 40139 Bologna, Italy

Debora Marangon
Institute of Psychiatry, Maggiore della Carità Hospital of Novara, C.so Mazzini 18, 28100 Novara, Italy

Bettina K. Doering, Antonia Barke and Thilo Friehs
Clinical Psychology & Psychotherapy, Department of Psychology, Philipps-University Marburg, Marburg, Germany

Maarten C. Eisma
Department of Clinical Psychology and Experimental Psychopathology, University of Groningen, Groningen, The Netherlands

Muna Bhattarai
Hope International College, Kathmandu 44600, Nepal

Khomapak Maneewat and Wipa Sae-Sia
Faculty of Nursing, Prince of Songkla University, Hat Yai, Songkhla, Thailand

Johanna König, Kristin Fenske, Johannes Hertel and Kathleen Zymara
Department of Psychiatry and Psychotherapy, University Medicine Greifswald, Ellernholzstraße 1-2, 17489 Greifswald, Germany

Andrea Block
Department of Psychiatry and Psychotherapy, University Medicine Greifswald, Ellernholzstraße 1-2, 17489 Greifswald, Germany
Department of Health Sciences, Institute of Sociology of Health and Physical Activity, University of Potsdam, Potsdam, Germany

Mathias Becker and Harald Jürgen Freyberger
Department of Psychiatry and Psychotherapy, University Medicine Greifswald, Ellernholzstraße 1-2, 17489 Greifswald, Germany
Department of Psychiatry and Psychotherapy, Helios Clinic, Stralsund, Germany

Sandra Van der Auwera and Hans Jörgen Grabe
Department of Psychiatry and Psychotherapy, University Medicine Greifswald, Ellernholzstraße 1-2, 17489 Greifswald, Germany
German Centre of Neurodegenerative Diseases (DZNE), Site Rostock/Greifswald, Greifswald, Germany

Henry Völzke
Institute for Community Medicine, University Medicine Greifswald, Greifswald, Germany

Ralph J. Johnson III
Departments of Myeloma, TMC Catholic Chaplain's Corps, and Houston Hospice, University of Texas–MD Anderson Cancer Center, Unit 439, 1515 Holcombe Blvd, Houston, Texas 77030, USA

Maha H. Aljuaid
King Abdullah International Medical Research Center, Nursing Department, King Abdulaziz Medical City, Ministry of National Guard Health Affairs, King Saud bin Abdulaziz University for Health Sciences, Riyadh, Saudi Arabia

Ahmad M. Deeb
King Abdullah International Medical Research Center, Research Office, King Abdulaziz Medical City, Ministry of National Guard Health Affairs, King Saud bin Abdulaziz University for Health Sciences, Riyadh, Saudi Arabia

Maamoun Dbsawy
King Abdullah International Medical Research Center, Intensive Care Department, King Abdulaziz Medical City, Ministry of National Guard Health Affairs, King Saud bin Abdulaziz University for Health Sciences, Riyadh, Saudi Arabia

Daniah Alsayegh and Moteb Alotaibi
King Abdullah International Medical Research Center, Mental Health Department, King Abdulaziz Medical City, Ministry of National Guard Health Affairs, King Saud bin Abdulaziz University for Health Sciences, Riyadh, Saudi Arabia

Yaseen M. Arabi
King Abdullah International Medical Research Center, College of Medicine, King Saud Bin Abdulaziz University for Health Sciences, Riyadh, Saudi Arabia
Intensive Care Department, King Abdulaziz Medical City, National Guard Health Affairs, Riyadh, Saudi Arabia

Lu Niu and Liang Zhou
The Affiliated Brain Hospital of Guangzhou Medical University (Guangzhou Huiai Hospital), 36 Mingxin Road, Liwan District, Guangzhou 510370, China

Cunxian Jia
School of Public Health, Shandong University, Jinan, China

Zhenyu Ma
School of Public Health, Guangxi Medical University, Nanning, China

Guojun Wang and Zhenjun Yu
Xiangya School of Public Health, Central South University, Changsha, China

Izumi Chihara, Ryusuke Ae, Ritei Uehara, Nobuko Makino, Yuri Matsubara, Teppei Sasahara, Yasuko Aoyama, Kazuhiko Kotani and Yosikazu Nakamura
Division of Public Health, Center for Community Medicine, Jichi Medical University, 3311-1 Yakushiji, Shimotsuke, Tochigi 329-0498, Japan

Yuka Kudo
Division of Public Health, Center for Community Medicine, Jichi Medical University, 3311-1 Yakushiji, Shimotsuke, Tochigi 329-0498, Japan
Department of Neuropsychiatry, Keio University School of Medicine, 35 Shinanomachi, Shinjuku-ku, Tokyo 160-8582, Japan

Douglas Archibald and Clare Liddy
Department of Family Medicine, University of Ottawa, Ottawa, ON, Canada
Bruyère Research Institute, 85 Primrose Avenue, Ottawa, ON K1R 6M1, Canada

Julia Stratton and Douglas Green
Department of Psychiatry, University of Ottawa, Ottawa, ON, Canada

Rachel E. Grant
Faculty of Education, University of Ottawa, Ottawa, ON, Canada

Erin J. Keely
Department of Medicine, University of Ottawa, Ottawa, ON, Canada
Ottawa Hospital Research Institute, Ottawa, ON, Canada

Han-Ting Lin and Chi-Huang Lai
National Defense Medical Center, School of Public Health 4325R, No. 161, Section 6, Min-Chuan East Road, Neihu District, Taipei City 11490, Taiwan, Republic of China

Wu-Chien Chien
National Defense Medical Center, School of Public Health 4325R, No. 161, Section 6, Min-Chuan East Road, Neihu District, Taipei City 11490, Taiwan, Republic of China
National Defense Medical Center, Graduate Institute of Life Sciences 7115R, No. 161, Section 6, Min-Chuan East Road, Neihu District, Taipei City 11490, Taiwan, Republic of China
Department of Medical Research 7115R, National Defense Medical Center, Tri-Service General Hospital Taipei, No. 325, Section 2, Cheng-Kung Road, Taipei City 11490, Taiwan, Republic of China

Huey-Jen Perng and Chi-Hsiang Chung
National Defense Medical Center, Graduate Institute of Life Sciences 7115R, No. 161, Section 6, Min-Chuan East Road, Neihu District, Taipei City 11490, Taiwan, Republic of China

Chung-Ching Wang and Wei-Liang Chen
Department of Family and Community Medicine, National Defense Medical Center, Tri-Service General Hospital Taipei, No. 325, Section 2, Cheng-Kung Road, Taipei City 11490, Taiwan, Republic of China

Omar Omar and Nourehan ElAzab
Weill Cornell Medicine-Qatar, Doha, Qatar

Ziad Kronfol
Weill Cornell Medicine-Qatar, Doha, Qatar
Weill Cornell Medicine, 445 E 69th St. Suite 432, New York, NY 10021, USA

Batoul Khalifa
Qatar University, Doha, Qatar

Brigitte Khoury and Sariah Daouk
American University of Beirut, Beirut, Lebanon

J. P. deWitt and Daniel Eisenberg
University of Michigan, Ann Arbor, USA

Mathieu Nacher, Gulen Ayhan and Célia Basurko
Centre d'Investigation Clinique CIC INSERM 1424, Centre Hospitalier de Cayenne, 97300 Cayenne, French Guiana

Romain Arnal
Service de Psychiatrie, Centre Hospitalier de Cayenne, 97300 Cayenne, French Guiana

Florence Huber
Hôpital de Jour Adultes, Centre Hospitalier de Cayenne, 97300 Cayenne, French Guiana

Agathe Pastre and Vincent About
Unité de Consultations Ambulatoires Carcérales, 97300 Cayenne, French Guiana

Louis Jehel
CESP- INSERM U1178 Equipe IPSOM, Centre Hospitalier Universitaire de Martinique, BP632, 97261 Cedex fort de France, France

Bruno Falissard
CESP/INSERM U1018 (Centre de Recherche en Epidémiologie et Santé des Populations), 75679 Paris cedex 14, France

Lukas Peter, Hartmut Lehfeld and Salina Brar-Reissinger
Clinic Nuremberg, University Clinic for Psychiatry and Psychotherapy, Paracelsus Private Medical University, Nuremberg, Germany

Günter Niklewski
Clinic Nuremberg, University Clinic for Psychiatry and Psychotherapy, Paracelsus Private Medical University, Nuremberg, Germany
Faculty for Social Sciences, Technical University for Applied Sciences Georg Simon Ohm, Nuremberg, Germany

Kneginja Richter
Clinic Nuremberg, University Clinic for Psychiatry and Psychotherapy, Paracelsus Private Medical University, Nuremberg, Germany
Faculty for Social Sciences, Technical University for Applied Sciences Georg Simon Ohm, Nuremberg, Germany
Faculty for Medical Sciences, University Goce Delcev, Stip, Macedonia

Harald Zäske
Department of Psychiatry and Psychotherapy, Medical Faculty, Heinrich-Heine-University, Düsseldorf, Germany

Marco Sarchiapone
Department of Health Sciences, University of Molise, Via Francesco De Sanctis, 1, 86100 Campobasso, Italy
National Institute for Health, Migration and Poverty, Via di S. Gallicano 25/a, 00153 Rome, Italy

Carla Gramaglia
Department of Translational Medicine, Azienda Ospedaliero Universitaria Maggiore della Carità, University of Piemonte Orientale, Via Solaroli 17, 28100 Novara, Italy

Vesa Paavonen
Faculty of Medicine and Life Sciences, University of Tampere, PB 100, FI-33014 Tampere, Finland

Esa Leinonen
Faculty of Medicine and Life Sciences, University of Tampere, PB 100, FI-33014 Tampere, Finland
Department of Psychiatry, Tampere University Hospital, PB 2000, FI-33521 Tampere, Finland

Kaisa E. Luoto and Olli Kampman
Faculty of Medicine and Life Sciences, University of Tampere, PB 100, FI-33014 Tampere, Finland
Department of Psychiatry, Seinäjoki Hospital District, Huhtalantie 53, 60220 Seinäjoki, Finland

Lars H. Lindholm, Antti Koivukangas and Antero Lassila
Department of Psychiatry, Seinäjoki Hospital District, Huhtalantie 53, 60220 Seinäjoki, Finland

Anja Friedrich, Merle Claßen and Angelika A. Schlarb
Faculty of Psychology and Sports Science, Department of Psychology, Clinical Psychology and Psychotherapy of children and adolescents, Bielefeld University, Universitätsstraße 25, 33615 Bielefeld, Germany

Takashi Nakamae and Jin Narumoto
Department of Psychiatry, Graduate School of Medical Science, Kyoto Prefectural University of Medicine, 465 Kajii-cho, Kawaramachi-Hirokoji, Kamigyo-ku, Kyoto 602-8566, Japan

Kenji Fukui
Health Care Center, Kyoto Prefectural University of Medicine, 465 Kajii-cho, Kawaramachi-Hirokoji, Kamigyo-ku, Kyoto 602-8566, Japan

Damiaan Denys
Department of Neuropsychiatry, Academic Medical Center, University of Amsterdam, Meibergdreef 9, 1105, AZ, Amsterdam, the Netherlands
The Netherlands Institute for Neuroscience, an institute of the Royal Netherlands Academy of Arts and Sciences, Meibergdreef 47, 1105, BA, Amsterdam, the Netherlands

Chao-Ming Hung
Department of General Surgery, E-Da Cancer Hospital, I-Shou University, Kaohsiung, Taiwan

Ying-Chun Li
Institute of Health Care Management, National Sun Yat-Sen University, Kaohsiung, Taiwan

Han-Jung Chen and Kang Lu
Institute of Health Care Management, National Sun Yat-Sen University, Kaohsiung, Taiwan
Department of Neurosurgery, E-Da Hospital, I-Shou University, Kaohsiung, Taiwan

Cheng-Loong Liang and Yu-Duan Tsai
Department of Neurosurgery, E-Da Hospital, I-Shou University, Kaohsiung, Taiwan

Po-Chou Liliang and Kuo-Wei Wang
Department of Neurosurgery, E-Da Cancer Hospital, I-Shou University, Kaohsiung, Taiwan

Kuan-Yu Chu
Taoyuan General Hospital, Taoyuan City, Taiwan
Department of Fine Art & Culture Creative Design, Hua-Fan University, New Taipei City, Taiwan
College of General studies, Yuan-Ze University, Taoyuan City, Taiwan

Chih-Yang Huang
Department of Fine Art & Culture Creative Design, Hua-Fan University, New Taipei City, Taiwan.

Wen-Chen Ouyang
Jianan Psychiatric Center, Tainan City, Taiwan
Department of Psychiatry, College of Medicine, Kaohsiung Medical University, Kaohsiung, Taiwan

Kathrin Bauernhofer, Daniela Bassa, Paulino Jiménez, Manuela Paechter, Ilona Papousek, Andreas Fink and Elisabeth M. Weiss
Department of Psychology, University of Graz, Universitätsplatz 2/DG, 8010 Graz, Austria

Markus Canazei
Department of Psychology, University of Innsbruck, Bruno-Sander-Haus Innrain 52f, 6020 Innsbruck, Austria

Hille T. de Vries
Academic Medical Center, University of Amsterdam, Meibergdreef 9, 1105, AZ, Amsterdam, the Netherlands

Sanjana Pampati, Zaineb Alattar and Carlos Mendes de Leon
University of Michigan School of Public Health, 1415 Washington Heights, Ann Arbor, MI 48109, USA

Evette Cordoba
University of North Carolina Gillings School of Global Public Health, 135 Dauer Dr., Chapel Hill, NC 27599, USA

Madiha Tariq
Arab Community Center for Economic and Social Services (ACCESS), 2651 Saulino Ct., Dearborn, MI 48120, USA

Index

www.ingramcontent.com/pod-product-compliance
Lightning Source LLC
LaVergne TN
LVHW080705210926
848485LV00003B/420

* 9 7 8 1 6 3 9 2 7 4 3 6 9 *